Dedicated to all alternative practitioners

Acupuncture in Practice

Luc De Schepper
M.D., Ph.D., Lic. Ac., C.Hom., D.I.Hom.

FULL OF LIFE PUBLISHING
500 N.Guadalupe St. G441
Santa Fe, NM 87501

1st printing

Library of Congress Catalog Card Number 94-071178

ISBN 0-942501-03-9

Printed by Community Press, Provo, Utah
Full of Life Publishing, Santa Fe, NM 87501

Note to Reader and disclaimer:
The information in this book is presented for information purposes only. All treatments, therapies, exercises or energetic interventions of any nature should be undertaken only under the direct guidance and care of a properly and legally, fully trained health care professional specializing in the services rendered. Nothing desribed in this book should be construed by any reader or other person to be a diagnosis or treatment for any disease or condition. Neither the author nor publisher can accept any responsibility for any ill effects resulting from the use or misuse of the information contained herein. Any uses or misuses of the information presented here for educational purposes are the responsibility of the reader.

Cover and design by Yolanda De Schepper

Other books by the same author:

"Acupuncture Within Everyone's Reach," 1980 (Dutch language)

"Acupuncture for the Practitioner," 1985 (out of print)

"Candida, the Causes, the Symptoms, the Cure," 1986

"Peak Immunity," 1989

"Full of Life," 1991

"How to Dine Like the Devil and Feel Like a Saint," 1993

"Human Condition: Critical," 1993

"Musculoskeletal Diseases and Homeopathy," 1994

Acknowledgements

I could not have written this book without the help and understanding from all my patients who have entrusted their care to me. I am greatly indepted to them. I owe a lot to my teachers in the Dutch Doctors Acupuncture Association, Amsterdam, Holland and to the many great teachers of the French Acupuncture Association, Paris, France. Names like Nogier, Niboyet, Mussat, Lebarbier, Kespi and my all-time favorite Borsarello are always engraved in my memory. And most important, without the support and artistic talents of my beloved wife, Yolanda, and the great typing efforts of mom Betty, this book would not have been possible.

"A doctor is somebody who puts medications of which he knows little in a body of which he knows less" (Voltaire)

Contents

The Qi 1

TRADITIONAL CHINESE MEDICINE (TCM)

The concept of Qi is essential in acupuncture: the whole of Traditional Chinese Medicine is based on it; hence TCM is often called "Energetic Medicine". It is not the only energetic medicine. Homeopathy, brought to humankind by Samuel Hahnemann (°1755-†1843), stresses the overall importance of the strength of "Qi or Vital Energy." It is interesting to compare TCM with Western Medicine.

Western Medicine can be considered a medicine of matter. The Western Doctor studies the symptoms presented by patients, combining them with the results found by the inquiry and the clinical examination. Guided by the previous findings, he will start a series of para-clinical examinations: lab-tests, X-rays, and, in extreme cases, surgical exploration (biopsy, laparatomy, etc.). Whatever the method used, the goal is to discover a material modification: too many red blood cells, alterations on X-rays, structure modifications found by laparoscopy, or albuminuria. Western medicine tends to overemphasize the analytical side, as if the human body could be broken down into a definite set of facts and drawers. By reducing the body to *Gray's Anatomy,* modern medicine fails to see that the Vital Energy (Qi) has no material existence and, therefore, cannot be dissected like other parts of the body. Western medicine regards pathology as the disease itself and seeks to remove it, thinking, thereby, that they are curing the patient. This folly continues today.

On the other hand, TCM views the patient quite differently. Of course, the acupuncturist listens carefully to every complaint of the patient, and it is no exaggeration to state that for him it is even more important to pay attention to any symptom the patient has. In fact, what will appear as puzzling symptoms to the Western doctor will give a clear and understandable picture to the acupuncturist. Often I have seen in my office patients who were diagnosed as "neurotic" and "nervous", simply because the variety of symptoms could not be understood by their Western doctor. For the acupuncturist and homeopath alike, *strange, peculiar and uncommon* symptoms will be a guide to healing, rather than a hindrance. These symptoms vary from individual to individual and are important since they will show the kinks in the patient's defense armor where the disease will enter, hook itself and become chronic.

The goal of the acupuncturist and alternative physician is different. Guided by the symptoms and the various specific steps explained in later chapters, he will try to find the disturbance that is the origin of these symptoms. Acupuncture goes to the root of the problem and is an outspoken causal medicine, contrary to what most patients and doctors believe. How often do we hear the patients ask: "But is acupuncture really curing or is it just relieving the pain?" Sad to say, this seems to be the method modern Western medicine often prefers. Giving a fancy name to the disease and treating the superficial symptoms like pruning sick leaves from the sick tree, Western medicine almost always falls into the trap of *suppression.* By suppression I mean that a disease manifestation is disappearing before the disease itself is cured. Often the first manifestations of an internal disorder develop on the externals, i.e., the skin and the mucous membranes (the internal skin).

Numerous examples of Western suppression of disease can be found. Anything that has been lasered or burned (warts, polyps, etc.) returns, if you are lucky, since Nature tries again, against human "better" judgment, to push the disease out of the body. How many cortisone creams (this poison is available over-the-counter!) have been tried in vain to eradicate poorly understood rashes. How many children got asthma after being treated with cortisone creams for eczema? Western medicine accepts this alternation as a "fait accompli," yet this therapeutic act is actually causing it. Vaginal discharge is another favorite for medical suppression. The suppositories and creams used to treat it are nothing but a therapeutic act against the natural flow of cure. Treatment should be directed at eliminating and, therefore, increasing this flow, since the body tries to get rid of toxins. Even in breast cancer treatment (or other cancers, for that matter), we often see the same thing. Patients who undergo mastectomy with radiation and chemotherapy come down with, a couple of years later, a spread of the tumor to the liver or other organs. "We were too late," proponents of this therapy will claim. Has anyone ever stood still and looked at this and reasoned that the suppression of the cancer was so powerful that the only choice was the invasion of other organs? Do not interpret this statement as signifying that I wish to forget everything I have learned in medical school. Pathology does have a role in the restoration of health. But to entirely rely on pathology and think that by knowing all its secrets the whole truth of the living being will be revealed, is a folly in the greatest sense of the word, a folly, indeed, that is all too often adhered to in modern times. It is, however, a tool, but by no means the leading element in the search for restoration of health.

Have you ever thought why what we were doing in Western medicine 20 years ago has almost vanished today? Proponents of this science call this progress. In reality, it was one of the many "hit and misses" of modern medicine. So inconstant and variable is allopathy that, should a Western trained doctor die today and come back to life fifty years from now and attempt to continue his profession, he would have to graduate all over again. Not so for the acupuncturist or homeopath, who could come back two hundred years from now and be very proficient. Why? Because these true sciences are based on infallible laws which can withstand the length of time: 5,000 years for acupuncture and 200 for homeopathy!

WHAT IS QI?

In the Western world, this word is rarely heard without being followed by an adjective: electric energy, atomic energy, thermal energy, all forms of energy that can be transformed into each other. These forms of Qi are, of course, known by the Orientals, but they are only manifestations of an

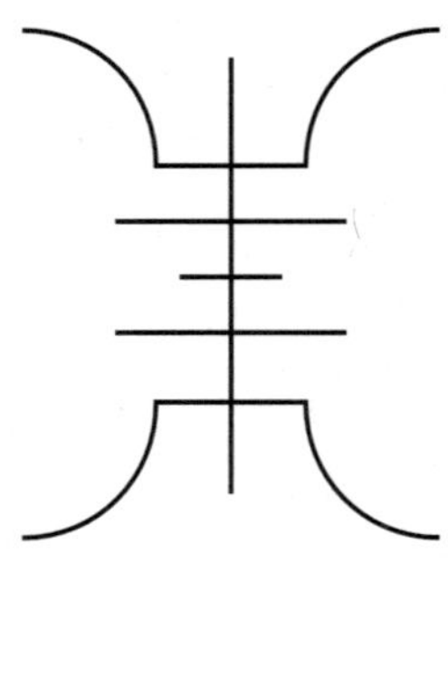

Figure 1

essential principle: energy. Qi differentiates the human being from inert matter; man thinks, works, reflects while absorbing energy from the earth and heaven. For the Chinese, man is a tree of which branches and leaves receive the energy from heaven, while its roots are connected with the deep energies from the earth (Figure 1).

Naturally, there is only one energy, but it can manifest itself in different forms:

The Ancestral or Heridity of Qi
The Iong (Yong) or Food Qi
The Wei or Defense Qi

THE ANCESTRAL OR HEREDITARY QI

This is the Qi transferred from the parents of the individual, it is the energy locked in the chromosomes. It can give us a bad or a good start in life. Arthritis, for instance, which is deficient Kidney Yin, is often found in the early family history, mostly on the mother's side. It creates a weak terrain for the individual, who will become susceptible to all diseases linked to deficient K Yin. It can be considered the first form of Qi and is stored as deeply as possible, for its protection, in the K Yin. This form of Qi is very precious, because the amount received at birth will only decrease throughout life, due to external perturbations, but also during the aging process. Every disease in life will decrease the quantity of this Qi, and at the end of life, the Ancestral Qi is exhausted. What is also particular about this Qi is that it is the only form of Qi that is difficult to increase or restore. An attempt can be made to tonify *"the magic triangle"*: GV4 and B23 bilateral.

The Ancestral Qi starts in the Kidneys (combination of Yin-Yang root) and will penetrate either in the Heart or the Lungs to circulate with the Yong Qi in the Energy cycle. A second tract is from its departure in the Kidneys through the Wonder meridians, Tchong Mo, Jenn Mo and Du Mo. Through multiple branches of Tchong Mo, this Qi will connect with the skin, tissues and interosseus spaces, circulating like the Wei Qi, outside of the meridians. When an exterior stress factor attacks an individual with good defense Qi (or Vital Energy), the disturbance will be superficial. However, if the exterior attack is strong and/or the defense Qi deficient, the disease process will progress into deeper layers. At that point, the Ancestral Energy will link with the Wei Qi to take command of the defense. Together they will try to fend off the enemy in order to avoid penetration of deeper, precious organs. More will be discussed in Chapter 4, "Wonder meridians."

THE YONG QI

The Yong — or Food — Qi is provided by exterior sources: the alimentation, but also the respiration. This Yong Qi, originates in the stomach after transformation of solid and liquid food stuffs. This energy circulates everywhere, in the organs and meridians, and makes the tour of the organism in 29 minutes. The Yong Qi does not circulate in the *Tmm or Tendino-muscular meridians*, located at the most external level of the skin. According to chapter 16 of *"Ling Tchrou"*, the Yong Qi accomplishes 50 cycles, approximately one every half an hour. But, as indicated by Soulie de Morant, this Qi stagnates partially in each organ for two hours. (Figure 2)

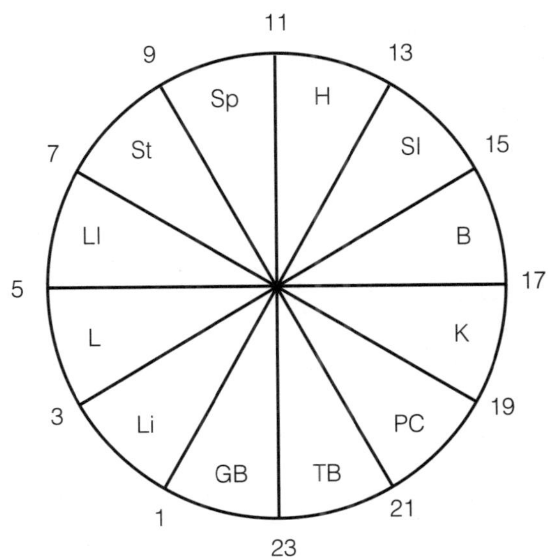

Figure 2

The acupuncturist is able to diagnose the Yong Qi qualitatively and quantitatively. The Yong Qi is of bad quality when symptoms such as maldigestion, diarrhea, vomiting and losing weight appear. This corresponds in the Ko cycle of the 5 elements to an attack on the stomach, or spleen, or liver, or small intestine. The quantity of the Yong Qi is measured by taking the pulses. Either the acupuncturist feels the pulse under slight pressure as a thin thread (the Yong Qi starts diminishing) or he feels the pulse only by pressing hard (the Yong Qi is extinguished). To restore the Yong Qi, the acupuncturist will reinforce the stomach ($St36^t$ and $CV12^t$) and the middle burner ($TB3^t$ and $St30^t$).

Needless to say, it is very important to have quality and quantity of both— respiratory and food Qi. And here begins our frustrating struggle for health. Nowadays, preservatives and hormones seem to be more important to our food providers than what good old Mother Nature offers us. Our air becomes polluted by cars, atomic and electrical plants. All this is done in the name of progress, but this "horn of plenty" already has too many rotten apples.

Nevertheless, whatever the quality, we can only hope that the defense mechanisms of our bodies can fight this sometimes unequal battle! All too often, I see patients overwhelmed by toxic substances, and the terrible picture of breathing through a mask has become reality for some unfortunate patients. Through respiration and alimentation, a certain quantity of Qi penetrates our system. The food will undergo several splittings in pure and impure Qi: the pure, going to the tissues, and the impure, eliminated by our excretion systems—urine, feces, and sweat.

We can also imagine the importance of the diet of the pregnant woman. The fetus, still intra-uterine, depends on what his mother provides. We all know the saying: "When you are pregnant, you have to eat for two." Unfortunately, this is understood by most mothers as to increase the quantity of food, while they should be concerned especially with the quality of it. The importance of diet is now more and more stressed in the Western World, when doctors found out that it had an influence on the formation of the brain of the unborn child.

THE WEI QI (DEFENSE QI)

The human being, subjected to constant attacks from the exterior, possesses a superficial energy, the first barrier of defense: the Wei Qi. Its principal function is to avoid penetration of Perverse Qi towards the organs and try to keep the disturbance to a superficial or local lesion. It runs in the most superficial meridians, the Tmm. During the day, this Wei Qi runs in the Yang meridians, during the night, the greatest concentration can be found in the Yin meridians. Like the Yong Qi, the Wei Qi has 50 cycles in 24 hours, but 25 will be in the Yang, and 25 in the Yin (Figure 3).

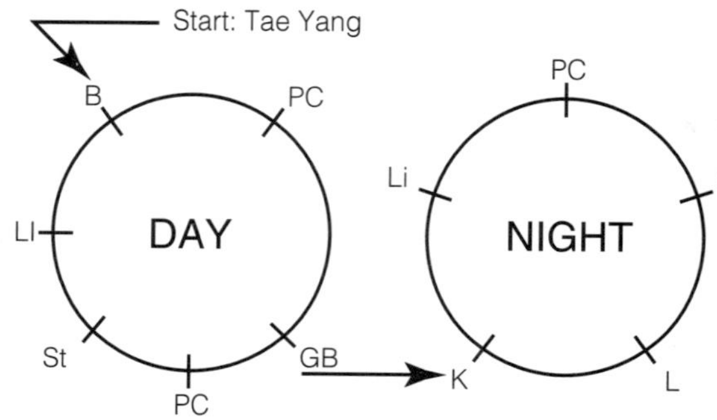

Figure 3.

But nothing is absolute. During the day the deeper or Yin regions must equally be protected. Hence, a certain amount of this Qi can be found at all times in any place. As we will see later, (Chapter 4, on the Different Channels) this Wei Qi is brought in the deeper areas by the divergent meridians. When we have a penetration of an "Exterior Excess," the Wei Qi will try to repulse this Excess, manifested by symptoms such as fever, sweating and intermittence of symptoms, typical of the battle between the Wei Qi and the Perverse Qi. This is the principal role of our Wei Qi: protection against any aggression, not only against the *Six Excesses* (Dampness, Dryness, Summer Heat, Heat, Cold and Fong), but also against the *Seven Emotions* (See Chapter 14).

Repetition of the same disease picture or a patient who catches every cold that is going around, must call our attention to a possible deficiency of

Wei Qi. It is necessary at that time to increase the amount of Wei Qi, in order to support the deficient organ; e.g., when we see a child with repetitive colds, increase the Wei Qi by puncturing: $L9^{t}$, $St36^{t}$, $TB3^{t}$ and $B67^{t}$. Also the points KING have a great reputation of drawing Wei Qi. So you must tonify these points (if they are not dispersing in the seasons) to bring Wei Qi in organs or a meridian. Another way of engaging Wei Qi is to tap lightly the skin with a special. little hammer on which surface are small needles located (Plum Blossom hammer). Acupuncturists who plant many needles in a locus dolendi, do nothing else but attracking Wei Qi to that area, which explains the short-lasting results of this superficial method.

KI - Magic triangle GV4 B23 Bilateral

Zong Qi - St 36 CV12 TB3 St30

Wei Qi - L9 St 36 TB3 B67

The Concept of Yin and Yang

2

CHARACTERISTICS OF YIN AND YANG

Yin and Yang are two terms constantly found in any explanation of TCM. In a very simple way, we could say that they correspond to negative (Yin) and positive (Yang). But they mean so much more. Any object, person, taste, feeling, etc., can be defined as being Yin and Yang. But be careful! When we mention Yin or Yang, that only means *preponderant* Yin or Yang: there is neither absolute Yin nor Yang. While they are each other's opposites, they are each other's complement: the one cannot exist without the other. They are both necessary. But we have to keep in mind that everything is relative! A certain object can be named Yang at one point, but Yin if we compare it to another object. For instance, the abdomen is Yang compared to the lower extremities, but it is Yin if we compare it to the upper extremities. We easily recognize coupled notions such as systolic-diastolic, inspiration-expiration, miosis-mydriasis, etc. A balanced system of opposite reactions exists in the human body. The Yin and the Yang must be in equilibrium: to maintain proper health, both must exist in the appropriate proportion. Disease is nothing else than a disequilibrium between the Yin and the Yang. This does not mean, as Western reasoning would presume, that health is the sum of 50% Yang and 50% Yin. Three thousand years ago, the Chinese expressed this as:

- The Yang unit is made of three thirds: $\frac{3}{3} = 1$ or 3.
- The Yin unit is made of two thirds: $\frac{2}{3}$ or 2.

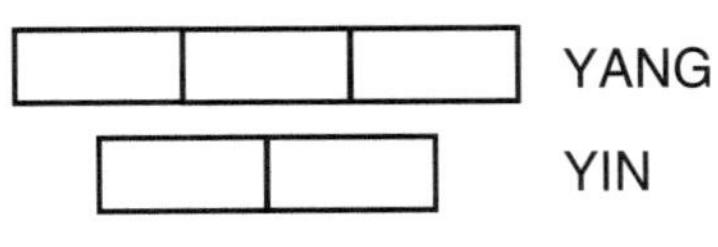

Figure 4

So Yang is uneven, Yin even. Hence for the Chinese, health is the alternation of Yin-Yang of $\frac{2}{3}$ Yang and $\frac{1}{3}$ Yin, and $\frac{2}{3}$ Yin and $\frac{1}{3}$ Yang, or $\frac{2}{3} + \frac{1}{3}(+) = \frac{2}{3} + \frac{1}{3}(-)$. Therefore, the Yin (or **blood**) and Yang (or **energy**) are distributed to the organs (kidney, heart, spleen, and liver) and hollow organs (stomach, colon, bladder and gallbladder) in the following way:

Stomach: 50% blood, 50% energy = + -
Spleen: 2/3 blood, 1/3 energy = -
Heart: 2/3 energy, 1/3 blood = +
Small Intestine: 2/3 blood, 1/3 energy = -
Bladder: 2/3 blood, 1/3 energy = -
Kidney: 2/3 energy, 1/3 blood = +

DAY

Pericardium: 2/3 blood, 1/3 energy = -
Triple Burner: 2/3 energy, 1/3 blood = +
Gallbladder: 2/3 energy, 1/3 blood = +
Liver: 2/3 blood, 1/3 energy = -
Lung: 2/3 energy, 1/3 blood = +
Large Intestine: 50% blood, 50% energy = - +

NIGHT

As we can see, in the day there is a slight dominance of blood, at night a slight dominance of energy. But there are five positive (energy) elements, five negative (blood) elements and two elements have as much blood as energy. In other words, there is a perfect balance. Always remember how the Yin and Yang are divided in the different organs and hollow organs. Be aware, that a Yang meridian according to its topography, such as the Small Intestine, contains more blood than energy! The same goes for the Bladder.

This all brings us to the different essential characteristics, when we mention Yin and Yang:

OPPOSITION - COMPLEMENT - EQUILIBRIUM - RELATIVITY

Let us consider the Yin and Yang in some examples: in time, in the seasons, in space and in the daily use.

THE YIN AND THE YANG IN TIME

In nature there is a succession of cycles: days follow nights, days follow each other, so do months, years and seasons. We can translate these cycles into the concept of Yin and Yang.

- The night is the darkness, the cold period, the state of sleep, hence related to the Yin.
- The day is the light, the warmth, the state of alertness, hence related to the Yang.

Let's put these notions on a circle. At the top, which is Yang as opposed to the bottom, Yin, we find the maximum Yang: **midday**. At the bottom, we find the maximum Yin: **midnight**. Going from the bottom to the top, the Yang increases while the Yin decreases; this is the **morning** portion of the day.

Going from the top to the bottom, the Yang decreases while the Yin increases. This corresponds tothe time period: **noon-midnight.**

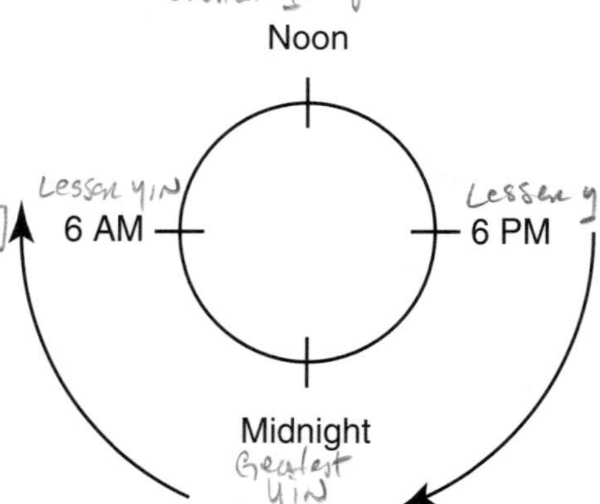

Figure 5

To summarize: (See Figure 5)

MIDNIGHT:	Fullness of Yin and minimum of Yang.
NOON:	Fullness of Yang and minimum of Yin.
6:00 PM:	Equilibrium between increasing Yin and decreasing Yang
6:00 PM:	Equilibrium between increasing Yang and decreasing Yin

THE YIN AND THE YANG IN THE SEASONS

What is true for the days, is also true for the seasons. At the top of the circle, we put the summer, at the bottom the winter.

SUMMER:	Fullness of Yang and minimum of Yin.
WINTER:	Fullness of Yin and minimum of Yang
SPRING:	Increasing of the Yang, decreasing of the Yin.
FALL:	Increasing of the Yin, decreasing of the Yang.

One of the important notions about the Yin-Yang is its *relativity*. Hence, we can combine the previous findings in the following matter:

Yin-winter plus Yin-midnight or midnight in the heart of the winter will give the maximum Yin or Tai Yin. Yang-summer plus Yang-midday or noon in the middle of the summer will give the maximum Yang or Tai Yang. (For more explanation, see "Dialectic on the Acupuncture Points," Chapter 11)

THE YIN AND THE YANG IN SPACE

Three important facts are to be remembered. The Yin is *below-at the interior-rest*. The Yang is *above-at the exterior-movement*. We see instantly some very practical deductions: heaven is Yang, earth is Yin. Man is in contact with both, through GV20 and K1, respectively. If we consider the microcosm that the human being is, then the head is the Yang, the lower extremities the Yin. All these are important notions and are the basis of reasoning frequently used in acupuncture.

THE YIN AND YANG IN DAILY USE

Previously we said the Yang is the Exterior, the Yin the Interior. The same reasoning tells us the Yang goes to the exterior, which is *expansion*, the Yin goes to the interior, which is *condensation*.

Examples can be taken from all daily events at every level, universal as well as atomic. We will always be capable of finding this duality, in variable proportions.

Some daily examples are listed below.

YANG	YIN
- The back	- The front of the body
- The limbs	- The trunk
- Skin	- Mucosae
- Fu organs	- Tsang organs
- Head	- Feet
- Light, warm	- Dark, cold
- Creativity	- Passivity
- Positive, fullness	- Negative, emptiness
- Centripetal	- Centrifugal
- Man	- Woman
- Active	- Passive
- Noise	- Silence
- Red	- Black
- Laughing	- Crying
- Left	- Right
- Dryness	- Dampness
- Baldness	- Abundant hair
- High	- Low
- Inspiration	- Expiration
- Miosis	- Midriasis
- Contraction	- Dilatation
- Movement, day	- Rest, night
- Triangle	- Circle
- Acidity	- Alkaline
- Delivery	- Pregnancy
- Hypertension	- Hypotension
etc.	etc.

The examples are unlimited, and one should be able to recognize in every situation, activity, mood, emotion and object the proportion of Yin to Yang. It should be remembered that the Yang is the active, driving force: **the Qi or Yang moves the Blood or Yin**. This is a fundamental law in acupuncture: emptiness of Yang will lead to a stagnation of the Yin, since there is not enough Yang to move it. In every clinical situation where we have a stagnation of Yin (the characteristics are explained in later chapters), therapy should include an increase of the Yang in the stagnated area. Even the various energies discussed in Chapter 1, conform to the Yin-Yang duality:

- ❑ The Wei or defense mechanism, which includes a notion of movement and mobility, since it goes where the aggression occurs, is Yang. Hence, we find this energy in the most external or superficial meridians: the Tmm.
- ❑ The Yong Qi (food, respiration) is more materialistic, hence more Yin.
- ❑ The Ancestral Qi, linked to the genes, is stored in the most Yin part of the body (the Kidney organ according to the Chinese) and therefore, is the extreme Yin Qi.

It is important to remember that the Yin and the Yang are constantly *interacting* upon each other.

- ❑ The Yang moves the Yin.
- ❑ The Yin controls the Yang and prevents its escape.

For example, deficient Li Yin will lead to an escape of the Li-Yang, manifested by irritability, anger, insomnia, stroke, hypertension and vertigo.

As we have seen in all these previous examples, the Yin and the Yang cannot be separated. They form one entity and are never absolute. In Chapter 7 (the *Eight Conditions*), we will see that the use of the Yin-Yang notion in our Chinese diagnostic is a must.

Human Contact = Between Heaven & Earth - GV20 KI 1

The Five Elements 3

LAWS IN THE FIVE ELEMENTS

Matter is Yin, Energy Yang. What is immobile, stable and little active, is "matter," as opposite to the very active, mobile "energy." But matter is not inert or static: it is dynamic and in continuous evolution. There are five characteristic moments in its evolution. The Chinese word for "five elements", WOU HING, means "what changes constantly." These five elements are not only characteristic, but also interact through a cycle of activation and a cycle of inhibition. What are these elements?

FIRE - EARTH - METAL - WATER - WOOD

These five elements are five totalities with five organs (Figure 6) and five hollow organs. All the influences that stimulates man will converge towards these five organs. Every organ is coupled to a hollow organ:

Heart .... Small Intestine (S.I.)
Spleen .... Stomach (St.)
Lung .... Large Intestine (L.I.)
Kidney .... Bladder (B)
Liver .... Gallbladder (GB)

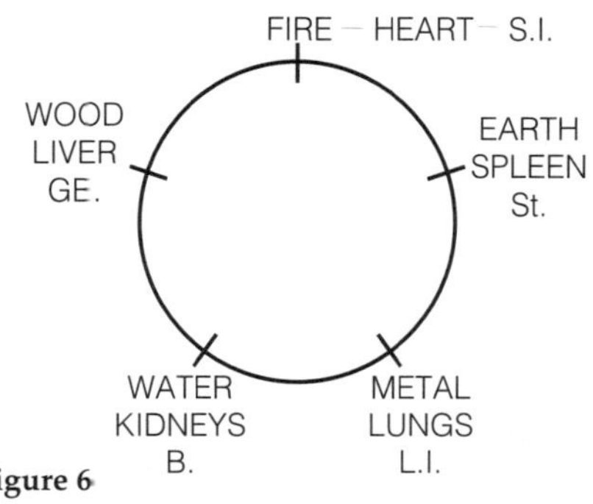

Figure 6

Normally, the Earth element should be placed in the center, but for reasoning purposes, it is put on the circle. The Pericardium (PC.) and the Triple Burner (TB.) are normally not a part of the Five Elements. Only recently historically have they been integrated in this cycle. They both were placed in the Fire element: PC. coupled to the Heart, TB. to the Small Intestine. The hollow organs being Yang, contain food stuff and their physiological role is one of a place of passage and destruction. The Yang destroys where the Yin conserves, and the Yang is movement while the Yin is rest or stagnation. Several important laws will dominate these five elements: the Sheng or generation cycle, the KO or destruction cycle and the anti-Ko cycle.

THE SHENG CYCLE

These five elements are by no means inert or immovable. They activate and destroy each other continuously, creating a certain equilibrium. In the Sheng cycle, a certain element activates another one, which in turn, activates the next one. This always occurs clockwise (Figure 7).

- Fire activates the Earth.
- Earth activates Metal.
- Metal activates Water.
- Water activates Wood.
- Wood activates Fire.

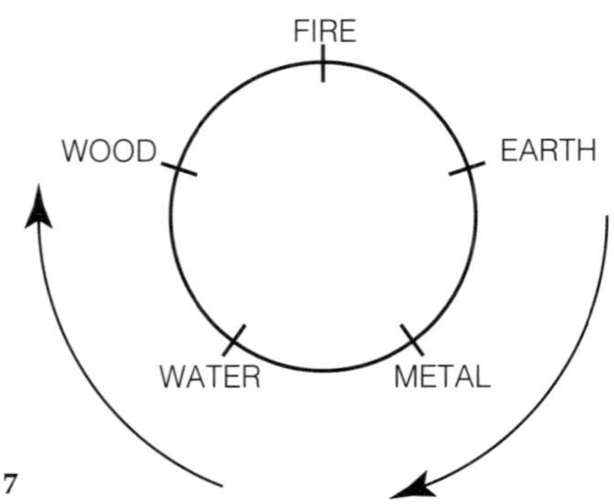

Figure 7

It needs to be well understood, that each organ does not provide energy to the next organ in the cycle; rather it activates or stimulates the organ that follows in the Sheng cycle. For instance, the Lung activates the functioning of the Kidney, it does not supply energy to the Kidney. The Lung meridian does not descend till the Kidney and therefore, cannot furnish energy to this organ. This gives us the following rule:

"Each organ activates the element that follows and is activated by the organ that precedes it."

All this may not be clear at first sight, but a few examples will clarify this frequently-used concept in acupuncture.

- ❏ Fire activates or produces Earth: the Fire burns everything to ashes, which will be mixed with the Earth.
- ❏ Earth produces Metal: the metals are found in the earth and are produced there.
- ❏ Metal produces Water: any metal at a certain temperature becomes liquid.
- ❏ Water produces Wood: any wood or vegetation needs water for its growth.
- ❏ Wood produces Fire: the first fire was made with the help of wood.

The relationships between the hollow organs are different. They are not ruled by the laws of activation and inhibition as the organs are. They are only bound to an organ. Why? Because these hollow organs are mainly places of passage of food, where energy and blood are extracted. Hence, we have a system of five organs and a system of six hollow organs, whose physiological role is to provide energy to the corresponding organ. Each organ, programmed by its Ancestral energy, will receive its energy from its paired hollow organ; it will metabolize and distribute this energy to all the cells of the human organism.

THE KO CYCLE

To keep an equilibrium in this world, there is no production without destruction. (Figure 8)

- ❏ Water destroys the Fire: this is self-evident.

- ❑ Wood destroys the Earth: the word "destroys" should be replaced by "hides or covers"; the earth is covered by the vegetation; the stronger the vegetation, the less earth is seen.
- ❑ Fire destroys the Metal: self-evident.
- ❑ Earth destroys the Water: we should say "absorbs" instead of destroys. When it rains, most of the water is absorbed by the earth. It is important to state here that the above explanations are only symbols to help the student memorize these important laws.

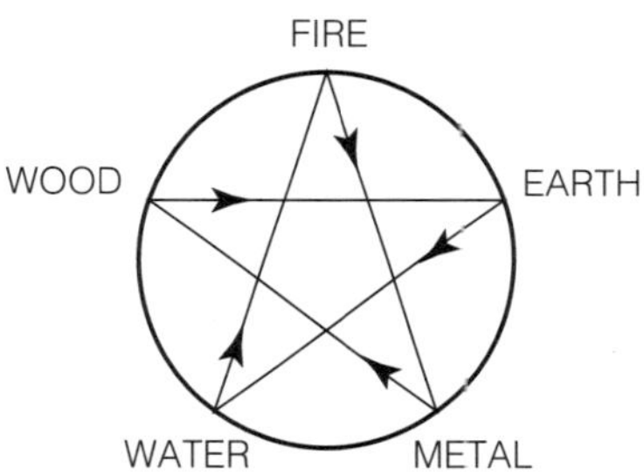

Figure 8

THE ANTI-KO CYCLE

This is the opposite of the Ko cycle: a certain element becomes so strong and excessive that it reverses the Ko cycle (Figure 9).

For example, in excess of the Earth, two elements are threatened: Water, according to the Ko cycle, but also Wood, according to the anti-Ko cycle. Hence, therapy must tonify both these elements, Water and Wood.

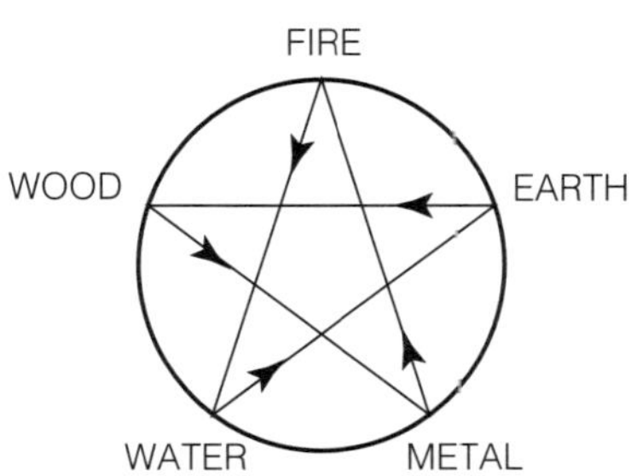

Figure 9

CATEGORIES IN THE FIVE ELEMENTS

We have put the Five Elements on a circle to facilitate our reasoning. Different categories can be linked to these elements. These correlations are so often used in acupuncture that they have to be known by every acupuncturist. We have seen that the energy passes from one organ to another, completing a cycle in one year, after staying in each organ for about one season. Each organ belongs to a season, but also to other useful characteristics such as tastes, odors, meats, vegetables, emotions, etc. The fifth season, or the Long Summer, is a period divided in four smaller ones, each of 18 days. They are placed between the four main seasons, and correspond to a time period in which one season gradually changes into the next one.

In a certain season, the organ of that season will be dominant in energy, it will dominate the other organs. The Chinese compared this to a state of balance existing in a palace: there is the emperor (dominant in his season), his mother (this organ precedes him and is empty in energy after feeding the emperor with her milk), his son (the organ after him, energetic and the next emperor in line in the following season), the conquered enemy (the organ situated after the son, must be dominated by the emperor or he can take over according to the Anti-Ko cycle), and finally "the chief-of-staff" or "chief-adviser", whose task it is to assist the emperor in his excesses and weaknesses. He is dominated by the emperor, but if the emperor becomes incapable of doing his duty, the adviser will take the emperor's place (Figure 10).

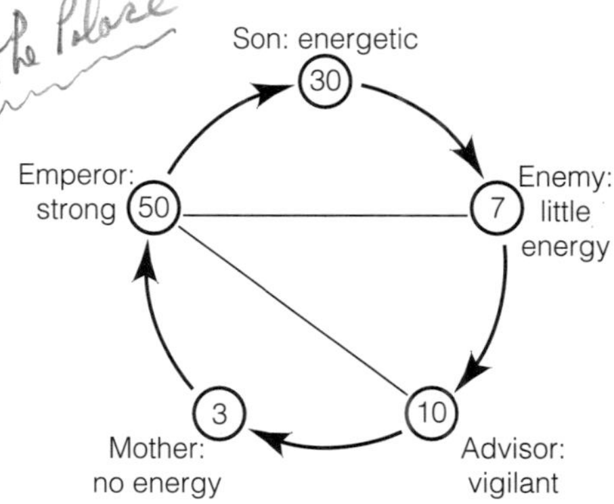

Figure 10

In the conditions expressed in percentages of Qi, shown in Figure 10, the So Ouenn says, "*The energies are in peace, disease cannot appear.*" The above diagram is important diagnostically and therapeutically. For example. If the liver is weak in the spring, the acupuncturist must tonify the liver, and disperse the two organs which possible can attack and dominate it: the adviser lung and the conquered enemy spleen. The quantity of energy will be spread badly among these organs, and a return of health can occur only by bringing these amounts in the appropriate proportion.

How does the acupuncturist know that an organ or the emperor is deficient in energy? There is of course the confirmation by taking the pulse, but it is safe for the beginner and the advanced acupuncturist, to confirm this weakness by clinical symptoms. Let's take again the example of the liver.

Symptoms of Liver Xu (Deficiency):

WOOD	
SPRING	"spring" diseases such as allergies, ulcers
FONG	likes running in wind
ACIDIDITY	cravings for sour things, oranges, lemons
WEST	
BLOOD	anemia
NAILS	brittle nails and deformed
EYES	decrease of visual acuity
TEARS	lack of tears
MUSCLES	muscular fatigue
ANGER	apathy
WALKING	walking fatigues easily
SHEEP	craves sheep
GREEN	
SPEAKING	abnormal autism

Symptoms of Liver Shi (Excess):

WOOD	
SPRING	
FONG	dislikes wind
ACIDITY	aversion for sour foods
WEST	
BLOOD	red face, polycythemia
NAILS	hard, deformed nails
EYES	tendency to conjunctivitis, irritation, redness
TEARS	abundant tearing
MUSCLES	spasms and contractures
ANGER	outbursts of anger, frustration and irritability
WALKING	wants to move, addicted to exercise
SHEEP	aversion for sheep
GREEN	
SPEAKING	logorrhea

I have outlined all the characteristics of the five elements in Table 1.

PRACTICAL EXAMPLES

- ❏ A patient has a flu in the fall, the season in which the lung is normally strong. This illness means that the lung is weak, the fire will be the most dangerous ("fire will melt the metal"). But the fong is the direct attacker (flu). The acupuncturist must defend the lung against the Heart fire and the Liver fong.
  1. Tonifie the Lung (L9t) and the alarm point, L1t.
  2. Defend against H-fire and Li-fong: L11d (Fong point) and L10d.
  3. Disperse the Li-fong (Li8d in fall) and Yu point of the liver (B18d).
  4. Disperse the H-fire (H3d in fall) and the Yu point of the heart (B15d).
  5. Disperse special points: B12d

Table 1 Characteristics of the Five Elements

Wood	Fire	Earth	Metal	Water
Spring	Summer	5th Season	Fall	Winter
Fong	Heat	Dampness	Dryness	Cold
Acidity	Bitter	Sweet	Pungent	Salty
West	South	Center	East	North
Blood	Psyche	Flesh	Energy	Will
Nails	Face Color	Lips	Hair-Body	Hair
Eyes	Tongue	Mouth	Nose	Ear
Eye Sight	Taste	Touch	Smell	Hearing
Tears	Sweat	Saliva	Mucus	Urine
Anger	Happiness	Worry	Sadness	Fear
Walking	Observing	Sitting	Lying	Standing
Sheep	Chicken	Beef	Horse	Pork
Green	Red	Yellow	Blue	Black
Speaking	Salivation	Swallowing	Coughing	Yawning

(Wind or fong point for the respiratory system) and GB 20d (fong point entering the body).

- During the fifth season (18 days) situated between the summer and the fall—the only period of the year that the Spleen is at its maximum energy—(while it has equal energy during the three other fifth seasons)a patient has liver problems and presents with fits of anger, irritability, muscle spasms, conjunctivitis, jaundice and digestive problems. A diagnosis of Emptiness of the Spleen Qi with Excess Liver Qi is established. The Liver attacks the Spleen.
  1. Disperse the Liver (Li4d in 5th season) and B18d (Liver Yu point).
  2. Tonifie the Spleen (Sp2t in 5th season) and Li13t (alarm point of Sp.).
  3. Protect the Spleen against the Liver (Sp1d).

For more insight in this therapy, see "Seasonal Tonification and Dispersion Points," Chapter 7.

TSANG AND FU ORGANS

As already mentioned before, there is a difference in structure and function in our organs. According to the number one law in acupuncture, we will have Yang (Fu) and Yin (Tsang) organs.

- The Fu organs are hollow and their essential role is one of transportation and transformation (this is movement, hence Yang).
- The Tsang organs are full (concentrated), and their essential role is storing of Energy (here is a notion of rest, matter, stagnation, hence Yin).

Running to and through these organs are the meridians or chings (kings), named for the organs to which they belong. The energy circulates everywhere but preferentially uses these pathways for their transportation according to a very precise pattern. The cycle of circulation of the Qi starts in the Lung meridian and continues in an alternation of a Yang with a Yin meridian:

LUNG—LARGE INTESTINE—STOMACH—SPLEEN—HEART—SMALL INTESTINE—BLADDER—KIDNEY—PERICARDIUM—TRIPLE BURNER—GALL BLADDER—LIVER

and from the Liver on starts a new cycle. We have 50 cycles in 24 hours, or one cycle every 29 minutes. The largest part of the Qi stays for two hours in each meridian (the meridian is in fullness), while the next two hours that same meridian will be in emptiness, or contains a minimum of energy. This is expressed in the Chinese Organ Clock. Starting with the Lung, this organ has its maximum energy between 3-5 a.m. The other maximum times of the organs can be found in Figure 2.

A few examples will clarify the importance of this clock. The moment that the energy is at its maximum in an organ will be the hours for that organ to be extremely sensitive, hence prone to disturbances. It is well known for instance, even in Western medicine, that an asthma patient will wake up or has a tendency to do so, between 3-5 a.m., just as the energy of the Lung should be at its maximum.

Other examples:

- ❑ The liver patient wakes up with a headache between 1-3 a.m.
- ❑ Heart attacks are frequently seen between 11 a.m. - 1 p.m.
- ❑ Kidney attacks, due to stones, often occur between 5-7 p.m.

But there is a second relationship in this organ clock: the Midday-Midnight relationship. Each organ has a relationship with the diametrical opposite organ:

Midday-Midnight Relationship

GB-H	Li-SI	L-B	LI-K
St-PC	Sp-TB	H-GB	

This has important symptomatic and therapeutic consequences. It is not rare to see a patient late at night with Gall Bladder pain, accompanied by palpitations—disturbance in an organ will always lead to disturbance in the Midday-Midnight relationship. The therapeutic consequences can be found in Chapter 4. A special word about the Pericardium and the Triple Burner: these are two functions rather than organs. They correspond to:

- ❑ Pericardium: the meridian of circulation but also of the sexual functions.
- ❑ Triple Burner: the meridian of metabolism, of solids and liquids.

All these Tsang and Fu organs are coupled in a Yin-Yang relationship, also called the Mother-Son Relationship:

Mother-Son Relationship

L-LI	St-SP	PC-TB	GB-Li
	H-SI	B-K	

Putting these organs in the Five Elements as seen in Figure 11:

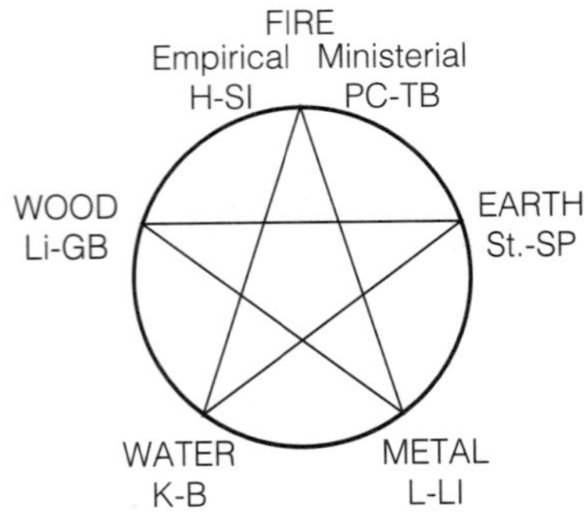

Figure 11

Adding the other categories into this picture will give us now the full value of the Five-Element theory. A few examples will clarify this theory.

- ❑ A patient's eye problem is related to a disturbance in the Liver, will aggravate in the spring due to fong, and causes tearing of the eyes; the fong brings the allergies, causing sneezing (anti-Ko cycle), and a feeling of fatigue in the muscles.
- ❑ A patient who is an obsessive compulsive worrier, a perfectionist, hypochondriac, can develop a stomach ulcer, aggravated in the post-summer (falling of the leaves) and in the spring (Ko-cycle). This Stomach patient is skinny (decrease of the volume of the muscles) and has no tone in his muscles.
- ❑ The asthma patient frequently alternates his asthma attacks with eczema attacks. The worst season will be the fall, and it is well know that these patients are prone to depression and hard to live with. They typically have a white face color (extremely pale).
- ❑ The Kidney patient is fearful, chilly and indecisive. He frequently complains about backaches (bones) or arthritis, loss of head hair, ear ringing

and palpitations (Ko-cycle).

LOCATION OF THE TONIFICATION AND DISPERSING POINTS IN RELATION TO THE FIVE ELEMENTS

Remember two important laws:

> "The tonification point of a meridian is always the Mother Element point of the concerned meridian."
>
> "The dispersion point of meridian is always the Son Element point of that meridian."

Some examples and Figure 12 will clarify this important notion.

The tonification point of the Fire-meridians (PC-H) is the Wood-point: H9 and PC9. It is a misconception of the beginner-acupuncturist to think that he needs in this case a point of the Liver meridian. We have to consider the Mother-point (Wood in this case) of the concerned element (Heart in this case): we stay within the same meridian. The dispersion point of the Fire-meridians (PC-H) is the Son-point, or, in this case, the Earth-point. Again we stay within the same meridian: PC7 and H7.

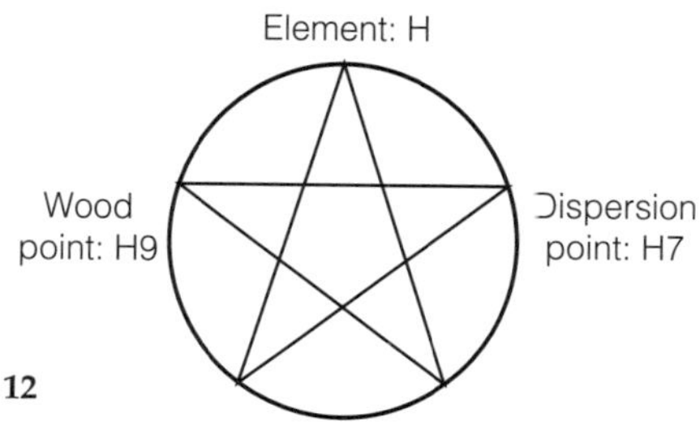

Figure 12

❑ *What meridians are influenced by puncturing the tonification point?*

Stimulating the tonification point of a meridian has an influence not only on that concerned meridian, but on all the meridians in relationship with the punctured meridian, which are:

- **The Mother-meridian**
- **The Son-meridian**
- **The Midday-Midnight relationship**
- **The Husband-Wife relationship**

Every meridian has two mothers and two sons because they are placed in two energetic cycles: the Five-Element cycle and the Great-Energy cycle (Chinese Clock). Let us look again at the example of the H-meridian.

The Mother-meridians of the H are: Sp (Chinese Clock) and Li (Five-Element cycle). The Son-meridians are: SI (Chinese Clock) and Sp (Five Element cycle). Summarized: *tonification of a meridian tonifies that meridian and the four surrounding meridians.*

This tonification Qi must be delivered by some other meridians. This Qi comes from the Midday-Midnight relationship and from the Husband-Wife relationship. For the H-meridian we have the GB and the L; tonification of the H will disperse these meridians.

❑ *What meridians are influenced by puncturing the dispersion point?*

The dispersion point of meridian is the Son-point of that meridian. In case of the H-meridian, the Earth-point (H-7) is the dispersion point. Puncturing this point disperses the H-meridian, but also the two Mother and Son points. They are, respectively: Sp and Li, SI and Sp again. The excess Qi taken away from the meridian flows to the Midday-Midnight relationship and the Husband-Wife relationship.

HUSBAND-WIFE RELATIONSHIP

Husband	Wife
H	L
Li	Sp
K	PC

BATTLE BETWEEN THE WEI QI AND PERVERSE QI IN THE DEEP ORGANS

CIRCULATION OF WEI QI IN THE DEEP ORGANS

The Wei Qi will circulate in the deep organs according to an annual rhythm: it will follow the Sheng cycle, going from the Liver, to the Heart, the Spleen, the Lung and the Kidney. When the Wei Qi circulates in a normal fashion according to this cycle, man is in perfect health. But the Liver energy can be disturbed if there is an abnormal cold spring or too hot, like an early summer. What is happening if this perverse energy (cold or heat in this case) is strong enough to overcome the Vital Energy (the sum of Wei, Iong and Ancestral QI) of the patient? This perverse Qi goes from the Liver to the Spleen, to the Kidney, to the Heart and finally will reach the Lung. At this point, when the perverse Qi arrives in the dominating organ according to the Ko-cycle, the life of the patient is in danger. How can we avoid this?

There is only one rule: act on the organs according to the Ko-cycle! E.g.,when the Liver is in emptiness, the Lung will be in excess . Hence, first disperse the Lung, and then tonify the Liver. In case of excess of the Liver, there will be deficiency of Qi in the Lung. In this case, first tonify the Lung, then disperse the Liver. The same law is applied for the hollow organs.

PATHWAYS OF PENETRATION OF THE PERVERSE QI IN THE DEEP ORGANS AND HOLLOW ORGANS

There are several ways that the perverse Qi can penetrate in the organs.

Direct way of food intake

This happens at the occasion of a food poisoning or severe food indigestion. Once the perverse Qi, has invaded an organ, the body will try to reject it. To penetrate an organ, the perverse Qi followed a certain path:

❑ Perverse Qi→ Hollow organ→ Organ.

To leave the organ, several pathways are possible:

❑ Organ→ Hollow organ→ diarrhea or vomiting.

❑ Organ→ Hollow organ→ Primary Channel Yang.

❑ Organ→ Divergent Meridian.

❑ Organ→ Organ→ Organ→ etc., according to "5 elements".

Through the Primary Yang Channels

The perverse Qi follows the route:

❑ Tmm→ Primary Yang Channel→ Hollow organ→ Organ.

To leave, the exact opposite path is followed. Another possibility, is following a Divergent meridian: at that point, symptoms will become intermittent (See "Divergent Meridians," Chapter 4). A last possibility is following the 5 element cycle:

❑ Organ→ Organfi Organ→ etc., according to "5 elements".

Through the Primary Yin Channel

As in the previous case, the perverse Qi invades consecutively the Tmm, the Primary Yin Channel, the Organ and terminates in the Hollow organ. Hence, the perverse Qi does not stay in the Organ, only passes through, to finish up in the Hollow organ.

The Perverse Qi leaves according to several possible circuits:

❑ Hollow organ→ Organ→ Primary Channel Yin.

❑ Hollow organ→ Organ→ Divergent Meridian.

4 The Different Channels: Characteristics and Therapy

THE PRIMARY CHANNELS (SEE FIGURE 13)

CHARACTERISTICS

The Primary Channels (King or Ching) are the most important meridians. It is the image of the principal river, connecting the different parts of the country, while receiving and splitting in different little streams. They cannot be materialized but can be shown indirectly: puncturing a point on the meridian often causes a sensation on the rest of the meridian. They have a very deep and a superficial part. The superficial fraction follows the limbs and goes more specifically from the elbow to the fingers and from the knee to the toes. This element contains the sixty-six important Su-antique points. The deep component runs from the shoulder or pelvic region to the elbow or knee. At the level of the trunk is the deepest section of the Primary Channel, connecting with the Tsang-and Fu organs. There are twelve meridians, bilateral: six Yang, six Yin, six at the superior limb, six at the inferior limb. The Yin meridians run in the Yin-zones: the front, the lower part, the inner or medial side of the limbs. The Yang meridians travel throught the Yang-zones: the back, the upper part, the exterior or lateral part of the limbs. As mentioned before, *the quantity of Yin and Yang in an organ has nothing to do with the topography of the corresponding meridian.* The Kidney and Lung are organs, containing high energy (very Yang!) although the meridians are located in the Yin-zones! (See "Characteristics of Yin-Yang," Chapter 1).

Each meridian is named for the Tsang-or Fu organ to which it is linked. The Yang meridians descend, the Yin ascend. Each Yang meridian is coupled with a Yin one. The Qi circulates in these meridians according to a certain pattern. The cycle starts in the meridian of the Lung, and the flow of the Qi will alternately go through two Yin and two Yang meridians:

L — LI — St — Sp — H — SI — B — K — PC — TB — GB — Li — L

The Qi follows the whole meridian, not only the superficial and the deeper part, but goes also to the organs. When the Qi arrives at the meridian of the Li, the cycle will start all over again. We have observed in the organ clock that the energy circulating in these organs, changes in quality and quantity. This energy is a mixture of Yong, Ancestral and seasonal Qi, always flowing centripetal for Cheou Yang and Tsou-Yin, Centrifugal for Cheou-Yin and Tsou-Yang. It speaks by itself, that the best moment to tonify a meridian is when it contains the maximum energy, while dispersion will be most successful, when the energy is minimal in the meridian. Unfortunately, modern life schedule does not always allow us to follow this important rule, although I would recommend it in a difficult case.

For further reasoning and working knowledge, it is much easier to adopt the Chinese terms:

- meridians of upper extremities are TSOU
- meridians of lower extremities are CHEOU

There are three levels for the Yin and Yang:

TAE-YANG or strongest Yang
CHAO-YANG or middle Yang
YANG-MING or weakest Yang
TAE-YIN or strongest Yin
CHAO-Yin or middle Yin
TSIUE-YIN or weakest Yin

Combining these terminologies, we have the new names for our meridians, which express immediately location, qualification (Yang or Yin) and the degree of energy, running through.

UPPER EXTREMITIES

CHEOU-TAE-YIN or Lung
CHEOU-CHAO-YIN or Heart
CHEOU-TSIUE YIN or Pericardium
CHEOU-TAE-YANG or Small Intestine
CHEOU-CHAO-YANG or Triple Burner
CHEOU-YANG-MING or Large Intestine

LOWER EXTREMITIES

TSOU-TAE-YIN or Spleen
TSOU-CHAO-YIN or Kidney
TSOU-TSIUE-YIN or Liver
TSOU-TAE-YANG or Bladder
TSOU-CHAO-YANG or Gall Bladder
TSOU-YANG-MING or Stomach

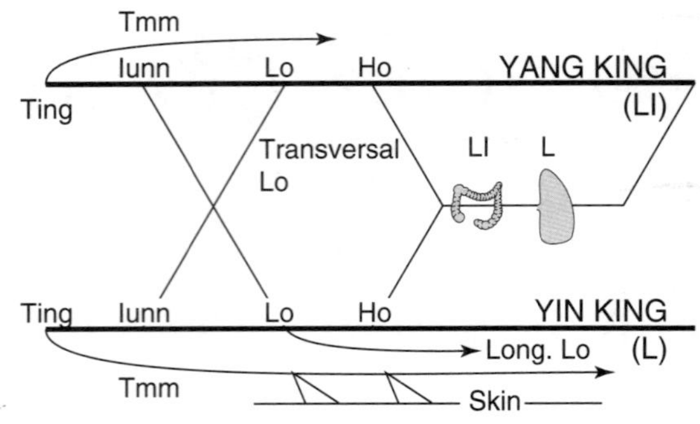

Figure 13

THE SU-ANTIQUE POINTS

As we see in Figure 13, the Su-antique points, sixty-six in total, are located on the superficial part of the meridian, between the Ting and Ho points. They are located between the fingers and the elbow, and between the toes and the knees. They are the most important points in therapy in acupuncture, and, therefore, a thorough understanding and description are necessary. They are on each meridian respectively: Ting, Tong, Iu (Shu), King and Ho.

Ting Points

They are the first or last points of the meridians, very important for therapeutical use, since the Yin flows into the Yang and vice-versa. The location in the five elements is different for the Yin and the Yang meridians.

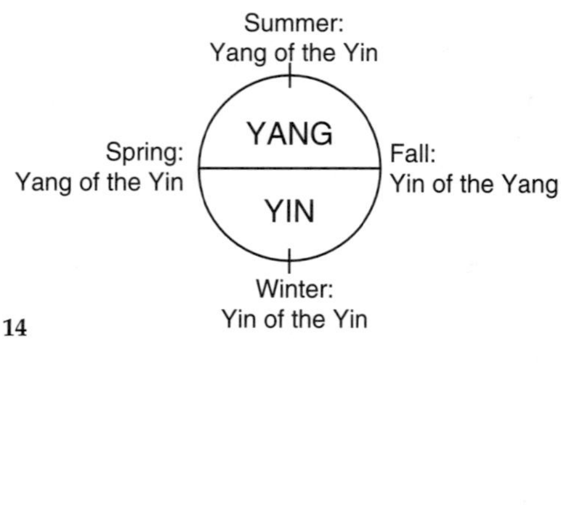

Figure 14

Yin-meridians: the Ting-point corresponds to wood-wind or spring. In the universe, the spring is the period where Yang penetrates into Yin: it is the Yang of the Yin. (Figure 14).

Since the Ting-point corresponds with the spring, the Qi of the coupled Yang-meridian communicates with the Qi of the Yin-meridian, exactly what happens in the Universe. Once the Ting-point is located on the Yin-meridians, the other Su-antique points are found easily. (Figure 15).

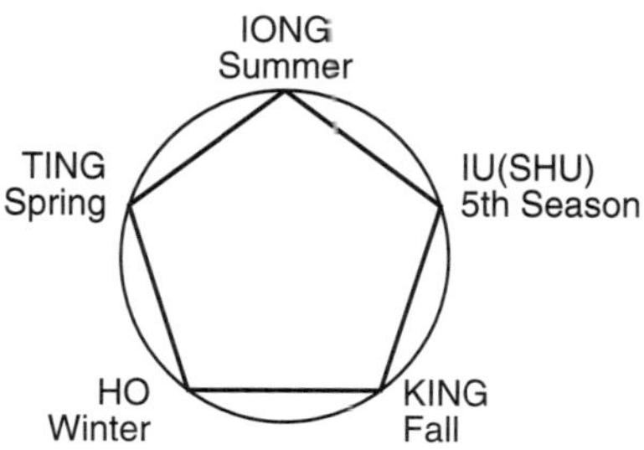

Figure 15 YIN MERIDIANS

Yang-meridians: The Ting-point corresponds with metal-dryness or fall. In the Universe, fall is the period where the Yin penetrates the Yang: it is the Yin of the Yang. (Figure 15) Hence, we can say that at the Ting-points of the Yang-meridians the Qi of the coupled Yin-meridian will communicate with the Qi of the Yang-meridian. The schema for the Yang-meridians is seen in Figure 16.

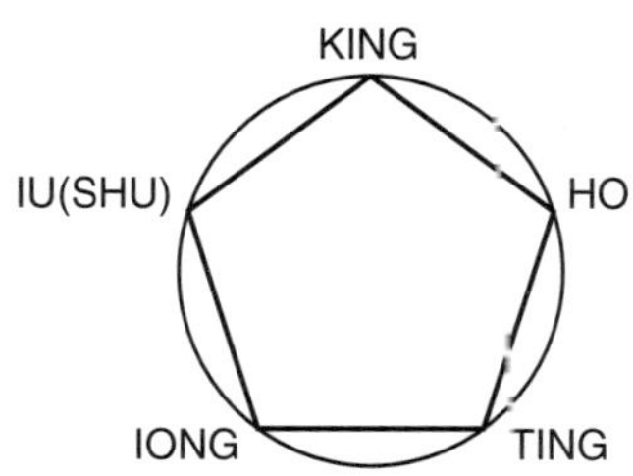

Figure 16 YANG MERIDIANS

There are several important aspects of the Ting-point:

- ❏ It draws the Qi from the Exterior in the meridian, important if we want to bring the essential (Wei and Yong) Qi in the meridian.
- ❏ It draws the Qi of the meridian towards the extremity. E.g., to draw the Qi of the B-meridian towards the foot (in case of torticollis), puncture B67, the Ting-point.
- ❏ It is the departure point of the Tmm: puncturing will avoid the penetration of the Perverse Qi in the meridian.
- ❏ It is punctured in the treatment of the Divergent Channels, on the opposite side. (See Chapter 4, Paragraph V)
- ❏ Puts the Energy into movement.

Iong Points

They are situated in the metacarpophalangial joints and the metatarsophalangial joints. Starting from the extremity, they are the second points. Figure 15 shows us that they correspond for the Yin-meridians, with fire-heat-Small Intestine-summer. We will use this point to bring Heat in a Yin-meridian. For the Yang-meridians, they correspond with water-Kidney-winter. They are used to bring to or disperse Cold from the Yin-meridians. (See Figure 16).

These points *accelerate* the Qi in the meridian. E.g., to accelerate the Qi in the B-meridian, puncture B66. Another example. We want to bring Qi towards a certain region of the body: the nose, in case of sinusitis. We use the tonification point and the acceleration or Iong point of the LI: LI2 and LI11 (in the Fall).

Iu or Shu Points

They are points that *transport or distribute* the Qi—Essential, Wei and Perverse Qi. For the Yin-meridians, they correspond with earth-spleen-Stomach-5th season. We will use these points to disperse the Perverse Qi dampness from the Yin-meridians. For the Yang-meridians, they correspond with wood-Gallbladder-Liver-spring. They will be punctured to disperse the wind or fong.

Important aspects of the Iu points are:

- ❏ In the Yin-meridians, the Iu point is also the Iuun point; in the Yang meridians, the Iu and Iuun points are different.

- ❑ It is the point where the Wei Qi as well as the Perverse Qi will penetrate; hence, this point has great therapeutical value. When the Perverse Qi attacks our system, it will penetrate first in the Tmm.

In the case of severe attack or deficiency of Wei Qi, this Perverse Qi will spread in Primary meridians via the Ting-point. (It is the only common point between the Tmm and their Primary vessels.) This Perverse Qi will continue its course via the Iong point to be absorbed in the Iu point. (See Figure 17)

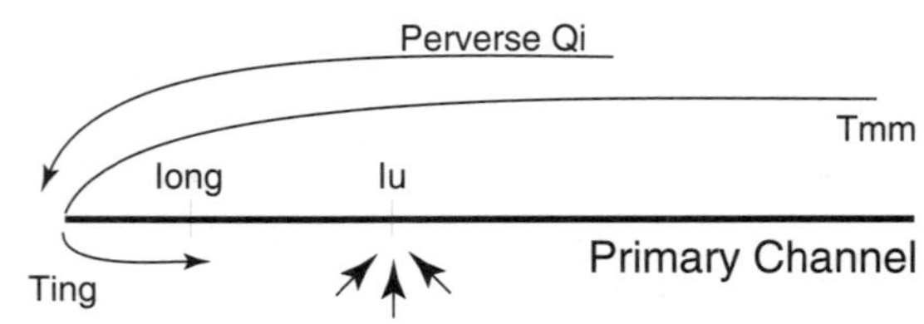

Figure 17

King Points

At the level of the King points, the flow of the Qi is strong: they are points of *transmission* and *collecting* of Qi. They put the energy in reserve. From the King points, there is transmission in two directions: the meridians and the bones-articulations. King points are situated at the articulations of the wrist and ankles. For the Yin-meridians, they correspond with metal-Lung-Large Intestine-fall. We will use these points to bring or to disperse dryness in a Yin-meridian. (See Figure 15). For the Yang-meridians, they correspond with fire-Heart-Small Intestine-summer. They will be used to bring heat or disperse heat in a Yang-meridian. (See Figure 16)

Important aspects of these points are:

- ❑ For the Yin-meridians: the Yang Qi decreases from the Ting point on and becomes zero at the King point; the Yin Qi increases from the Ting point on and reaches its maximum at the King point. (Figure 18). We have the opposite for the Yang-meridians. In other words, from the point King on, the Qi is Yin in the Yin-meridians, Yang in the Yang-meridians.
- ❑ The perverse Qi Dampness fixes itself in the bones and the muscles; it is absorbed at the Iu point and deviated to the bones and muscles at the King points. In case of the Yin-meridians, when the bones, muscles and articulations are attacked, puncture the King points to block the penetration of the Perverse Qi. In the case of the Yang-meridians, puncture these points to accelerate the transmission of Qi.

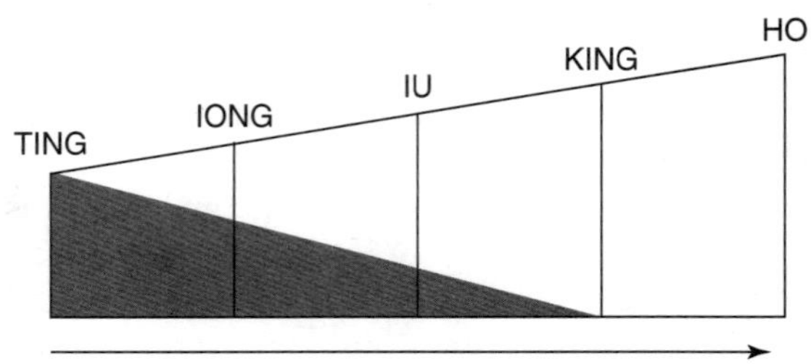

Figure 18

Ho Points

These points are situated at the elbows and the knees. They are the border points between the superficial and deeper part of the meridian. For the Yin-meridians, they correspond with the water-Kidney-Bladder-winter. They will be used to bring cold or disperse cold in the Yin-meridians. For the Yang-meridians, they correspond with earth-Stomach-Spleen-long summer. They will be used to disperse dampness in the Yang-meridians.

Important characteristics:

- ❑ Situated between the superficial and the deeper part of the meridian, they are points of entrance or exit of the Qi. In centripetal meridians, they are a point of exit of the Qi.

- It is at these points that the Qi is transmitted to the deeper areas (Tsang and Fu organs). Puncturing these points will have a deep action. They are also called reunion points.

THERAPEUTICAL TECHNIQUES

Tonification and Dispersion

See chapter 7 on the *"Eight Principles"* and Addendum 1 at the end of this chapter.

"Grande Piqûre"

This technique is one of the most important in the treatment of pain, especially traumatic pain. On what principle is this technique based?

The two symmetrical branches of the same meridian (left and right) are connected through secondary vessels. Normally, an excess in one branch is diverted and channeled to the contra lateral branch. This way, the transport of the Qi is balanced and there will be no pain. However, under certain conditions (i.e., trauma), this equilibrium is broken so that the excessive Qi cannot flow to the collateral branch.

For example, we have an excess in LI Channel right (causing pain), and extending over a certain length of the channel. Frequently, it is linear pain. The technique will bring the excess of one channel into the deficient contra lateral channel by tonification of the Lo-point of the deficient, non-painful channel. In this case, we will tonify LI 6 on the left, the non-painful side. If there are more meridians involved of the same nature (Yang or Yin) in the trauma, the Group Lo point will be utilized. Assuming that the trauma involves the Li and SI channel on the right, the Lo point of the Cheou Yang Channels, TB8t on the left will be tonified. (Figure 19)

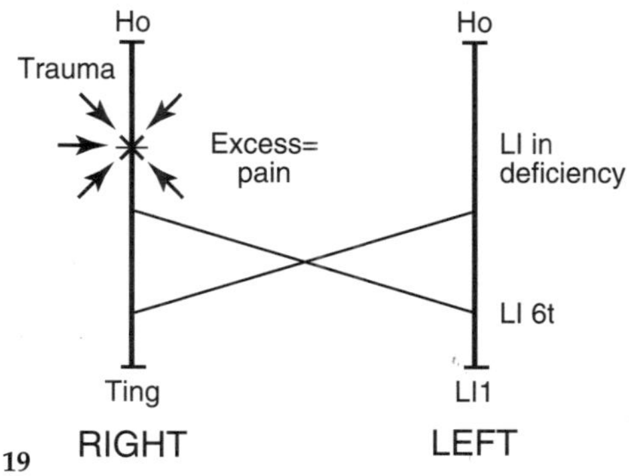

Figure 19

"Grande Piqûre" Combined with "Midday-Midnight" Law

Excess Qi in the meridian is drawn not only to the contra-lateral equivalent channel, but also to its coupled meridian, according to the Day/Night relationship which can be found in the Chinese Organ Clock (Figure 11). Referring to the above example, therapy would be: LI6t left and K4t left (LO point of the Kidney). In case of a Group-Lo point, the opposite Yin-Yang Group-Lo point on the other extremity is used to enhance treatment. Using the previous example, we stimulate TB8t left and Sp6t left. A Yang Group-Lo point above, requires a Yin Group-Lo point below.

"Petite Piqûre"

This technique is used in case the pain zone has the form of a small spot and is non-linear. For example, trauma on LI channel, right side: the pain is felt on the right side, concentrated in one spot, and not extended over the length of the channel.

The therapy consists of puncturing three points in a specific order:

- Puncture a point of the LI channel, the closest one above the pain center.
- Puncture a point of the Li channel just below the pain center.
- Puncture the pain center itself. An exception to this technique is facial paralysis: puncturing the non-painful

side in tonification is indicated in this situation. Failure to do so will result in an aggravation.

Yu-Mo Technique

This technique uses the Back-Yu points (Associated Points) and the Front-Mu points simultaneously. Both points are areas where the Qi of the organs connects and flows through. In chronic diseases involving an organ, these points become tender and painful upon pressure and are, therefore, very useful diagnostically. Controversy exists as to what stimulating technique to use for these points. It is better to rely on the ancient texts which dictate that the Qi enters throught the Mo points and leaves through the Yu points, going from Yin to Yang. Puncturing the Mo-points is supposed to bring Qi to the diseased organs (tonification), while the Back-Shu point is dispersed in order to drain excess in an organ or heat in the corresponding organ. This technique is very powerful, and it is known that some ancient masters used this technique solely and with great efficiency.

To summarize, there are three possibilities to act upon an organ directly: by puncturing the Hu or season tonification point, Mo and Ho points. The Mo point always is located in the front, and is a point of concentration of the Qi. To strengthen this organ and its meridian without simultaneously strengthening the organs surrounding the one being stimulated, it is preferable to use the Front-Mo points. For example, to treat a bitter taste in the mouth due to a deficiency of the Gall Bladder, one could use either the seasonal tonification point of the GB or the Mo point (GB24t). The preferred point in this case is GB24t, since tonifying the seasonal tonification point of the GB, will also tonify Li, TB, B and SI (according to the Five Elements and the Chinese Organ Clock).

The Back-Yu points have a calming and dispersing effect. This calming effect is less intense than the puncturing of the seasonal dispersion point of the corresponding meridian. Hence, in the case of incorrect diagnosis, the disturbance of Qi will be less severe if the Back-Yu points were punctured.

Source-Lo Technique

This technique uses the Source point of meridian and the Lo point of the meridian involved in the "Brother/Sister relationship." The points are used to regulate a disease involving both channels. For example, St primarily affected by a disease is called the "host", the Sp (the Yin Primary Channel in the Yin/Yang relationship), is called the "guest". Applying this technique requires puncturing of the source point of St (St42) and the Lo point of the Sp (Sp4). A major contra-indication of this technique is when the cause of the disease is an Exterior Excess (e.g., cold, heat, etc.). For instance, dampness attacks the St. Use of this technique will bring the Dampness in the Sp and cause disastrous results for the patient! The Source-point (point where the original Qi is located) will indicate the health of the channel. The Lo-point is the departure point of the Transversal and Longitudinal Lo-vessels.

While applying this technique, two important questions can be asked:

Where does the Qi go in case of dispersion of the Lo-point, and where does the Qi originates from in case of tonification of the Lo-point?

When dispersing the Lo-point, the Qi goes to:

- ❑ The Source-point of the meridian in the Yin-Yang relationship.
- ❑ To the same meridian of the other side.
- ❑ To the Day/Night relationship of the involved meridian.

E.g., dispersion of L7d: the Qi goes to LI4, to the L meridian of the other side and to the Bladder meridian (according to the Chinese Clock).

When tonifying the Lo-point, the Qi comes from:

The same sources as mentioned above, but the situation is reversed.

Four-Needle Technique

This technique is used according to the Five Elements. The purpose is to tonify an element in deficiency or to disperse an element in excess. Two cycles are used:

- ❏ The Sheng-cycle (inter promoting law)
- ❏ The Ko-cycle (counteracting law)

a. Deficiency of an Element (XU)

The general rule is that in case of Xu or Shi of an element, we have to act first according to the Ko-cycle. For example, Xu of the Liver is diagnosed. Two points need to be dispersed. First, L8 (King point of the Lung). The L normally controls the Li, but here due to the deficiency of the Li, the L overpowers the Li and takes the place of the Li. At the same time, we stay within the involved meridian (Li), and disperse its Ko-element or King point: Li4d.

The second part of the therapy consists of tonifying the Xu meridian: tonification of an element is using its Mother-Point! We have two mothers. First, the Element Mother of the Liver is the Kidney: K10t (Ho point); then the mother-point of the meridian itself, Li8t (Ho-point). To summarize: to strengthen the deficient Li, we use 4 needles: L8d, Li4d, K10t and Li8t. At first sight, this technique seems very attractive. However its use is limited to the season of the concerned meridian. In the above example, we use this technique only in the Spring. Preference has to be given to the seasonal points (Figure 20).

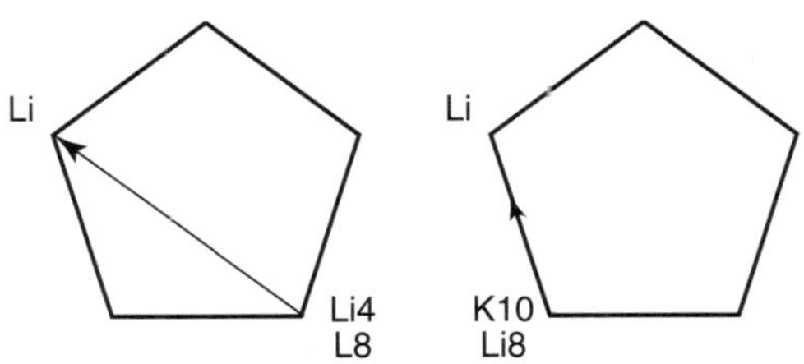

Figure 20

b. Excess of an Element (SHI)

First act on the Ko-cycle: L8t and Li4t; then disperse the meridian using the Son-element points: H8d and Li2d (Figure 21).

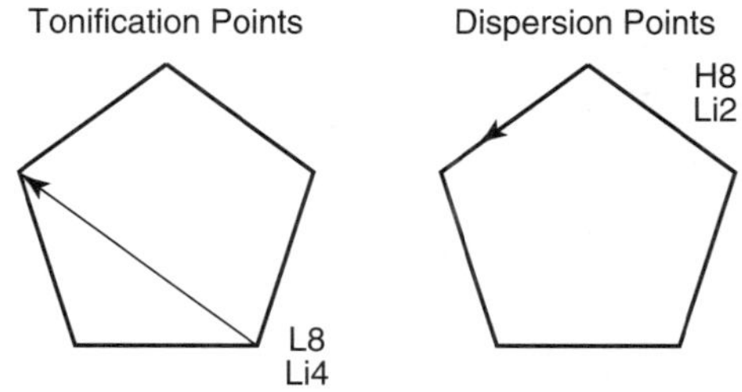

Figure 21

The technique has the same limited used as mentioned in the Xu of an element.

Use of the Penn Points

Often in practice, a desperate patient will come with a problem that is very important to him and his family. "When I go to the warm climates on our vacation (and God knows how much we need this if we are not living in California), right away I get a rash which does not leave me for the entire vacation. Do I have to give up this kind of vacation (sigh of the wife is heard), or can you help me?" (hopeful look of the wife)

The Penn points will be an excellent weapon. Each organ, whether Tsang or Fu, is represented during the entire year by a point which acts directly on it. These are called the "Penn points" or "Protection points" (the latter name relates to its function). These points are listed in Figure 22.

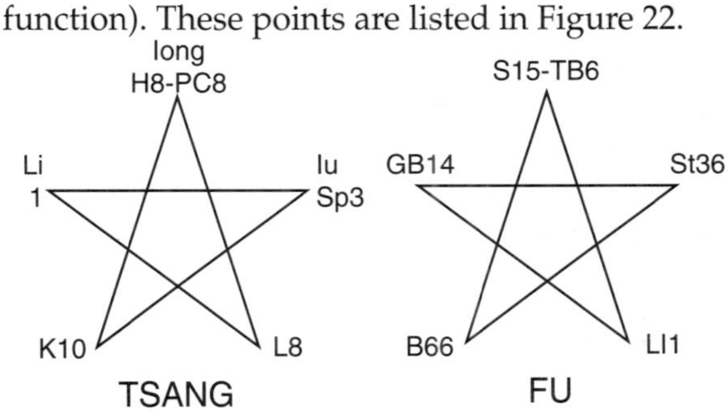

Figure 22

How are they used?

There is an important law that explains their use:

> "When an organ (Tsang or Fu) is attacked by another organ excess, or any characteristic belonging to the Five Elements (color, sense, meat, climate, etc.), then we disperse the Penn-point of the attacker."

A few examples will clarify this law.

- ❑ Neck pain due to Cold. Bladder is the attacked meridian, cold is the attacker (K-B). B is Yang, so we stay in the Yang and we disperse the Yang part of the Cold (B): B66d.
- ❑ Pain in the thigh following the GB meridian, caused by the cold. Attacker: cold; attacked meridian: GB (Yang); Therapy: B66d (Penn point) and GB43d (Cold point of GB).
- ❑ Diarrhea, due to too much cold or raw food. Attacker: Cold; attacked organ is LI (Yang). Therapy: B66d (Penn and LI2d (Cold point of LI).
- ❑ In the example mentioned before, rash due to the Heat of the sun. Attacked organ: skin or Lung (Yin); attacker is Heat. Therapy: Penn-point, H8d and L10d, Heat point of the L.
- ❑ Fong allergies, attack on the skin (rash). Attacker: Heat. Attacked organ: skin (L, Yin). Therapy: Li1d (Penn) and L11d, Fong point of L.
- ❑ Sciatica due to Cold, following B meridian. Attacker: Cold; attacked meridian: B. Therapy: B66d (Pen-point but also at the same time Cold point of B).
- ❑ Sciatica due to Dampness: B40d and St36d.
- ❑ Sciatica due to muscular activity: B65d and GB41d.
- ❑ Paralysis a frigore" (Bell's palsy). Attacked meridian: St. Attacker: Cold. Therapy: B66d and St44d.
- ❑ Protecting the patient against cold and bronchitis. Attacker: Cold; attacked organ: L(Yin); therapy: K10d (Penn, we stay in the Yin) and L5d (Cold Point of L).
- ❑ A patient has diarrhea every time he eats herring. Attacker: salt (Winter); Attacked organ (LI; Therapy: B66(Penn) and LI 2 (salt point of LI).
- ❑ A more local problem in the area of Los Angeles is the "smog", irritating the eyes. Attacker, the smog brought by the Wind; attacked organ: eyes (Li); therapy: Li1d.

Conclusion: we can use the Penn-points as therapeutic points, once the disease has invaded the meridians or organs, but we can also use them in order to avoid the disease, as preventive therapy. Of course, using these points is not sufficient as therapy. Since an excess has been able to penetrate, the organ has to be in deficiency. Tonifying the empty organ and dispersing the attacking organ (Ko-cycle) using the seasonal points, is a necessary step in the treatment.

Different Methods To Disperse A Full Meridian

Example: a patient suffers from a sciatica, following the B-meridian on the right side.

- ❑ Use the season dispersion point on the right side.
- ❑ Use the contra-lateral Lo-point: B58 in tonificationor use of the Group-Lo point, GB39t on the left side.
- ❑ Use the coupled homolateral Primary Channel, Shao Yin or K: K3 and K4 in tonification, on the right side.
- ❑ Use of the Midday-Midnight rule: tonify on the same side (right, in this case), the corresponding organ in the Chinese Clock: L7t, Lo-point, or L9, tonification point.
- ❑ Use the Mother-Son law. To disperse a meridian, use its Son-point: K2 in dispersion on the right side.

- ❑ Use the Husband-Wife Relationship: disperse TB10 on the right side.

Use of a Taste in Dispersing or Strengthening An Organ

a. Physiology of the Tastes

The first transformation of the food happens in the Stomach, where it is split into pure and impure Qi. The impure Qi is sent down, and the pure Qi goes to the Spleen, where a second division takes place. The pure Qi goes to the Lung, the impure will form the tastes (Figure 23).

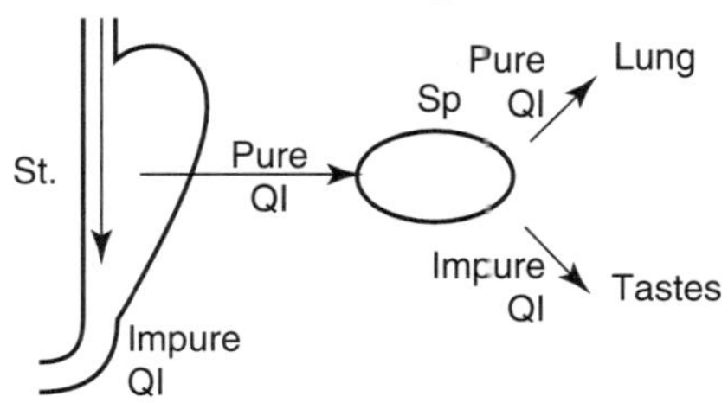

Figure 23

b. Characteristics of the Tastes

According to the Five Elements, to each organ belongs a taste:

Sour: Li, Bitter: H, Sweet: Sp, Pungent: L, Salt: K.

The tastes are classified as Yin or Yang according to different criteria:

- ❑ Quantitatively: food rich in taste is Yin, that which is less rich is Yang in the Yin; strong odors are Yang, less strong are Yin in the Yang ("Su Ouenn" Chapter 5).
- ❑ Qualitatively: the pungent and sweet tastes are Yang; salt, sour and bitter are Yin ("Su Ouenn" Chapter 5 and Figure 24).

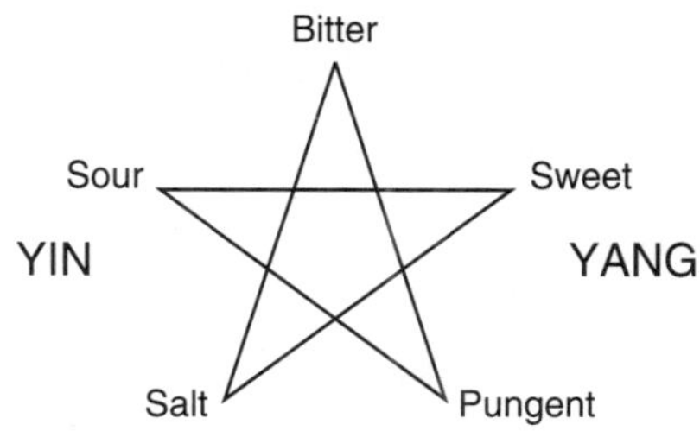

Figure 24

How will the knowledge of tastes help us in the diagnosis of an Excess or deficiency of an organ?

- ❑ Recent craving for a taste indicates a deficiency for the corresponding organ. For example, craving for sweet indicates a deficient Sp.
- ❑ Recent refusal of a certain taste indicates excess of the corresponding organ.

Each taste has specific characteristics ("Su Ouenn," Chapter 22):

Sour: immobilizes, collects.

Sweet: tonifies.

Bitter: consolidates.

Salt: lubricates.

Pungent: disperses, facilitates the circulation.

How can tastes help us in the tonification and dispersion of an organ? Tastes used in small quantities, will nourish the corresponding deficient organ. Tastes used in greater quantities, will cause different reactions. When taken during a short period of time, they will disperse the corresponding organ; taken for a longer period, they will disperse the organ in the Ko-cycle. Example: Too much sugar, taken over a long period of time, will contribute to a loss of head hair, sensitivity to Cold, impotence, etc. (K Deficiency, according to the Ko-Cycle).

The nature of the tastes can also be used to tonify or disperse: some tastes tonify the Yang, others tonify the Yin. (Figure 23). In chronic disturbances, to treat properly, one has to introduce the "assistant" taste (Long Shu Chapter 56):

"It is the taste, belonging to the organ in the Ko-cycle, and it will strengthen the action of the tonifying taste."

For example, the assistant taste for the Spleen is salt, belonging to the Kidney in the Ko-cycle. Other assistant tastes are:

Li: sweet; H: pungent; L: sour; K: bitter.

THE TENDINO MUSCULAR MERIDIANS (TMM) OR TCHING KANN

CHARACTERISTICS

These channels are the most superficial ones and have no direct connection with the organs. The Qi in these meridians is the Wei or Defensive Qi, indicating the main function of these Tmm channels. The direction of the Wei Qi in these Tmm has no importance: the only requirement is that there is enough Wei Qi present. Wei Qi circulates in the Yang during the day, in the Yin during the night. The Tmm channel has only the Ting point in common with the Primary channel. Hence, puncturing this point will be of great importance in the therapy. (Figure 25)

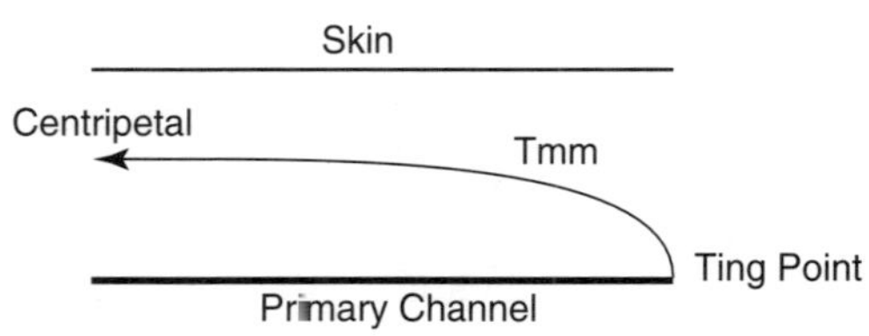

Figure 25

According to the So Ouenn, two important laws will guide us in the Tmm therapy:

> "When the Primary channel is Empty of Qi, the corresponding Tmm is Full"; and "When the Primary channel is Full of Qi, the corresponding Tmm will be empty."

The Tmm are broad areas, rather than lines, more or less following the course of the Primary channels. At the end of their course, the Tmm unite with each other in a particular zone, concentrated around an acupuncture point. These points are called the "meeting points" of the Tmm. When the Perverse Qi has penetrated the Tmm, we puncture these points in order to avoid the invasion of this Pernicious Qi in the other branches of the same group; e.g., invasion of Cold in the B-meridian, causing sciatica. We puncture the meeting point of the leg Yang channels SI18, to avoid spreading of Cold in the GB and St-meridian.

The other meeting points are :

Three arm Yang channels (LI-SI-TB): GB13;
Three arm Yin channels (L-H-PC): GB22;
Three foot Yin channels (K-SP-Li): CV4.

Rather than puncturing these points, we surround these points with three needles covering the area around them.

INDICATIONS OF THE TMM

- Dermatoses: eczema, sunstroke, warts, urticaria, pruritus.
- Muscular involvement: contusio, trauma (sprained ankle, tennis elbow, etc.).
- Neuralgia: herpes, zoster, zona ophtalmica, sciatica.
- Any superficial pain.

SYMPTOMS

- Fullness: hyperesthesia, hypersensitivity, superficial pain and dermatoses.
- Emptiness: hypo-esthesia and baldness of an area.

THERAPY

In case of Fullness:

- ❏ Disperse the locus dolendi (dispersing of the excess).
- ❏ Disperse the Ting point (brings Wei Qi).
- ❏ Use the season tonification point.
- ❏ Disperse the meeting point of the concerned meridians.

In case of Emptiness

- ❏ Plum blossom or rolling drum technique over the diseased area (brings Wei Qi in that area).
- ❏ Disperse the Ting point (to keep the point open).
- ❏ Use the season dispersion point

NOTE: the Ting point is the only point of connection between the Tmm and the Primary channel; hence, we must always disperse it!

THE LO-VESSELS

CHARACTERISTICS

The Longitudinal Lo-vessels all start from the Lo point. The general direction is *centripetal*, although there are two exceptions: *GB and L are centrifugal.* These vessels go directly to the organs, but their course is not as deep as that of the Primary vessels. This explains why a disturbance of a Longitudinal Lo-vessel is easily corrected. A disturbance is always due to an external excess (cold, heat, dryness, etc.). The Lo vessels are 16 in number:

- ❏ 12 split from the Primary channels
- ❏ 2 start from the Wonder meridians, Conception Vessel; (C.V.) and the Governor Vessel (G.V.), from CV15 and GV1 respectively.
- ❏ One start from the Spleen, Sp21 and is called the "Great" Lo, because it is a group of small vessels, with ramifications on the chest and the whole body. Its role is to control the whole Lo network.
- ❏ One start from St1.

In the case of the Transversal Lo-vessels, there is a disturbance of Internal Qi involving two vessels with a Yin-Yang relationship.

In the Nei King, we read: "When a Lo-point is in fullness, we see it easily." An exterior excess attack will have success only if the general resistance or body Qi (especially the sum of Wei and Yong Qi) is decreased. This attack leaves the Lo-vessel full, with a very sensitive, swollen Lo-point. It will be necessary to disperse the Lo-point.

It is also said in the Nei King, "When a Lo-point is in emptiness, the point is invisible." After the first attack of the excess which leaves the Lo-vessel in fullness, the excess goes on to overwhelm the Primary Channel, leaving the Lo-vessel in emptiness, as the second stage of the illness.

INDICATIONS

Longitudinal Lo-vessels

Essentially, the Longitudinal Lo's are disturbed by the action of Perverse Qi. This Perverse Qi can successfully attack our body only when there is a deficiency of Essential Qi. The Pernicious Qi causes first a Fullness, then an Emptiness of the Longitudinal Qi when it penetrates the Primary Channel.

In case of excess, the Lo-point will be sensitive. Since the Lo-vessels are more superficial than the Primary Channels, a disturbance of the Lo-vessels will be less harmful than an attack on the Primary vessels.

Transversal Lo-vessels

Their role is strictly limited to a function as regulators between coupled meridians when there is a disturbance of essential Internal Qi. WARNING! In case of an attack by an exterior excess, this technique cannot be used, since this will bring the Perverse Qi in the healthy coupled meridian.

They all have an identical trajectory: starting from the Lo-point of the meridian, they go to the Source-point of the coupled meridian. It is important to notice that disturbances of the Primary channels always change the pulses, while disturbed Secondary channels do not change them at all.

SYMPTOMS

Longitudinal Lo-vessels

See list at the end of this chapter (Addendum 2).

Transversal Lo-vessel

These vessels do not have their own symptomatology, since they borrow the points of the Primary channels. Their symptoms will be those of excess or deficiency of the Primary channels. They play strictly the role of regulators between the coupled meridians. In other words, they are the vessels passing the excess energy from one meridian to its coupled meridian.

THERAPY

Longitudinal Lo-vessels

- ❑ In case of fullness:
  - Disperse the Lo-point;
  - Puncture the season tonification point (Xu of Essential Qi) in the involved meridian; and
  - Tonify the Iu (Shu) point and the Ting point to bring more Wei Qi
- ❑ In case of emptiness:
  - First protect the healthy coupled meridian by tonifying the Lo- and Source points of the coupled meridian;
  - Then tonify the Lo-point of the attacked meridian; and
  - Puncture the Iu point of the Empty vessel.

For example, Xu of the Lung Lo-vessels; first LI6 and LI4 in tonification, then L7 and L9 in tonification.

Transversal Lo-vessels

- ❑ Fullness
  - Disperse the Source point of the Full meridian; and
  - Tonify the Lo-point of the coupled meridian
- ❑ Emptiness
  - Tonify the Source-point of the Empty meridian; ; Disperse the Lo-point of the coupled meridian.

THE EXTRA-MERIDIANS

There are eight Extra meridians, coupled two by two in a Yin-Yang relationship. One Extra meridian, Tchong Mo, is discussed in Chapter 9. These vessels do not have transport points (Ting, Iong, Iu, King, Ho), but are put into action by stimulation of their *confluent* point or *opening* point. They are activated when they are needed; if the Primary Channels show an Excess or Deficiency, the eight Extras are ready to "stand by". They help regulate the flow of the Qi in the Primary vessels. Other names are "Wonder meridians", "Curious vessels" ("Méridiens Curieux" in French), "Extraordinary meridians," "Secondary Vessels," or "Miscellaneous." They are called this way, because they have no relationship or link with the Organs-Hollow organs or Yin-Yang union. They are connected to a special system, compromised of:

The nervous system
The skeleton
The circulatory system
The genito-urinary system
The hepato-biliary functions

These Extra meridians are neither organs nor hollow organs, yet sometimes they behave as such. It bears to express here that when we speak about "organ" in Traditional Chinese Medicine, we speak about the Energy of that organ, which leaves that organ in its season, and not about the organ itself.

Four Extra channels will appear for the Yang disturbance, four others for the Yin disturbance. They are like small rivers ready to drain or supply the large (Primary) channels with Qi in case the latter cannot handle it. They are able to remove exogenous pathogens and can supplement the body with Qi and blood. An important rule to remember is to *never begin therapy in a new patient by using these Extras*. Resistance to any further therapy might be the consequence! First always use the Primary Channels; and only in case of negative results should the confluent point be opened. Soulié De Morant, the father of acupuncture, expressed this clearly:

> *"If there is no positive response when treating the Primary Channels, only then use the confluent or master points of the 8 Extra meridians."*

The main energy, circulating in these meridians, is the Ancestral Qi, but often we find a mixture of Ancestral, Iong and Wei Qi in the 8 Extras, running in the same or opposite sense. There is place enough for all these kinds of Qi in these meridians, as we could compare them to lakes in which the Primary channels irrigate. However, the direction of the flow of Energy is always from the lower towards the upper body. The Wonder meridians are in connection with the Primary channels through their points of origin and the reunion points. As we will see below, these meridians have a close relationship with the Kidney and Bladder. This should not surprise us as we have already noted that the Ancestral Qi originates in the Kidney-organ.

INDICATIONS

Indications involving the different Extras are listed in Chapter 9 on Tchong Mo. Use of these vessels in the treatment of a local excess is discussed in Chapter 7 on the "Eight Conditions." Besides the functions expressed above, the Extra meridians:

- ❏ Regulate life changes (they all originate in the Kidney-organ).
- ❏ Regulate the Blood and Qi in the 12 Primary channels.
- ❏ Have a supervising role over certain functions; e.g., Du Mo regulates the Yang Qi, Jen (Ren) Mo, is the master of concentration of the Yin Qi.
- ❏ Are used, as Soulié De Morant expressed it, "When the 12 Primary channels failed in therapy."
- ❏ Are used when the patient's Energy is depleted and too many needles would further weaken his Vital Qi.

SYMPTOMS

In general, when an Extra meridian is involved, we see the following signs:

pain-contraction-stiffness

· The first couple is comprised of Du Mo and Yang Chiao Mo (Keo) with their respective Confluent or Master points, SI3 and B62. Du Mo, "Sea of Yang", governs all the Yang channels; Yang Chiao Mo puts the Yang into movement and accelerates it. Frequent symptoms are stiffness and pain along the spinal column, stiff neck, trismus apoplexy, convulsions, Parkinsonism and other illnesses of the CNS, irritability, opisthotonos, redness and pain at the inner canthus, hallucinations and surexcitation. When Yang Keo is attacked by

Perverse Qi, the kidney area is painful, "as being hit by a hammer." Yin and Yang Keo bring the liquids to the eyes. In case of disturbance, and there is fullness of Yang, the eyes can't be shut and tear abundantly.

· The second couple involves Dai Mo (Tae Mo) and Yang Wei Mo (Yang Oe) with their confluent points GB41 and TB5. Dai Mo is the only Extra in connection with the Exterior and promotes the circulation in the pelvis and legs as well as nourishing the hepatobiliary system. When Dai Mo is affected, the patient has the strange sensation of "sitting in water." Yang Wei Mo links all the Yang meridians together and is called the preserver of Yang. Below the girdle formed by GB26, 27 and 28, GB41 has an action on the opposite side; e.g., GB41 punctured on the left side has an action on the right shoulder. Dai Mo starts in the point bearing its name: GB26. Frequent symptoms are leucorrhea, prurigo, tinnitus, dermatoses (eczema), shoulder pain, contractions, pain in abdomen and sides, weak feeling in legs, and dysmenorrhea. According to the So Ouenn (Chapter19), "Dai mo is the cause of paralysis of the legs." Many of these symptoms are signs of acceleration of the Exterior. A Yang Wei Mo disturbance causes chills and fever and sensitivity to weather changes.

· The third couple is made up of Ren Mo (Jen Mo), and Yin Chiao Mo (Yin Keo) with their respective confluent points L7 and K6. Ren Mo is the Director vessel and governs all the Yin channels. It is also called the "Sea of Yin". Yin Chiao Mo accelerates the Yin, puts the Yin into movement and brings fluid to the eyes. Leucorrhea, sterility, frigidity, menstrual disturbances, renal colic, renal stones, cystitis, retention of urine, nocturnal emission, menopausal problems, fibroids, cysts, and enuresis; also, others such as asthma, chronic bronchitis, and insomnia. Problems of the eyes (pain, tearing, closed eyes and itching), spasms of lower limbs, sleepiness and pain in lower abdomen can be related to disturbance in Yin Tchiao Mo.

· The fourth couple is composed of Tchong Mo and Yin Wei Mo (Yin Oe) with their respective confluent points Sp4 and PC6. Tchong Mo is discussed in Chapter 9. Yin Wei Mo links all the Yin channels. If these Yin (=Blood) Energies can't circulate freely, there will be circulation troubles and pains in the heart region. Frequent symptoms for Tchong Mo are aerophagia, abdominal distention, constipation, gynecological syndromes, menstrual irregularities. A disturbance in Yin Wei Mo causes cardialgia (this is an essential symptom!) and oppression in the thorax. The patient is irritable and prone to anger attacks. At the same time he sighs continuously and is full of fears. In this case, K9 will be punctured. Other symptoms are summarized in the chapter on Tchong Mo.

THERAPY

The first point to puncture when using the Extras, must be the confluent point; failure to do so leads to a loss of the special action of this point. To improve the action of the confluent point, the confluent point of the coupled Extra is also stimulated.

When the therapeutic session is ended, the last needle to take out is the one of the opening point of the involved Extra meridian, in other words, the first point you needled. Not too many other points may be punctured when using these opening points in order to keep the special action of the master point.

OTHER POINTS OF THE EXTRAS AND CONNECTING POINTS ARE:

- Du Mo: points of GV, CV1, and B12.
- Ren Mo: points of CV, B28, and St1.
- Tchong Mo: K11 - K21, CV1, CV7, and St30.
- Dai Mo: GB26, GB27, GB28.
- Yang Chiao Mo: B61-62-59-1, GB20, GV16, ST4-3-1, SI10, and LI15-16.
- Yin Chiao Mo: K6, K8, and B1.
- Yang Wei Mo: B63, GB35, GB21, GB13, SI10, GV15-16, and St8.
- Yin Wei Mo: K9, CV22-23, Sp12-13-15-16, and Li14.

DIVERGENT MERIDIANS OR TCHING PIE

Other names are Collateral meridians and "Méridiens Distincts" in French. There are twelve Divergent channels, each corresponding with a Primary Channel. The starting point of these meridians is located near the big joints, e.g., knee and hip. From there, they penetrate into the depth passing through their corresponding organ and through the organ in the Biao-Li connection. Further, they pass through the heart zone and appear in the exterior zones around the neck (Li zones) in the vicinity of the Sky-Window points (Figure 26).

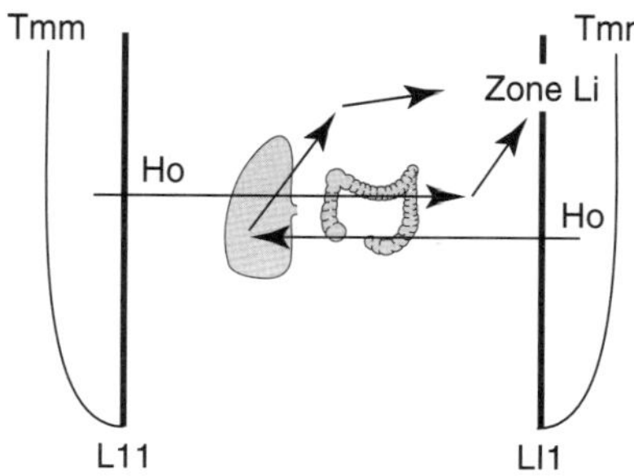

Figure 26

From the Li zone on (always situated on the head), the Tching Pie will go exclusively into the Yang meridians of the head. Hence, they form a link between the two Primary Yin/Yang channels. As we see in Figure 25, the Yang returns to the Yang, The Yin travels to the Yang, and the Yang never goes to the Yin! The Pernicious Qi will use these meridians as a vehicle to penetrate the coupled organs, but will not stay long in them. The Excess is pushed back by the Wei Qi which is also brought into the depth of the organism through the Divergent channels. This is the main function of the Tching Pié: delivering Wei Qi to the deepest parts of the human body, so that the battle against Pernicious excesses can continue beyond the surface.

The constant battle between the Wei Qi and the Excess at the level of the organ produces the "intermittent" symptoms, so typical for invasion of these meridians. The Tching Pié will also be responsible for bringing the Qi, and especially Yin Qi to the head and areas which are not traversed by other meridians. Hence, the only way of bringing Yin Qi to the head is to employ the Divergent meridians of the Yin meridians. There are no Yin meridians on the head which is paradoxical, since a Yin-Yang exchange has to take place at this level. Especially the Tching Pié of the Spleen, Liver and PC (they all possess 2/3 Yin versus 1/3 Yang) will bring Yin Qi to the head. The others have too little Yin to be of any benefit in this situation.

Let's present a clinical example. Trigeminus neuralgia on the left side. This is a Yang Excess at the head. We bring the Yin to the head by dispersing the Ho point of the Sp, Sp9, the Liver or Li8d, and the Pericardium or PC3d. As a last step we will tonify St1, TB23 and GB1 on the opposite side (left). To complete the treatment, we will stimulate the Ho point of the corresponding meridian in the Yin-Yang unity. E.g., when there is a block in the Spleen, organ or meridian, we will also stimulate the Ho point of the Stomach, St36.

Where do the two Tching Pié unite at the Zone Li?

Pair	unite at zone Li
L-LI	LI20
St-Sp	St1
H-SI	Unknown
B-K	B1
PC-TB	TB23?
GB-Li	GB1

INDICATIONS

Disturbance of these vessels occur much more often than one might think. Not much is provided by the ancient texts regarding the symptomatology of the Divergent meridian when they are attacked. The main characteristics of an attack in these channels are:

INTERMITTENT SYMPTOMS, UNILATERAL PAIN, SYMPTOMS OF THE DISTURBED ORGAN.

Example: Sciatica, following the bladder meridian, unilateral, intermittent and symptoms of cystitis.

THERAPY

The French call it "Piqûre a l'Opposé", puncturing the opposite side. The name is related to the tonification of the Ting-point of the involved channel of the opposite side; e.g., in case of invasion of the GB Divergent meridian, right side, tonify GB44t left. Why? Because we cannot puncture and disperse the attacked side, since that side of the body shows an emptiness of Qi. There is no use in withdrawing Qi from our patient when there is already so little Qi. What needs to be done is to increase the patient's Wei Qi in order to battle the excess Qi or Perverse Qi. The Wei Qi is increased by puncturing the Ting-point on the healthy side.

Another point to always stimulate and tonify under these conditions is GV20. Tonification of GV20 lifts the Qi to the upper part of the body.

The last point in the therapy is the sedation of the two meeting zones. The Tching Pié of a Yin and Yang Primary Channel meet each other at an inferior and superior meeting point. These meeting points are listed below.

To summarize: Ting-point of the opposite side in tonification, GV20 in tonification and dispersion of the lower and upper meeting points of the coupled involved meridians or organs. (Figure 27).

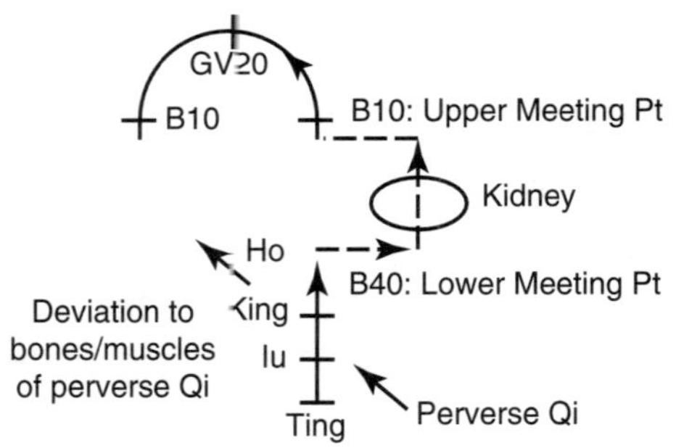

Figure 27

We can see that the perverse Qi attacks the Kidney meridian in the Iu point. If the Wei Qi is sufficient, the Perverse Qi will be deviated to the bones and muscles. With deficient Wei Qi, the Perverse Qi traverses the meridian till the Ho point, goes in the lower meeting point, passes through the organ (Kidney in this case) and will join GV20 through the upper meeting point of the affected side to pass through the meridian of the opposite side.

Meeting points of the Divergent channels

Couple M.P.	Inferior Meeting	PointSuperior
B - K	B 40	B 10
GB - Li	GB 30	GB 1
St - Sp	St 30	B 1
H - SI	H 1	B 1
TB - PC	TB 16	TB 16
LI - L	SI 18	SI 18

THE SIX LEVELS OR THE GREAT MERIDIANS

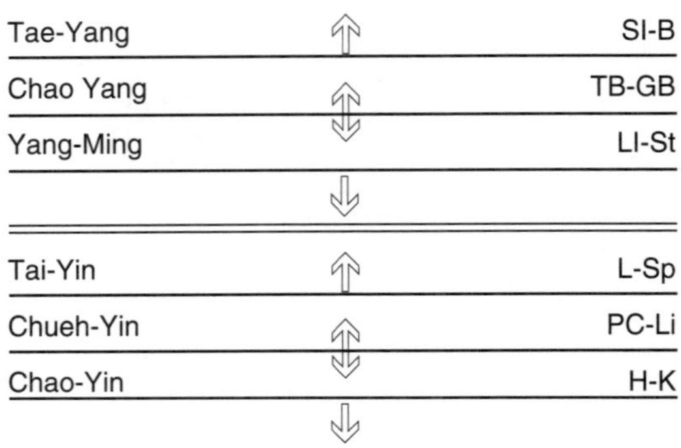

The meridians are organized in different levels to form a barrier of defense against Exterior Pernicious Qi. Each level opens to the interior or exterior while the two hinges of the Yang and the Yin open to both sides. Two Primary channels form one great meridian. Going from the exterior to the interior we have the following levels:

Three of these levels have a special importance since they represent a *hinge* with special pathology.

- Chao-Yang: hinge of the Yang
- Chueh-Yin: hinge of the Yin
- Yang-Ming: hinge of the Yin-Yang

Tai Yang and Tai Yin open to the exterior, while Yang Ming and Chao Yin open to the interior. The Perverse Qi always penetrates from the exterior to the interior, hence Tae-Yang, the most superficial level, will be attacked first, and Chao-Yin, the deepest level, will be reached last. However, the Perverse Qi can penetrate directly in the Yin level. This happens when the essential Qi and Wei Qi of the patient is weak and empty. Depending upon the strength of the Excess (Shi syndrome) or the quantity of the Essential and Wei Qi (Xu syndrome) in the body, the excess will penetrate the different levels and cause specific symptoms. These symptoms will be a guide to the practitioner to recognize the intensity of the disease and to evaluate the prognosis. The deeper the excess has penetrated, the worse the prognosis.

The basis of the treatment in acupuncture is to bring the excess from the interior to the exterior. (*Healing from the inside to the outside, a principle common to all scientific medicines*). For instance, a patient presents with a Tai Yin syndrome, characterized by bloating, nausea, morning diarrhea, thirstlessness and cold limbs. After treatment he presents with constipation, thirst and fever. These last symptoms belong to Yang Ming, hence the disease went from Yin to Yang, or from more precious organs to less important organs. It is a proof that the therapy was correct and the prognosis is favorable. The different great meridians with their symptomatology are discussed, followed by their therapeutic measures.

TAI YANG SYNDROME

Cause	Symptoms	Pulse	Tongue
Wind-Cold	Fever and chills, sensitivity to Cold, running nose, waterish liquid, no sweat, stiff neck and arthritis pain	Floating & slow	Thin, white moist fur
Wind-Heat	Fever, thirst, yellow mucus from the nose, and headache	Floating & fast	Moderate pink with yellow fur

SHAO YANG SYNDROME

The Perverse Qi has broken through the first barrier but has not reached the interior, causing very typical symptoms. The most important is the appearance of fever, sign of the Fire attacking the Fong. (Figure 28) Involvement of TB and GB

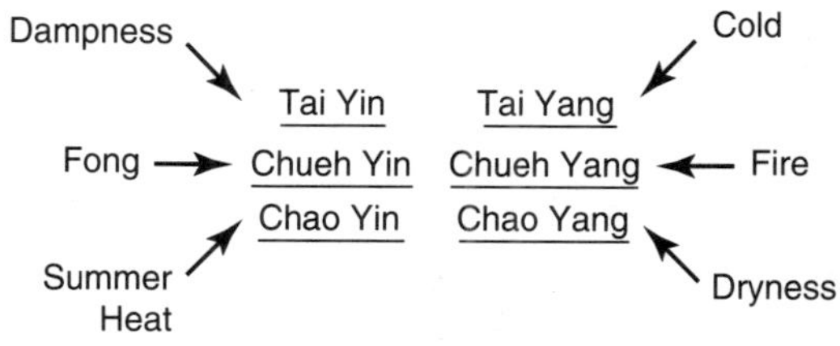

Figure 28

causes bitter taste in the mouth, dry throat, stabbing pain in the sides and chest, and alternating fever and chills. The pulse is rapid and tight, while the tongue is red and yellow-coated.

YANG MING SYNDROME

The Perverse Qi (Heat-Dryness) has not been halted at the level of Tai Yang and will penetrate first in the meridians Yang Ming, and then in the organs (LI and St.). Hence, the diseases of Yang Ming present symptoms of the meridians and organs. Meridian symptoms are strong fever, abundant perspiration, strong thirst and sensitivity to heat. Organ symptoms are abdominal distention, belching, gastric pain, cervical adenitis, foul breath, nausea and vomiting, restlessness and sinusitis. The pulse is deep and rapid, while the tongue is covered with a thick, greasy fur in the Middle Burner when the organs are involved.

TAI YIN SYNDROME

The syndromes of Tai Yin are of nature Yin, caused by the perverse energy Cold. Once the Cold concentrates in the Spleen, it transforms into Dampness. Symptoms are caused by weakness of the Spleen, attacked by Dampness. Deficient Spleen Yang Qi causes diarrhea, heavy feeling and numbness in the limbs, fatigue, no thirst, vomiting, sallow complexion, anorexia, hemorrhages, prolaps uteri, varices and hemorrhoids. Both, the diseases of Yang Ming and Tai Yin are caused by a weakness of the Yang energy of the Middle Burner. A differentiation between Yang Ming and Tai Yin is easily made:

Yang Ming:	fever and thirst; deep, strong pulse
Tai Yin:	no fever and no thirst; slow, weak pulse

CHUEH YIN SYNDROME

Chueh Yin is situated between the interior and the exterior. Chapter Five of the Su Wen mentions: *"The symptomatology of the hinge of the Yin is very complex due to a mixture of the Yin and the Yang Qi; normally at this level, there is more Xue than Qi."*

Two different aggressions are possible: Cold and a mixture of Cold and Heat. Each will bring its specific syndrome.

❑ Cold attack: since this level has more Yin than Yang, the Cold will encounter very little Yang to balance it. In order to avoid penetration of this Excess, our therapy has to bring more Yang to this level. Icy cold limbs and a soft and fine pulse are often found.

❑ Heat mixed with Cold: this attack is possible when there is an emptiness of Yin. The Heat usually attacks the upper part of this level, Cheou Chueh Yin or PC, whereas the Cold will attack the lower part, Tsou (ZU) Chueh Yin or Li. Symptoms found here are dysentery, tenesmus ani, thirst, thoracic oppression, and heart pain. Nausea, vomiting and hunger are more an expression of liver involvement.

CHAO YIN SYNDROME

Since this level has more Qi than Xue (the K Yang gives its Yang to the Heart Yang), an attack of Cold is only successful when there is deficiency of Yang at this level. Symptoms are cold, icy limbs, sensitivity to cold, tendency to sleep, undigested food in stools, arthritis pain and a very small fine pulse.

Once the level of progression of the disease is recognized, the different therapeutic steps are described in ancient Chinese techniques and will be discussed in this chapter, step by step.

ANCIENT THERAPEUTIC TECHNIQUES

The different levels form a fortress in the human body against exterior Excesses. Each of these Excesses has a predilection for one of these levels. This is represented in Figure 27. If all these meridians, grouped two by two, are well balanced in Qi and Xue, then Pernicious Qi will not be able to invade.

What happens if the first barrier of defense (Tai Yang and Tai Yin) has been broken through?

This *first level* has more Yin than Yang (more Xue than Qi) although Tai Yang consists of only Yang meridians! Cold (Yin) usually attacks this level, and in a healthy individual, this Yin is countered by the Yang. Thus, this barrier is only broken in case of deficiency of Yang or Qi. The special technique applied in this case is the perspiration technique (Nei King Chapter 23): it brings Wei Qi to the upper level where it will neutralize the Perverse Qi (Cold).

Where do we find our therapeutical points? Since the first level is formed by Tai Yang and Tai Yin, it will be only normal that the points for this technique are found on these meridians. Since L and Sp (respectively masters of the Qi and Blood) are energetically more important than SI and B, they will form the root of our therapy.

The therapy consists of *three different steps*. The first step is to increase the Wei Qi which prevents the Perverse Qi from penetrating the deeper layers. As we have seen before, the third antique point (Iu or Shu) has both of these characteristics: L9 in dispersion will be the first step in our therapy.

The second step is bringing more Qi (Yang) to the first level, since a Deficiency of Qi made it possible for the Excess to penetrate. This is done by root therapy. Sp1 in tonification draws the Yang Qi of the Yang Ming level to the first barrier.

The third step is dependent on the nature of the Excess. In case of Heat, we disperse the fire points of L and Sp: L10 and Sp2. In case of Cold we tonify the above-mentioned points. If the treatment works, the patient often experiences increased perspiration, giving the name to this technique. In case the perspiration is too abundant, puncture Sp6.

Perspiration Technique:
L9d and Sp1t, L10t or d,Sp2t or d

The *attack of the second level* will result in a typical symptom: fever—the result of the Fire attacking the Fong, is the sign of invasion of the Perverse Qi in the second level. Therapy will try to bring the Excess from the interior (second level) to the exterior: this is called *regularization.*

The Source point brings the Excess from the interior to the exterior: GB42d. The Gall Bladder is coupled to the powerful organ, the Liver, whose main function is the storage of the Blood. This Blood contains the white blood cells, defenders of our immune system. Bringing the Excess from the GB to the Li will allow the immune system to destroy it. The Lo-point of the GB, GB37d will bring the Excess to the Li. The next action is strengthening the Li by puncturing the Shu point, Li3t, and applying the Back Shu-Front Mu technique, B18 and Li14.

The last step is a tonification of PC6t in order to activate the Yin of the Li.

Regularization Technique:
GB 42 d, GB 37 d, Li 3 t, B 18 and Li 14, PC 6 t

The *third level* is the last defense barrier to be broken. Once this ultimate defense line has been broken though, the way will be open for the Excesses to invade the different organs. Organ involvement according to the Ko-cycle is inevitable at this moment. (Figure 29)

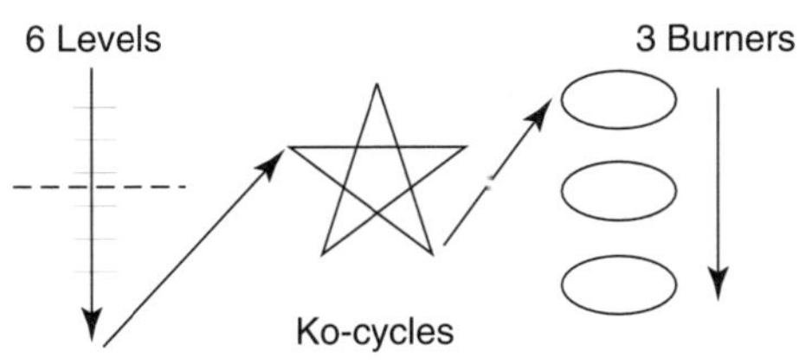

Figure 29

Therapy must prevent the Excess from going deeper, in other words, slowing down this process. Slowing down in Traditional Chinese Medicine means use of cold. The best defense at this stage is the refrigeration or input of cold. Increasing the cold means increasing the Yin and decreasing the Yang.

Increasing the Yin is done by puncturing the cold points or Iong points of the Yang meridians, LI2t and St44t. To reinforce the action we create a stagnation of the Blood by draining the Fire of the Li (which stores the Blood) and cooling the vessels, (PC): Li2d and PC8d (Figure 30).

Refrigeration Technique
LI 2t, St44t, Li2d, and PC8d

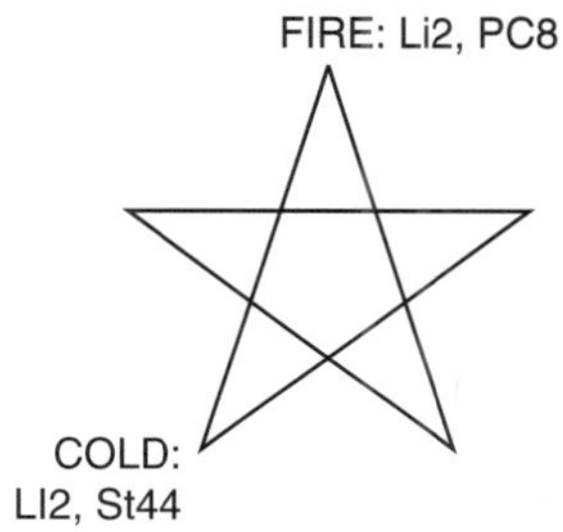

Figure 30

PATIENT CASE IN CONNECTION WITH DISTURBANCE OF A LEVEL

Mr. Clive, 37 years old, came on consultation with a complaint of hot flashes, ascending from CV12 to the face (CV24). The problem started six months ago when he stopped smoking cigarettes.

1. *Inquiry:*
   - Headaches: not serious, related to studying.
   - Thirst and appetite: very good appetite, likes cold drinks.
   - Stool: tendency to constipation.
   - Urination: yellowish
   - Sleep: sleeps only four to five hours a night, does not feel the need for more rest; sometimes he passes a day without sleep without being affected by it.
   - No chills or fever, no eye or ear problem.
   - Chest normal.
   - Abdomen: good digestion, sometimes ab-

dominal distention.

- Habits: he stopped regular smoking six months ago but he uses daily great quantities of marijuana and is a regular user of alcohol.
- Previous history: Clive travels a lot (India, Spain, England); on his trips he contracted malaria, hepatitis twice and cholera.
- Psychological structure: easily angry, outgoing, talkative.
- Other important symptoms: bitter taste in the mouth, cervical adenitis, likes to eat hot Mexican food, eats it daily; no gum bleeding or nose bleeding, foul breath, pain in the sides, increasing when he sneezes; cold feet and varicose veins.

2. *Appearance:*
   - Face: the whole face looks red.
   - Tongue: large, flabby, dry, aspect and presence of cracks. especially in the Upper Burner, greasy fur in the Middle Burner.
   - Appearance: tendency to obesity, hair loss on the head.

3. *Listening:*
   - Voice: normal strength.
   - Respiration: normal
   - Cough: normal

4. *Palpation:*
   - Pulse rate: normal
   - Strength: left stronger than right (Yang tendency).
   - Missed pulse beats: none
   - Organ pulses: he consulted in the Winter, the season organs being K/B; Sp pulse was weak, H pulse strong.
   - Mu points: Li14 very sensitive
CV12 sensitive
St25 sensitive
   - Back Shu points: B20 and 21 sensitive

5. *Conclusions.*

a. According to the Eight Conditions

Hot flashes in the face means Excess of Yang, the Yang is not descending properly while there is a deficiency of blood (yin) at the head.

Question: Is this a local Yin deficiency, type Sky-Window point SI17 or a total Yin-or Blood deficiency?

This is a blocking of the Yin at the neck since there is only cerebral fatigue (the headaches appear when his is studying). In case of total Blood deficiency, there would be a total exhaustion which is not present, since he sleeps very little.

Another symptom of this local Yin deficiency is the head hair loss (Su Ouenn Chapter #65): "When the Blood and Qi are in equilibrium in Tchong Mo, there is abundant hair growth; on places where there is a lot of Blood, there will be abundant hair growth." An example of the last statement is seen in women. There is no beard growth, but there is hair growth in the lower part of the body, since the pelvis is the Yin of the Yin Zone.

We also observe that there is a stagnation of the Yin in the lower part of the body: cold feet and varicose veins.

CONCLUSION: Yang Excess in a Yang person, stagnation of Yin the lower part of the body and non-distribution of the Yin to the head.

b. According to the Theory of Zang Fu

There is clearly a stagnation on the level of Yang Ming: foul breath, the hot flashes starting at CV12, MO point of the Stomach and Middle Burner, cervical adenitis, tendency to constipation and a greasy fur on the tongue at the level of the Middle Burner. It is obvious that there is an invasion of Heat in the Middle Burner. What is the cause?

This can be found in the habits of the patient. He smokes marijuana, one ounce a month, eats hot Mexican and Indian food daily, and is a regular consumer of alcohol. All this creates intense Heat in the Middle Burner, drying up the liquids and exhausting the Yin (dry tongue, red face, very little sleep, etc.)

This intense Heat inhibits a good functioning of the Spleen, especially its transformation and transportation functions. As a result, there is a tendency towards obesity and greasy fur on the tongue. This deficiency of the Sp. leads to secondary excess Liver Qi. Alcohol and marijuana use also increases the Heat in the Li, decreasing the Li Yin. The patient is easily irritated, suffers somewhat from insomnia, has a bitter taste in the mouth, and pain in the sides which increases with sneezing.

Why does the pain increase when he sneezes? Sneezing is a consequence of a Fong attack on the Lung. The pain in the sides indicates a Li stagnation: there is a Li Yang excess. The Li is connected with the Lung (Li14 with LI, internal connection). The sneezing will increase the intra-thoracic pressure, and since there is an excess, any increase in pressure will aggravate the condition. (See "Eight Conditions")

> Li14 was sensitive: indicates the Li Yin deficiency.

6. Therapy

- St25t, St36t and LI11t opens the level Yang Ming to the interior and lifts the obstruction.
- PC6d: digestive barrier.
- TB5d: drains the Yang excess in the head, bilateral.
- St37t: brings the Yang excess down.
- SI17t: Sky-Window point, brings the Yin to the head.
- K 6t and Sp6t: increases the Yin and puts it into movement.
- Li14t and Li2d: increases the Yin of the Li and drains the Fire of the Li.
- CV12t: Mo point of the Middle Burner.

ADDENDUM 1

TONIFICATION	DISPERSION
SU OUENN (Chapter 20): -to tonify, one must puncture in the direction of the stream of the Qi of the meridian.	- to disperse, one must puncture in the opposite direction of the stream of the Qi.
SU OUENN (Chapter 26): -to tonify, one must puncture at the superficial level; puncture in the beginning of an expiration and take the needle out at the beginning of an inspiration.	-insert the needle during an inspiration, withdraw during an expiration.
SU OUENN (Chapter 53): -puncturing a pt. in emptiness will leave the needle cold: after withdrawing the needle, one must close the hole with the fingertip.	-puncturing a pt. in fullness will heat the needle; at the insertion of the needle, one enlarges the whole by handling the needle.
SU OUENN (Chapter 54): -to tonify the emptiness, one must wait to withdraw the needle until the needle gets hot and until the pt. also has the sensation of heat, because at this moment the Yang Qi arrives.	-to disperse the emptiness, one must wait until the needle gets cold before withdrawing it. When the Qi is dispersed, the pt. will have this sensation of cold.
SU OUENN (Chapter 62): -to tonify, one must push and massage the point, before and after puncturing, to attract the Qi; insert the needle one time.	
NEI CHING (Chapter 1): -inserting the needle too easily means emptiness. One must withdraw the needle and massage the hole with the left hand; this way the body Qi will not disperse.	-difficult insertion in the skin means fullness of the Qi. At the withdrawl of the needle, one must not touch the punctured place anymore so that the perverse Qi can escape and the body can circulate.
NEI CHING (Chapter 73): -before puncturing, massage first the point; with the left hand stretch the skin and puncture with the right hand, turning the needle.	-one lets the needle turn between thumb and index to activate the arrival of Qi; one inserts fast and withdraws slowly.
GENERAL TEXTBOOK OF ACCUPUNCTURE OF YAN: -before puncturing one heats the needle in the mouth. One must massage the point. Ask the pt. to cough and insert the needle in 3 stages.	-insert the needle at the moment of inspiration and withdraw during an expiration.

ADDENDUM 2
SYMPTOMS OF THE LO MERIDIANS

Meridian	Pt.	Symptoms
L	.7	+ Lower end of radius and palms hot - Coughing, yawing with mouth wide open, constant desire to urinate
LI	.6	+ Dental caries, deafness - Teeth cold, diaphragmatic area feels blocked
St	.40	+ Sudden loss of speech, insanity psychosis - Feet flaccid and weak, flesh and skin on shins withered and shrunken
Sp	.4	+ Sharp pain in the intestines (stays at specific point) - Ascites, timpanites and swellings
H	.5	+ Chest and diaphragmatic area feel as if they are bearing a heavy weight and are uncomfortable - Inability to speak
SI	.7	+ Bones and joints flaccid and weak, elbow joint cannot move, paralyzed - Nodules between the fingers, excrescence or scabies with itch
B	.58	+ Clear nasal discharge, blocked nose, cold nose pain cervical spine - Clear nasal discharge, epistaxis
K	.4	+ Feeling of depression in the region of the heart, constipation - Pain at the waist (sore loins)
PC	.6	+ Painful heart, vexation - Stiffness and inability to turn the head
TB	.5	+ Restriction in movement of elbow joint - Elbow joint too flaccid, over-relaxed
GB	.37	+ Cold in extremities _ Legs weak, inability to walk or to rise after sitting down
Li	.5	+ Excessive erections, swelling of testicles - Genitalia itch violently
Sp	.21	+ Pain all over the body - Extreme weakness of the joints
CV	.15	+ Pain at the skin of the abdomen - Itch at the skin of the abdomen
GV	.1	+ Stiff neck - Heavy feeling of the head

Chinese Diagnosis 5

"A skillful doctor knows by observation, a mediocre doctor knows by interrogation, an ordinary doctor knows by palpation." (Zhang Zhong Jing)

As in other alternative medicines such as Homeopathy, the examination of the patient is very important: observations and questions succeed those asked in a regular Western medical diagnostic. The guidelines for the Chinese examination were written down in the ancient books, the Su Ouenn and the Nei King. Chapter 77 of the Su Ouenn, *"Five mistakes of Doctors"* is a prime example for us, practitioners to follow. All the principles established in these paragraphs are still valid, and most doctors don't pay enough attention to these pitfalls of the practice. Therefore, it is important to repeat these time-established rules.

- *"Doctors must know the social status of their patients: when the patient is rich, he most likely will suffer from organic disease; when he is poor, most illnesses will stem from lack of proper nourishment."* No matter what medical discipline we apply, medications, homeopathic remedies or acupuncture treatments, will not help since the Yong and Wei Qi will be deficient among these patients.
- *"Ask the patient about his life style: is he moderate or excessive in his habits; ask about emotional traumas and events: has there been severe anxiety, fear or anger?* " In our modern times, we will also ask about drug and alcohol use. Hahnemann, 200 years ago, aptly expressed it: *"Chronic diseases cannot be called chronic if they are maintained because of drugs, bad diet, bad environment..."* All too frequently, the practitioner fails to ask about the life style which can account for many failed cases.
- *"The great doctor must know first the normal pulses very well; only then can he know the correlation between the symptoms and the pathological pulse."* This rule is less followed by modern practitioners. Other diagnostic aids are available, and physicians are not limited to feeling the pulse as this was the case in ancient times.
- *"A good physician must be able to differentiate if a disease is caused by an Exterior Excess or by an emotional disorder. He must know that if the reason of the psychic imbalance persists (for instance an emotional shock), he can do nothing for this patient, because a calm mind is necessary for the normal circulation of the Yong and Wei Qi."* Again, an imbalance has become chronic in such a case because the exciting factor has not been removed. If a woman lives in a marriage with constant verbal or mental abuse, treatments will not

be able to correct her imbalance. However, homeopathy can, through the well-researched remedy, aid the patient in the above situation, by helping her to stand up for herself.

❑ *"When a doctor examines the patient, he must go back to the origin of the disease and follow the evolution. He must determine the indicated therapeutic technique: acupuncture, moxa or herbs."* This is the most common mistake by most doctors. They focus on the end results (diagnosing and treating the sick leaves) and forget the beginnings of the disease (the sick root). Homeopathy will also work with these layers of the patient. These layers are built during the patient's life time because of strong physical or emotional events.

Another myth in acupuncture, is to think that ancient practitioners and authors considered the pulse diagnosis as the absolute value for therapy. On the contrary. They insisted on the importance of an extensive inquiry in order to pick up the most *peculiar, rare and strange* symptoms. For the acupuncturist as well as for the homeopath, "that which is out of the common is usually a guide rather than a hindrance." Symptoms vary from individual to individual and peculiar, uncommon symptoms show the kinks in the patient's defense armor where the disease will enter, hook itself and become chronic.

What is the purpose of the diagnosis?

- ❑ To establish the site of the lesion: muscle, skin, organs, meridians; indicates *where to treat.*
- ❑ To establish the condition: Yin/Yang, Hot/Cold, Full/Empty; indicates *which kind of treatment* is necessary.
- ❑ To establish the cause: trauma, infection, external, internal, emotions, diet, life style, hereditary; can *prevent the disease from returning* if the causality was treated.

There are four principal categories of Chinese Diagnostics:

LOOKING
LISTENING AND SMELLING
INQUIRY
PALPATION

LOOKING

This is one of the most important steps in Chinese diagnosis. Different aspects will be screened: complexion of the face, the picture of the tongue, the spirit of the patient, his constitution and abnormalities found on the undressed patient.

COMPLEXION OF THE FACE

Each area of the face belongs to an organ (Figure 31):

- ❑ Nose, lips and the space between the commissura labialis and alae nasi belong to the Spleen.
- ❑ Left cheek: Liver.
- ❑ Right cheek: Lung.
- ❑ Chin: Kidney.
- ❑ Front: Heart.

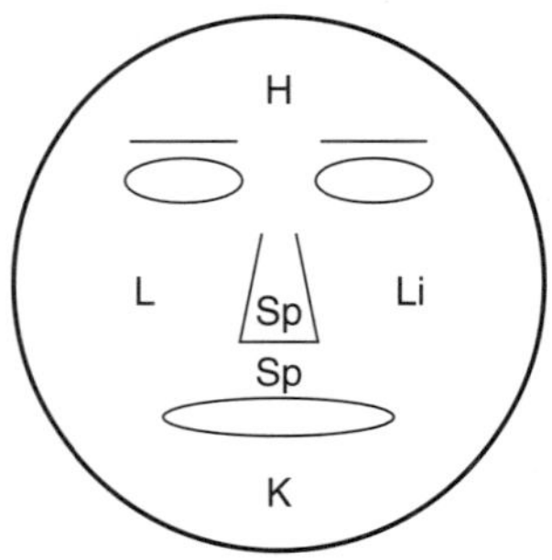

Figure 31

Knowing these areas, we look for discoloration in a certain part of the face and the dominant color in the face. Chapter 3 on the Five Elements mentions these colors.

More precisely we can say that a bluish-green discoloration of the skin is usually caused by stagnation or obstruction of Essential Qi or Blood, indicating the presence of Cold, stasis or illness in the liver. A yellow discoloration is seen in cases of dysfunction of the Spleen or in icteric patients, indicating the presence of Heat-Dampness. A sallow complexion is usually caused by disturbance of the Sp. Redness of the skin is caused by excessive filling of the skin capillaries, indicating the presence of Heat excess. White color or pallor usually indicates the presence of Cold or Xu of Blood and Essential Qi. Black or dark color of the skin is seen in severe chronic cases of Blood stasis, Cold and decreased Qi of the Kidney. In general, we can say that the five colors reveal illness in the corresponding viscera: green-blue, red, yellow, white and black suggest disease in the Liver, Heart, Spleen, Lung and Kidney, respectively.

Nei King Chapter 49, indicates that if "*the mother element presents the color of the son, the prognosis is favorable.*" For instance. The kidney corresponds to the color black and is the son of the lung which has the color white. If one sees the black color on the right cheek, then this is a good sign.

In the Su Ouenn, Chapter 10, it is written that the signs of death are reflected in the face by the following colors:

Green like grass.
Yellow like a rice paddy.
Black like ashes.
Red like blood.
White like a skeleton.

TONGUE PICTURE

Diagnosis through observations of the tongue was a late development in the history of Chinese medicine, although there were brief mentions of it in the Nei King and Nan King. It was not until the Yuan Dynasty (about 1200 AD.) that a book was published by Gniao with changes of the tongues related to infectious diseases. The tongue, being the opening of the heart, is a very important place to watch over bodily changes. Ideally, tongue picture diagnosis should be performed in bright sunlight in order to avoid false interpretations. Always examine the tongue from the tip to the back. Spicy foods can change the tongue picture, the same with cigarettes, coffee and black olives. Tongue diagnosis gives objective and important information, and gross changes can be distinguished rather easily. A "normal" tongue found in a healthy individual, is neither engorged (fat) nor constricted (thin). It has a moderate red color, is relatively wet and has no coating ("fur") or mostly a thin, white coating, showing life in the functions of the stomach. (moss or fur is nothing else but the vaporizing of a small amount of food that is not digested; this "dirty" Qi is combined with the Yang Sp. Qi to form the moss. In illness there is a change in the fur and in the character of the body of the tongue itself. When toxins are accumulating, the fur becomes thick, oily and yellow. Many organs are related to the tongue through their meridians—heart, kidneys, spleen, bladder, triple warmer, and liver meridians are all linked to the tongue. The tongue is divided into areas which correspond to the different Tsang and Fu organs. (Figure 32)

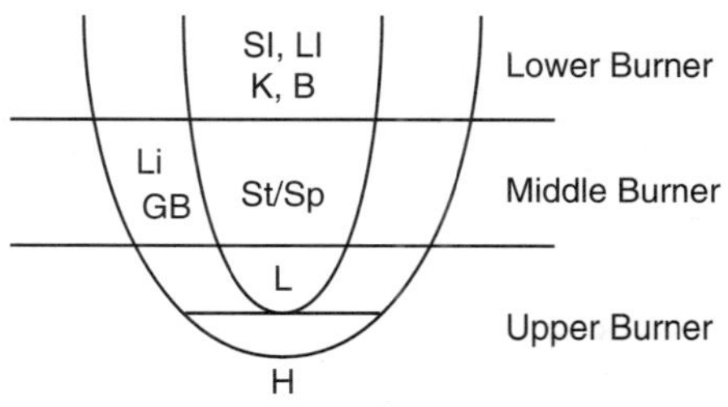

Figure 32

What can we learn from the tongue picture? Why is it so important?

- ❑ It is a valuable tool to distinguish the EIGHT ESSENTIAL CONDITIONS (see further in this chapter).
- ❑ Determines the prognosis of a disease (numerous examples are found, further in this chapter).
- ❑ Tells the progression of the diseases, whether the patient gets better or worse.
- ❑ Tells whether a disease is going to the interior or exterior.
- ❑ It will be used to confirm the diagnosis obtained by other means such as pulses and inquiry. I.g., deficient Yang Qi in the spleen, with morning diarrhea, cold limbs, undigested food, pale face, etc., will show a pale tongue.
- ❑ A tongue will show changes early on in the disease and can be used when

there are no symptoms yet or very few; vice versa, a tongue picture will show improvement *before* the subjective symptoms improve, showing the accuracy of the instituted treatment.

- ❑ It is most likely the most objective diagnostic tool, not influenced by outside environmental factors (Wind, Cold, Heat, etc.) acutely induced or by acute emotional shocks (i.e. sudden fear would turn the face white, but the tongue picture will not change). Of course, long-time exposure to those environmental factors and emotions would change the tongue in the long run.
- ❑ Tells how much Qi is in the body.
- ❑ Tells what organ is affected (see figure 32).

Examination of the tongue includes observation of four aspects:

BODY OF THE TONGUE
COLOR OF THE BODY OF THE TONGUE
TONGUE COATING
COLOR OF THE COATING

Body of the Tongue

A *"thick"* tongue (one which appears engorged, "fatter" than normal) indicates the presence of Dampness in the body or a Deficiency of Qi. If the tongue is thick and has a white, thin coating it denotes Deficiency of Qi. If the coating appears greasy, yellow and thick, it shows the presence of Dampness in the body. Tongue often has teeth marks.

A *"thin"* tongue (one which is narrow in diameter) suggests either a deficiency of Qi and Yin or only a deficient Yin.

- ❑ Deficiency of Yin and Qi: the tongue is thin and pale.
- ❑ Deficiency of Yin: the tongue is redder than usual.

Note also any cleavages of the tongue. This is either a congenital condition or an indication of Heat in the body. Eruptions of the tip of the tongue represent Heat in the Heart. Purplish eruptions on the sides of the tongue demonstrate congealed Blood or stagnation of Qi in the Liver.

A *"hard "* tongue indicates a disease of Chueh Yin; a red, hard and stiff tongue suggests severe heat in the organs; pain at the root of the tongue and head hair fall-out implies consumption of too many sweets; a swollen and cyanosed tongue and lips point to poisoning; a big, round flaccid tongue insinuates a weakness of the kidney meridian; trembling and quivering tongue shows that damp-heat has hurt the blood and Qi in alcoholics; a flaccid and motionless tongue denotes that heat has hurt the Yin; red scarlet tongue, quivering and pulled to one side is symbolic for wind in the liver or impending stroke; tongue pulled to one side, impaired speech, mouth and eyes pulled to one side is typically for a hemiplegia in capsula interna; a tongue that is contracted, and too short to come out of the mouth insinuates either cold contracting tendons and muscles (pale, white) or heat has injured the Yin (fluids), causing wind which prevents the tongue from coming out.

In general, in a strong body, the tongue is broad, thick and flat, with a slight white or yellow fur, and lively in color. In a weak body, the tongue is thin and pointed, often red or purplish at the edge, little fur or no fur.

Color of the Tongue

A *"red"* tongue indicates intense Heat in the body. A dry, red tongue in a person with ravenous appetite shows a lack of Yin with apparent Yang Excess. Light red throughout the tongue suggests a Deficiency of both Qi and Blood. Burning red tongue without fur and cracks denotes Deficiency of Yin and intense fire. A red, painful tongue implies invasion of liver Wind and Fire pressing towards the heart. A scarlet red tongue is significant for a Deficiency of Yin fluids.

A *"gray"* tongue insinuates Excess Heat. A pure gray tongue throughout with little saliva and dryness of the lips, is symptomatic for the Excess Heat hitting the three Yins directly. A gray tongue with burning lips implies an accumulation of toxins in the body.

A *"black"* tongue is characteristic for an illness of the spleen and/or kidney. Tip of the tongue black and dry represents the heart Fire burning itself, and the patient is not recoverable. A black, dried and cracked tongue insinuates a depletion of kidney Yin, and is extremely dangerous.

A *"purple"* tongue is significant for an illness of the heart and/or the kidneys. A dry, purple tongue in a patient with thirst, dry lips, clouding of consciousness and sleep talking hints at deficiency of water of the kidneys and phlegm fire in the upper burner. Purple, swollen and dry tongue is connotative for alcohol poison attacking the heart.

A *"pale"* tongue demonstrates a Deficiency of Qi and Yin, and represents emptiness and coldness. A pale, white damp tongue signifies a weak Sp. Yang energy (Earth not controlling Water, so the Sp. Yang is not transforming enough water).

Tongue Coating

A normal coating is thin and even, covering the entire tongue, or just the center, because it originates from the Sp/St. A thin coating indicates either a good prognosis, or a recent invasion of Excess, or a Sp/St. Emptiness which does not have the energy to bring up the "dirty" Qi. A thick, greasy coating is the mirror Phlegm in the body or the long-time presence of an Excess. The thicker the moss, the stronger the evil or pernicious Excess. No coating at all (so-called "stripped tongue) is caused by a Deficiency of Yin in the course of the long-time illness. A very wet tongue shows the presence of Cold or Dampness in the body; a very dry tongue, on the other hand, is caused by intensive Heat in the body which exhausts the liquids. Patches of moss on the tongue signify a lack of harmony in the Sp/St. entity. A greasy moss is common and insinuates presence of mucus. The more cracks in the moss, the heavier the disease. Causes are Empty Qi (pale color), Empty Yin (dry and pale) or Exterior Heat injuring the fluids (red, dry).

Check if the moss has a root or not. It is not rooted if the moss is growing like grass from the tongue and it appears that you can scrape it off. This reflects a St. Qi emptiness. A rooted moss is more healthy and represents a stronger St. Qi. Note if the moss is increasing or decreasing. If it is going from thick to thin, the pernicious excess is on the way out, and the prognosis is favorable. The applied therapy was correct or the Essential Qi of the patient was strong enough to overcome the excess. If the moss is going from thin to thick, the exterior excess is getting stronger, and is able to break through the defense barriers of the patient: unfavorable prognosis, requiring immediate action.

Color of the Tongue Coating

A thin white moss is normal and there is no imbalance in Sp/St. A white, moist coating reveals presence of Cold in the body. On the other hand, white-and-dry denotes the invasion of Cold, transforming steadily into Heat. A greasy, thick, moist and white coating reflects Dampness in the body. If the greasiness is not very wet or dry, it means stuck food in St. or intestines or the Yang Qi of the Sp. is not moving and transforming the food stuff properly. A yellow color always shows the presence of Heat. Also, a white moss symbolizes a new disease or a light one, while a yellow moss reveals a deeper and older illness. A yellow, moist moss looks like a contradiction because yellow is heat and moist is cold. However, this is typical when the outside Excess has just begun to invade the body and fluids are not injured yet.

A change from yellow to white is diagnostic for a good prognosis. From white to yellow shows that the disease is beginning to go to the interior. In the course of a disease, the coating can reveal different aspects. For instance, attack of Cold will show eventually the following different aspects, one after another: white and wet, white and dry, greasy fur, red tongue with yellow fur, red dry tongue and "stripped" tongue. As a rule of thumb, a thick moss is symptomatic for excessive evil (Damp-Heat), while a thin fur reflects less intense evil.

It is very important to observe the tongue closely, especially before meals, as food can change the color of the tongue itself or the color of the coating. In addition to request information from the patient regarding his or her food intake, the acupuncturist must also find out what medications the patient is taking, since this may affect the tongue picture.

SPIRIT OF THE PATIENT

There are four classes of mental symptoms. The most important ones are relating to the *WILL*. The most fundamental instinct of mankind is self preservation. Hence the deepest aberration would be suicidal impulses and attempts. The *Su Wen* states: *"To lose the spirit is death—to recover the spirit is life."* Loathing of life, complete indifference and fears of death, darkness, thunderstorms and animals also come under the will. The second group deals with the *EMOTIONS*. They include the loves and the hates, the apprehension, desire or aversion for company, weepiness, tidiness, low self-confidence and self-worth, loquacity, taciturnity and over-sensitiveness (easily offended). The third class belongs to the *INTELLECT*. They compromise the memory, mistakes, confusions and concentration. The fourth group are the symptoms relative to the *VITALITY*. They group symptoms from any conditions such like *"Ailments from."* Ailments from grief, anticipation, fright, anger, mortification, vexation, disappointed love, etc. Also sex reactions in so far they apply to the whole person: aversion to coitus, onanism, perversions, nymphomania, etc. For the first group of patients, the prognosis is guarded. The will to survive plays an important role in the healing process and depends upon a strong Roun or Li Qi (See Psychological Diseases). In general, when the patient is cooperative, has bright eyes, exhudes radiance, speaks and answers clearly, and has a normal respiration, the disease situation is shallow and recovery will be easy. When the patient shows no spirit, feels weak and defeated, the eyes don't shine, he has no interest, is somnolent, and talks slowly with a low voice, then the disease is deeper and more dangerous. This is the case especially when more than one of the above classes is involved.

CONSTITUTION OF THE PATIENT

An obese patient indicates the presence of Dampness and Xu of Qi in his body. A thin patient reflects a hyperactivity of Fire (of the Xu type). Deviation of the mouth is caused by pathogenic Wind in the channels or Xu of Yin and Blood. Paralysis of the limbs is due to Xu of Qi and Xue, caused by a dysfunction of the Spleen. This is called "central disease" since the Sp governs the limbs and will spread the Qi and Blood to the periphery.

PHYSICAL EXAMINATION

"Looking at the patient" will be incomplete if a full examination is neglected on the undressed patient. This includes the way the patient is walking: is he limping? Does he walk stiffly, or is he stiff when he starts walking and improves as he continues? Does he use one side of the body more than the other as is evident in muscular hypotrophy, etc. Examine the skin: dryness, greasy skin, rashes, abundant hair growth or lack of it, are all valuable features leading to a correct therapeutic action. Look for visible deformations: tumors, cysts, swollen lymph nodes, lipomas, bone deformations and abnormal muscular swellings. Explore for varicose veins and the capillary system in general: especially under the ribs, lumbosacral, nasal and peri-nasal and on the thighs, internal and external. Inspect the limbs and note abnormal coloration, coldness, perspiration, edema and aspect of the nails.

Examine the *eyes* for obvious strabismus, nystagmus and pupilary abnormalities. All meridians have connections to the eyes. *Nei Ching* , Chapter 80 states: *"The essential Qi of the 5 organs and 6 entrails has its concentration point at the eyes."* The pupil represents the essence of the bones or kidney. The iris symbolizes the essence of the muscles and tendons or the liver. The sclera (and the small capillaries running across it) represents the Yang. The eyes are the window of the soul and reflect the condition of the viscera. A patient's spirit is reflected in the eyes as well as his mental state. If the patient always moves his eyes, it signifies fear, indecision and insecurity (kidney or water problem). If he stares at things, the fire is in excess, denotative for a heart problem. Sadness in the eyes reveals a grief or lung problem. An angry look is symptomatic for liver or wood involvement. In general, the eyes as well as the tears, are controlled by the liver. Dull eyes are typical for Qi depletion. Ask about double vision: it represents liver and kidney Qi deficiency. Photophobia and swelling symbolizes liver fire. Photophobia alone shows weak Yin energy while night blindness suggests a liver Qi deficiency. Check on the eyebrows. If they meet across it is symptomatic for a hyperactive liver. Long eyebrows are a sign of happiness and longevity. Thickness shows strong vitality.

The *hair* is controlled by the kidney, Lung and Spleen. Kidney controls the thickness, Lung the shine, Spleen the dryness. Dry and lifeless hair demonstrates weak Qi and Blood. Dandruff or other scalp problems reflect a spleen problem. Gray hair (especially early onset) reveals a Liver Yin Deficiency. Explore the *ears*. The *Ling Shu* notes: *"The ear is the place where all the meridians meet."* The main 6 Yang meridians have a direct connection to the ear and although the main 6 Yin meridians do not pass directly through the ear, there is an indirect connection through the Divergent or Deep meridians. The classics say, *"the energy of the kidneys is connected with the ear—thus when there is harmony in the kidneys the ears can distinguish the five musical notes."* A normal ear should be thick and lustrous, showing a lot of Qi. If it is thin and dry, the reserve Qi is low. If the ear as a whole is white, it denotes an attack of Cold on the Kidney. If a person is over 60 years old and his ears are wrinkled, then he is sure to suffer from a major illness within 3 to 5 years. Investigate the *nails*. Generally speaking, diseases of the liver are observed in the nails. Healthy strong nails demonstrate a good liver blood condition. They are a measure of the prognosis. By pressing on the nails, they become white. By releasing the pressure, if they come back to the normal color, the disease is curable even though it is chronic. If not, the disease is severe and mostly incurable, even if it is acute. Thin nails are typical for Liver Qi Deficiency while thick, horny ones reveal Liver excess (except in older patients).

LISTENING AND SMELLING

Listen to the voice, respiration and cough. Smell the patient's urine and breath.

VOICE

The strength of the voice is a reflection of the quantity of Qi in the Lung. A loud and clear voice indicates a strong L, a feeble and low one a Xu of Qi in this organ. (See also previous remarks under "Spirit" of the patient). Stuttering indicates presence of Wind Phlegm in the collaterals, white muttering, weeping and laughing at the same time is considered excessive Fire in Heart and derangement of the mind. A quivering voice tells you about a Wind-Dampness attack while hoarseness is usually caused by an internal injury to the Qi. To each element in the Five Elements is linked a variance of the voice:

· Shouting:	Li
· Laughing:	H
· Singing:	Sp
· Weeping:	L
· Grieving:	K

A loss of voice is mainly caused by an attack from:

- ❏ Cold on a person with an empty Lung Qi.
- ❏ Wind-heat rising and obstructing (external or Liver heat).
- ❏ Phlegm obstructing the Heart orifice with loss of tongue movement and speech difficulty.
- ❏ Dryness in the Lungs, like in TB.
- ❏ Seen in an insufficient nourishment from the Spleen, the center does not disperse Qi to the periphery, as in a stroke.
- ❏ Caused by Kidney Qi Deficiency in which the Kidney water cannot ascend.

RESPIRATION

The respiration in acute and chronic lung diseases reveals important information. Shortness of breath indicates Xu of Qi of H and L; a coarse, asthmatic breathing with presence of Phlegm is more a reflection of the Heat-Dampness in the L, of the Shi type. A strong breathing is diagnostic for an External disease with strong fever. Asthmatic breathing can be empty or full. In fullness, the patient feels better when exhaling. There is a full and oppressed chest. In emptiness, the patient feels better after a long inspiration. This is due to a Kidney Deficiency. Sighing is meaningful "stuck" energy, especially the Lung Qi not descending properly. Wheezing and difficult breathing can come from disharmony in the lungs from perverse Cold, or phlegm fire rising up or perverse fluid rising up (L or K meridian problem). Spleen deficiency can allow phlegm to rise causing congestion and difficult breathing.

COUGH

Cough is obviously linked to pulmonary disorders, but disease of the 5 organs can exert an influence on the lungs and bring about cough. This is why it is important to differentiate main and secondary causes of cough. Listen to the cough and ask about the appearance of Phlegm. The Chinese physician distinguishes cough without sputum—Lung disorder or cough with sputum—Sp. disorder. Pulmonary cough is more a dry cough, splenic cough more a wet cough. Wind-Cold will trigger a choking cough with little sputum; Wind-Heat produces purulent, thick sputum. Xu of Yin of the L causes a dry cough, sometimes with blood in the sputum. Xu of Yang of the Sp will cause the presence of excessive sputum.

SMELL

Trung Y Hoc says, "*In healthy patients the energy has no smell. At the beginning of disease due to the perverse toxic heat, the patient exhales an "abnormal" strong and foul smell.*"In the less severe cases, the smell does not leave the patient's room. In severe cases the smell reaches the other room. In disorders of offensive cold, in the early stage, the essential energy is not yet affected, hence absence of smell. But when they progress deeper towards Yang Ming the smell appears. The 5 smells indicate body odor from each of the solid organs:

Liver	rancid
Hear	scorched
Spleen	fragrant
Lung	fleshy
Kidneys	rotted

An offensive smell of the urine indicates Heat in the body (Shi syndrome); an insipid odor is rather a Cold syndrome of the Xu type. A foul breath is a reflection of the Heat in the St., retention of food in the Middle Burner and stagnation at the Yang Ming level.

THE INQUIRY

Su Ouenn, Chapter 77:

> *While making a diagnosis, the physician should ask the patient if he is rich or poor. If he is rich, most of the diseases he will present will be organic diseases. On the contrary, if he is poor, he will present most frequently, with disorders due to lack of food.... Not to inquire about the social situation of the patient and not to treat the disease in time, is the first mistake of the physician. In making diagnosis of disease, it is necessary to ask the patient concerning his eating habits and place of residence—whether he had been suffering from extreme joy or extreme misery, which are harmful to his fire energy...extreme anger is harmful to the Yin and acute joy is harmful to the yang.*

It is important to look for the diagnostic impressions on the first clinical manifestations. For instance:

- ❑ If the patient complains about headaches, fears the cold and has fever, it is a sign that the disease is external.

- ❑ If he complains about abdominal pains, diarrhea and icy limbs, the disease is internal.
- ❑ If the patient present first signs of a mild disorder which develop into a severe disease, it is necessary to look for the main and secondary causes and observe how quickly the disease progresses in order to apply an appropriate therapy.
- ❑ If the signs of oppression and bloating occur *after* an asthma attack, the disease is in the lungs; if the oppression and bloating occur *before* the attack, the disease is in the spleen.

In Western medicine and acupuncture, the inquiry will be of extreme importance and must be complete.

AGE:

Provides information about menopause, loss of Qi (especially K Qi, since this Qi decreases with aging and every occurred disease).

PROFESSION:

Often indicates possible pathogenic factors (Six Excesses, Seven Emotions). Think about the high-powered executive who just lives for his work. He consumes fast foods and drinks coffee and alcohol to stimulate his flagging energy in order to obtain his goals. All this will have a nefast influence on his liver. This is a typical Nux Vomica or Sulphur type in homeopathy.

COLD AND HEAT:

Simultaneous presence of chills and fever means attack of Exogenous factors. Chills alone: either direct attack of exterior Cold on the organs or weakness of Yang Qi. Fever alone: Heat penetrated the Tai Yang stage and reaches the Shao Yang Stage. Alternating chills and fever denote primary symptoms of Shao Yang involvement. Aversion to cold (feeling cold and afraid of cold) represents an exterior syndrome while no aversion to cold shows an interior syndrome. A low grade, persistent fever is typical for a Yin Xu. A fever at a certain time of the day (tidal fever) is caused by Xu of Yin of that organ; e.g., afternoon-fever is due to a Xu of Yin of the L. Feeling hot in the daytime reveals a problem in Yang Ming. Feeling hot in the night suggests deficient Yin Qi.

PERSPIRATION:

Perspiration is the fluid of the Yin; when internal heat slowly increases, the Wei Qi cannot maintain its protective function and the pores do not close—the fluid of the Yin cannot be held in the body so Yin becomes deficient. The heavy sweating takes the Yang energy when it leaves because there is not enough Yin left in the Body to hold the Yang. Sweating during the day is caused by a Xu of Wei Qi and Yang Qi while at night, Xu of Yin and hyperactivity of Yang Qi is responsible. Perspiration with constant fever and no fear of cold signifies that the Perverse Qi is penetrating in the interior. Sweating on the forehead only indicates Stomach heat and a sign of Empty Yang. Continuous, abundant sweating reflects a Deficient L Qi. Sweaty hands and feet are symbolic for heat in the Yang meridian and weak Qi. Hot flashes at menopause with spontaneous, profuse sweating tells us about deficiency of Blood and empty fire rising or Yin Xu. Cold sweat (sweating without fever) is symptomatic for weak Yang Qi while sweating when there is fever is characteristic for strong Yang Qi. Profuse diaphoresis looking like oil dripping from the patient's body shows a loss of Yang or signs of extreme cold.

HEADACHE:

There are different types of headaches.

❑ *Headaches due to an attack of the primary and secondary meridians:*

Frontal is due to a disturbance in Yang Ming.

Vertex is due to a disturbance in Chueh Yin.

Occipital is due to a disturbance in Tai Yang.
Temporal is due to a disturbance in Shao Yang.
Dull, pressure or eyeballs alleviates: Xu type.
Violent, sharp and worse on pressure: Shi type.
Headaches with sensation of tightness: Tai Yin

❑ *Headaches due to internal disorders:* they will be intermittent, accompanied by vertigo and dizzy turns. They mainly result from an emotional imbalance like Liver Yang rising or K Qi/Blood deficiency.

❑ *Headaches due to attacks of Perverse Qi:* they are constant and accompanied by chills and fever. e.g. Wind-Heat causes a headache with empty feeling and dizziness while Dampness creates headaches with a sensation of bloating or bursting. In migraine, perverse Wind penetrates both liver and gallbladder and prevent normal circulation of Qi Headaches related to the menstrual cycle: before is related to stagnant Liver Qi, during indicates hot blood and after denotes Xu of Qi.

VERTIGO:

Can be classified in two groups:

- Vertigo with signs of fullness, due to Dampness preventing Yang from going up to the head.
- Vertigo with signs of emptiness, often due to Kidney Deficiency. K Yin Deficiency leads to Liver Yin Deficiency with escape of Liver Yang Qi, ascending to the head.

Various causes can be involved:

- Disturbance by external perverse Qi.
- Negative emotions like anger, frustration and irritability, causing Li Fire to ascend.
- Blockage by phlegm due to Sp. Yang Deficiency.
- Impure Yin, created by incorrect food and drinking, rises instead of Yang creating dizziness, with fatigue in the limbs.
- Blood Deficiency due to chronic loss such as after child birth, chronic bleeding ulcer or post-operative.
- Deficient K Yin due to excessive fear, phobias, sugar intake, standing and cold-exposure.

URINE:

Normal color is yellow. Dark yellow signifies excessive heat in the liver. Yellow and cloudy represents presence of Damp-Heat. Clear and white is diagnostic for K Yang Deficiency or a sign of Cold. Oliguria is due to Heat in the body drying up the liquids or Xu of B Qi. Polyuria and frequent urination at night is caused by a Deficient K Yang causing an apparent Yin condition; this K Qi does not help the Bladder in its function to store the urine. Incontinence or loss of urine on exertion, laughing, coughing is typical for a Sp. Qi Deficiency. Anuria is caused by a disturbance of Qi transformation in the Triple Burner, or by precipitation of Damp-Heat in the bladder, or trauma or renal stones.

STOOL:

Constipation is due to either to intensive Heat drying up the liquids, or Xu of Qi (senility, but also after delivery), or long-time illness (Xu of Yin). In the latter case, there is no urgency at all. A difficult expulsion of fecal matter with abdominal pains, relieved after bowel movements demonstrate a fullness; easy expulsion of matter with aggravation after bowel movements represents an emptiness. Loose stools which start when the menstrual starts and stop when the period stops are due to a K and Sp. Yang Deficiency. Chronic hemorrhoids that come and go are symptomatic for a Sp. Yang Qi Deficiency. Acute diarrhea is caused by Cold-Damp (watery stool, absence of thirst) or Heat-Damp (hot, fetid, bloody stools, thirst). Chronic is due to either Xu of Yang of the Sp (undigested food in the stool) or Xu of Yang of the K ("Five o' clock a.m." diarrhea, common in older people).

THIRST:

Too many people drink their "Eight glasses of water a day" out of habit, thirsty or not! This often leads to insomnia and strain on the kidney organ. People should drink according to their needs, not because they read it is "healthy" to drink eight glasses of water a day (it is not!). Desire to take hot drinks is a liver sign caused by Cold in the body. Desire to take cold drinks is caused by Heat in the body. No thirst or little when the patient is sick, is denotative of a Cold or Cold-Damp syndrome. If the patient is in good health and not thirsty, it is because the organic fluid is flowing normally. Note that excessive thirst, hunger and urination is called the "Three Consumption Disease" or diabetes.

APPETITE:

If a patient eats normally during a disease, Yang Ming is not affected. If the patient refuses to eat and drink, has constipation and belching, this means the energy of the stomach and intestines cannot circulate. If the patient likes to eat although he suffers from indigestion, this tells us that there is an energetic imbalance between the stomach and spleen—the stomach energy is stronger than the spleen. If the patient is always hungry, overeats a lot but remains skinny, it reveals a fire overheating the interior. Poor appetite is due to a deficient Sp Qi or deficient Qi or from Dampness-Cold or from obstruction in the stomach.

TASTES IN THE MOUTH:

- ❑ Sweet: Damp-Heat in the Sp.
- ❑ Bitter: Fire of Li and GB.
- ❑ Salty: Shi K Yin Qi.
- ❑ Foul: heat in Lung.
- ❑ Tasteless feeling: Dampness in St./ Intestines.
- ❑ Tasteless feeling with desire of salt: sign of Emptiness.

CHEST AND ABDOMEN:

❑ Spontaneous palpitations with restlessness can have different causes:

- Deficiency of body Qi.
- Yin Deficiency: caused by overwork, or excessive loss of fluids. as in sexual hyperactivity, delivery, dehydration, postoperative.
- Blood stagnation.
- Weak K Yang cannot hold the fluids and water rises.
- In fright palpitations there is a Deficiency of H Qi, leading to empty Sp/ St. Qi.

❑ Cardialgy: feeling of needles in the Heart shows involvement of Yin Wei Mo.

❑ Abdominal distention: is caused by a Xu of Sp Qi and is called Fullness of Yin when it happens right after the meals and Fullness of Yang when the distention appears two hours after the meals.

❑ Pain in the sides: stagnation of Li Qi.

EYES AND EARS:

- ❑ Red eyes and tears: ascending Li-Yang.
- ❑ Dry eyes and blurred vision: Xu of Yin of Li and K or Yin Chiao Mo (Keo) is affected.
- ❑ Cataract: Liver and Kidney Yin Deficiency
- ❑ Ringing in the ears and deafness: Xu of K-Yin, accompanied by vertigo and palpitations, >when ear is pressed. When tinnitus with constipation, loss of appetite, nausea, vomiting and <when pressing the ear: sign of fullness.

SLEEP:

insomnia takes place following a deficiency or after a disease with severe pain or emotional trauma, causing a restlessness of the spirit. Following are some of the causes of insomnia.

- ❑ Disturbance by Pernicious Energy, especially Wind-Cold and Wind-Heat.
- ❑ Impure Qi in the Stomach (late eating, bad diet habits).
- ❑ Stagnation of phlegm as in asthma.

- ❑ Spleen and Blood Xu causing difficulty falling asleep.
- ❑ H/K disharmony due to K Yin Xu (I.e. excessive fear).
- ❑ Liver Fire rising in anger, depression, alcoholics.
- ❑ Fire in Yang-Ming: the patient does not know if he slept or not.
- ❑ With excessive dreaming: mostly Li and K Yin Xu.

PAIN:

- ❑ Painful spots: differentiation according to the Eight Conditions.
- ❑ Painful or sensitive Back Shu points and Front Mu points: direct indication of the affected organ.

MENSTRUAL CYCLE:

- ❑ Amount
  - Profuse or prolonged bleeding is due to Qi Deficiency (pale red) or Heat in the Blood (dark red).
  - Scanty bleeding is due to Deficiency of Blood (pale blood) or blood/phlegm obstruction (blood with clots).
- ❑ Color
  - Very red represents Heat and Excess symptoms
  - Scarlet fresh red suggests Heat from Yin Xu.
  - Very dark red is typical for stagnant Qi and Blood or Heat in the Blood.
  - Clotting signifies Qi/Blood stagnation or Liver problem.
- ❑ Cycle
  - Late is typical for Yin/Blood Xu or sudden Cold.
  - Early is denotative for Qi Xu, K Yin Xu or Hot Blood.
  - Irregular is diagnostic for stagnation of Qi/Blood.
  - Amenorrhea (if not pregnant) reveals Empty, dried Blood (especially Liver involvement) or Blood stagnation (Cold, emotions) or Cold/Dampness (cold food or swimming in cold water can suppress the menses).
- ❑ Dysmenorrhea
  - SHI type: stagnation of Qi and/or Blood, stagnation of Cold or Hot Blood, due to emotions, cold and cold foods.
  - XU type: Qi and Blood Xu due to Li/K Yin Deficiency and also Tchong Mo and Ren Mo Dysfunction.
  - Pain before period demonstrates Blood/Qi stagnation.

LEUCORRHEA:
represents Sp. Deficiency, K Deficiency or Dampness/Cold/Heat/Toxins.

- ❑ White, thick suggests Sp. Deficiency or Li Qi blocked; white, thin with back pain, clear urine reveals K Deficiency.
- ❑ Yellow color signifies Damp-Heat.
- ❑ Reddish shows Li Damp/Heat (Yang Shi condition).
- ❑ Dead fish smell is characteristic for Cold-Damp.

MEDICAL HISTORY:

- ❑ Operations
- ❑ Diseases
- ❑ Medication intake

FAMILY HISTORY:
Indicates terrain and hereditary factors important in many diseases: heart, kidney, diabetes, epilepsy, impairment of hearing, hypertension, etc.

HABITS:
Smoking, drinking, and drug abuse (marijuana, heroin, etc.) all create Heat in the Middle Burner.

PSYCHOLOGICAL STRUCTURE OF THE PATIENT:
See Seven Emotions, Chapter 14.

TIME OF ONSET OF THE MAIN COMPLAINT:
In my 23 years of practice, one thing has always astonished me: that patients and physicians alike pay so little attention to the causes and effects of their diseases. The most important questions to ask when one gets sick are: *"When exactly did I get sick?"* and *"What happened in my life around that time?"* These will describe the beginnings or the *root* of the disease. Without treating and recognizing the root, no cure can be achieved. The patient and physician has to see the correlation between his symptoms and the occurrence of emotional factors, trauma, diseases, food or drug abuses, exceptional stresses, etc. In general, when symptoms are present less than six months we call the disease acute (Yang). More than six months represents a chronic (Yin) disease.

PALPATION

The palpation consists of two different steps, the abdominal palpation and the palpation of the pulses. Where the first one is easily acquired, the second one will require years of work with thousands of pulse taking. There is a proverb that says: "Treating a patient without taking the pulses is like navigating a boat without a compass." Nevertheless, since we no longer live in ancient times where the doctor could feel the pulses to rely on his diagnosis, only while the patient was sitting behind a curtain, a good diagnosis can be made even without taking the pulses.

ABDOMINAL PALPATION

Todo Yoshimasu, a Chinese medical sage, said: *"The abdomen is the basis of life and disease—therefore to diagnose the symptoms of disease, one should start with abdominal diagnosis,"* In general, if the patient's abdomen is flaccid and lacks suppleness, his vitality is weak. Whereas if it is supple and firm, his vitality is strong, even when his physical condition may not be. In a healthy person, there is no tenderness, the skin is tight and elastic, moist and thick. The epigastric part of the abdomen belongs to the Upper Burner, the umbilical part corresponds to the Middle Burner while the Lower part (under the navel) corresponds to the Lower Burner. Palpate with palm of the hand.

Check the umbilicus first. In general it is set in, deep and firm. The umbilicus is the center of energy in the body. Examine the thickness of the abdominal muscles. Thick, supple muscles and layers of subcutaneous fat are signs of a Full condition. Thin, flaccid muscles, with little fat, and cold limbs reveal an empty condition.

A swollen abdomen is either a sign of Fullness or Emptiness. Fullness when there is constipation, Emptiness if diarrhea or ascites. A hard and congested lower abdomen is symbolic for stagnant Blood or a phlegm disease. Of course other situations like obstructed bowels and pregnancy cause a hard abdomen. When the upper abdomen is full and bulging and the muscles below the navel are weak, it suggests a Shi Sp. and a Xu K. A Shi situation of upper and lower abdomen shows abnormal hardness which may be caused by an excessive, faulty diet. A Xu of the upper and lower abdomen is present in Deficient Yin diseases (usually involvement of Sp/K).

In a second step, the physician palpates the *front Mu points or Alarm points and the Back Shu points.* Each organ has a Front Mu point that is located, as its name indicates, on the front of the body, and more specifically, on the thorax and abdomen. When an organ is suffering (deficiency of Qi), the corresponding Front Mu point becomes painful spontaneously and/or upon pressure, drawing the attention of the patient to a disorder. They are like guards in our body, ready to warn us of every possible dysfunction. Often the points are located above the organ involved, but there are quite a few exceptions, as seen in the next table.

ALARM POINTS OF THE ORGANS

Lung: L1; Liver: Li14; Spleen: Li13; Heart: CV14;Colon: St.25; Gall Bladder: GB24; Kidney: GB25Pericardium, Influential point of Qi: CV17; Stomach: CV12

The Back Shu points are directly connected with the Qi of the organs and can become sensitive spontaneously or under pressure when that organ is affected.

BACK SHU POINTS OF THE ORGANS

B11: Bones; B12 Wind; B13: Lung; B14: PC; B15: H;B16: GV; B17: Blood; B18: Li; B19: GB; B20: Sp; B21: St.; B22: TB; B23: K; B24: Sea of Qi; B25: LI; B27: SI; B28: B

TRADITIONAL CHINESE PULSOLOGY

Taking of pulses, one of the most important steps in our diagnosis, is not an easy task. The purpose here is to discuss the most important aspects of Chinese pulsology. Deliberately, the twenty-eight different forms of pulses are not described, but rather a simple, practical methodology for approaching this part of the examination of the patient. The pulses are taken at the wrist, the area normal used for this purpose. But this is not the only place to look for pathological changes in pulses.

General Characteristics

It is best to take pulses early in the morning, before the patient has eaten, in an atmosphere of relative calmness and serenity, if possible. The doctor as well as the patient should have peace of mind. The patient must not speak, and the palpation should occur under moderate light, since sudden variations of the voice and light will change the characteristics of the pulses.

The position of the patient is very important. If we take the pulses the first session while the patient lies down, then it is absolutely forbidden to take the pulses of that patient on a second occasion, in a sitting position. The best position is the lying-down position.

There are situations where taking the pulses will be of no value. In the case of the last trimester of pregnancy, the pulse of the fetus will interfere too much with the pulse of the mother. In heart deficiency, the circulation of the blood is too weak to provide a reliable diagnosis. Amputation of a limb means blockage of one side. Taking the pulses is based on symmetry.

It is necessary to consider whether or not the fingertips or pulpae of the acupuncturist are in good condition. Amateur gardeners, guitar players, or harpists will loose their sensitivity when taking pulses. Avoid any hobby that will cause callus on the fingertips because it will build a barrier between skin and artery, making it hard for the touch to perceive the correct pulse reading of the patient.

The pulse of female patients changes during the menstrual cycle. Shortly before menstruation, we find a pulse "rolling as a pearl under the finger." The same pulse can be found during pregnancy. At the end of the menstrual cycle, due to a Xu of Blood, there is a weak pulse. From the seventh day of the cycle on, the pulse resumes its normal strength.

The pulses of the Fu reflect the physiological state of the Fu; e.g., the Spleen/Stomach pulse will be stronger in the post pandrial period. Another trap and example of this law is the empty pulse of the Bladder, so often felt in the examination room. We should remember that most patients empty their bladder just before being examined by the doctor. Hence, a weak Bladder pulse should not be corrected per se!

It should also be remembered that each pulse has its dominance in its own season. For example, the Liver pulse is dominant in the Spring, thus a strong Li pulse felt in this season should be considered as normal and needs no correction. Correction (dispersing) would only aggravate the patient's condition, enough to discourage the acupuncturist from ever taking the pulse.

Finally, the pulse rate can also change by medication intake, cachexia and recent travel.

Practical Schema for Taking the Pulses

Nobody should think that he will be proficient in taking the pulses after some years in practice. It takes thirty years and more and many thousands of patients, before we can even think of feeling the pulses as the masters practiced it in ancient times. But there are characteristics that can be found, sometimes almost immediately. That is what this chapter is about.

What are we looking for?

- ❑ Taking the peripheral pulses
- ❑ Taking the radial pulses: depth, pace, amplitude, strength, zones of pulses, other characteristics

The Peripheral Pulses

It is a mistake to think that pulses are taken only at the wrist. Pulses are taken at different levels of the body, reflecting the Qi of certain organs. We consider three different zones: superior level or the head, middle level (upper extremity), and lower level (lower extremity).

- ❑ Superior level:
  - Tang Yang (Extra point) represents the Qi of the front.
  - TB2I reflects the Qi of the eyes and ears.
  - St3 indicates the Qi of the mouth and teeth.
- ❑ Middle level:
  - L9 shows the Qi of the Lung
  - H7 reveals the Qi of the Heart.
  - LI4 reflects the Qi of the thorax and Large Intestine.
- ❑ Lower Level
  - Li3—Qi of the Liver.
  - St42—Qi of the Stomach; when the radial pulses are weak we look for St42. If that pulse is weak, too, then the disease is considered serious, for the St is "the Mother of the Tsang and Fu organs: The strength of this pulse determines the possibility of a cure. If the disease is grave and the St pulse is feeble, we will have difficulty obtaining a cure; but when the St Qi is strong, a cure will be possible.

The Radial Pulses

Each organ has its corresponding pulse, in the superficial zones for the Yang pulses, in the deep for the Yin ones. They are summarized below. There are three different levels where the pulse is felt: the CUN position, above the radialis artery; the GUAN or barrier position at the epicondylus radialis; and the CHI position above the latter.

Left			Right		
Superficial			***Deep***		
CUN	SI	H	Li	L	TB Superior
GUAN	GB	Li	St	Sp	TB Middle
CHI	B	K Yin	TB	K Yang	TB Inferior

Depth of the Pulse

"Floating pulse": the pulse is felt as superficial but fades under increasing pressure. This pulse is related to Exterior conditions; in other words, an attack of one of the Six Excesses (Dampness, Heat, etc.). An Exterior attack will cause symptoms such as chills, temperature, headache and floating pulse. If we do not find a floating pulse, then we can be sure that the disease is internal in origin.

"Deep pulse": this pulse reflects the location of the disease in the internal organs. It can be either deep and strong (Shi disease) or deep and weak (Xu disease, deficiency of Qi in the internal organs). A deep and slow pulse indicates the presence of

Cold, whereas a deep, fast one shows internal symptoms of Heat.

Pace of the Pulse

In a healthy person, there are five pulsations per one complete respiration. There should be two pulsations per one inhalation, two pulses per exhalation and one pulse for the repiratory pause: R/P=1/5.

A slow pulse is defined a R/P< 1/4 and shows the presence of Cold in the body. But there are two possible slow pulses: the true and apparent slow pulse. In the true slow pulse, the respiration is normal and the pulse is less than four for one respiration. In the "apparent" slow pulse, the respiration is fast, while the pulse has a normal rate; we only get the *impression* of a slow pulse since the respiration is fast. Clinical conditions of an apparent slow pulse are anxiety, diabetes, hyperventilation syndrome, hyperthyroidy, encephalitis and acetyl salicylic acid (aspirin) intoxication.

A fast pulse is defined as R/P>1/16 and shows the presence of Heat in the body. Again we have a true and an "apparent" fast pulse. In the first, we have normal respiration and fast pulse; in the latter, a fast respiration and normal pulse rate. Clinical conditions of an "apparent" fast pulse are obstructive lung disease and asthma with emphysema. This demonstrates the importance of a complete clinical inquiry.

Amplitude of the Pulse

The amplitude of the pulse reveals the quantity of Qi in the pulse. In a full pulse, there is an impression of length of duration and strong pulsations. Both characteristics are "conditions sine qua non." If more pressure is applied on the pulse and the strength is no longer felt, then this is not considered a "full pulse." This kind of pulse is associated with evolving disease with good reactions of the patient. Fullness of the pulse signifies the presence of an excess of some kind but can also be found in healthy, sportive individuals.

In a really empty pulse we feel the presence of largesse without strength. Through this characteristic, the differential diagnosis with a weak pulse can be made. A weak pulse has no largesse as in an empty pulse. Emptiness of the pulse signifies the presence of a deficiency in the patient.

Strength of the Pulse

Taking the pulses means also comparing the right pulses with the left ones. On the right side there is arrival of the Yin (decrease of Energy, going from the Fire to the Water). On the left side, there is the arrival of the Yang (increase of the Qi going from the Water to the Fire). Discussing pulses means elaborating about movement of the Qi; e.g., if the left pulses are stronger and harder than the right, there is a Shi of Yang Qi.

Diagnosis of a Zone Trouble

The two Cun pulses reflect the Superior Burner, the two Guan (barrier) pulses the Middle, and the two Chi pulses the Inferior Burner. Specifically, emptiness of the two Cun positions, Heart and Lung, means Emptiness of the Upper Burner. Looking at the law of the Elements, Heart and Lung are in opposition. Hence, if one is Empty the other is in Fullness. Emptiness of both pulses at the same time means disturbance at the level of a Burner. It means that the disease has penetrated into depth due to loss of resistance in the patient or due to the strength of the pathogenic factor. The prognosis is reserved in this case, and acupuncture treatment alone might be insufficient.

Other Characteristics of the Pulse

In a healthy individual, the pulse should not stop for fifty pulsations. One stop means injury of one organ, several stops denotes injury of several organs.

When the pulse at St9 is stronger than at L9, then the energy is at the Exterior. When the pulse felt at L9 is stronger than at St9, the Energy is at the Interior.

The pulse has to be in conformity with its season. Thus, the Liver pulse is strong in the Spring. When this is the case, the Qi is of good quality.

The Yin needs to go into the Yang and, viceversa, the Yang needs to flow into the Yin. If this is not the case, there is an absence of the two deep pulses at the barrier position. Often we see that this is the cause of serious diseases, such as severe depression. Therapy is puncturing of GV25

6 Differentiation of Syndromes According to the Theory of Zang and Fu

When I first was confronted with this theory years ago, the whole text seemed to be a mixture of esoteric poetry and fragmented ideas without any great therapeutic value. Better understanding and further study, however, changed my mind completely: it is one of the most exciting theories I ever came across, following to the letter the principles of Traditional Chinese Medicine. What is more, knowledge of the physiological characteristics of each organ allows you to recognize easily the disturbed organ involved.

In the next step, your findings are easily supported by one of the more accurate and objective diagnostic methods: the tongue picture. Taking the pulses is a very valuable though difficult step in the diagnosis, and it takes years to develop the kind of skill necessary to rely on its findings. In fact, it is the only step in the diagnosis where every acupuncturist can let his fantasy go, because it will be very difficult to contradict him. What we really want to learn from the reading of the pulses is explained in Chapter 5.

Basing your diagnosis on the tongue reading, however, can be taught in half an hour and the findings will be consistent with every acupuncturist. Once you have diagnosed the disturbed organ and the aggravating factor (food, Six Excesses. Seven Emotions), the therapy is a "piece of cake"! One need not know more than thirty to forty points to correct the problems, most of them being points of great energetic value, easy to locate and to remember.

Personally, what I find to be the greatest value of the Tsang Fu method is the fact that acupuncturists using this thought process, will come to the same conclusion, diagnostic and therapeutic. This chapter will describe the various syndromes for each organ, including causes, symptoms and therapy.

"KEY TO THE SOLUTION"

What seemed to be a chaos of ideas in the first place changed into a truly fine logical sequence of events when I had a better insight into the relationship of the various presented syndromes. I decided to call it the "key" to the solution. We know that as long as the Yin and Yang are in equilibrium, there is no disease. Every disease begins with an imbalance of Yin and Yang caused by the Seven Emotions (See Chapter 14), the Six Excesses (See Chapter 11), food intake (irregular, too cold, too raw, too much, etc.) and long-term illness.

This initial disease attack will decrease the Qi in general, and a certain part of the total body Qi will be consumed. The Qi showing signs of deficiency will manifest a weakening of its holding, transforming and moving functions. As we will see further, since the Lung is the master of the Qi, many symptoms of Empty Qi in this early stage relate to the Lung.

If the attack progresses unchecked, the most mobile, and hence most vulnerable, part will decrease and stagnate: the Yang Qi. The situation then becomes more severe. A decrease of the Yang Qi is generally considered more severe than a decrease of the Qi. Apart from the above symptoms, Yang deficiency will cause a weakening of the warming energy, and therefore, Cold symptoms (mainly involved are K- and Sp Yang) will appear. The Su Wen says: *"Decrease in Qi (Yang) will lead to decrease in Xue (Yin), and the stagnation of one will lead to stagnation of the other."* Inevitably, the decrease and stagnation of Yang Qi will lead to a decrease and stagnation of Yin Qi. Or a stagnation of Fire (Yang) leads to stagnation of Water (Yin). Stagnation of water is nothing more than formation of Phlegm, a process in which the Spleen plays a very important role. The Phlegm itself will obstruct the Primary Channels, injure and obstruct the organs and ultimately the Heart .

The above pathway described the consequences of the stagnation of the Yin. Alternatively, stagnation of Yang Qi will develop into Endogenous Heat (too much Yang concentrated in one place gives the extreme Yang excess, Fire). Endogenous Heat will always stir up the Wind (formation of Interior Wind), which will ascend to the head to give symptoms such as headaches, insomnia, hypertension, stroke, etc. The extreme Heat will injure the Yin and exhaust the fluids, leading also to the formation of Phlegm. In this way the vicious circle is closed(Figure 33).

Recognizing the symptoms will be fairly easy. A state of *emptiness of Qi* is characterized by:

- Physical and psychological fatigue.
- Pale face.
- Feeble or empty pulse.
- Weak voice.
- Abundant perspiration.

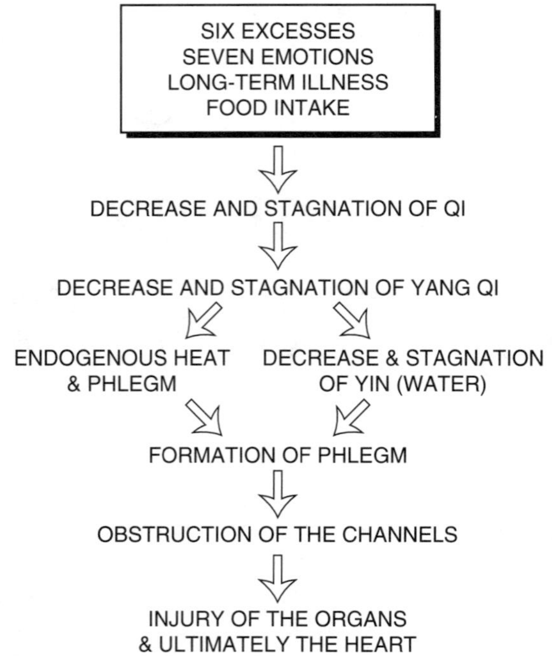

Figure 33

- Pale tongue and
- Reluctance to speak.

If we have palpitations: emptiness of Qi of the Heart is involved. If we have intermittent shortness of breath: emptiness of Qi of the Lung. If we have sexual disturbances: emptiness of Qi of the Kidney.

When we add to the three signs of emptiness symptoms such as:

- Sensation of tingling and
- Menstrual cycle disturbance

then we have an *emptiness of Blood.*

LUNG

There are several reasons for starting with this organ. First, the Lung is considered the *Master of the Qi*. It commands the Qi, dispersing and causing it to descend throughout the body. As the Lung is located in the Upper Burner, the Qi is normally descending. The same applies to all the organs located in the Upper and Middle Burner. Psychological factors (frustration, anger, etc.) as well as Excesses, can prevent the descending of this Qi and create a new form of Qi, *Rebellious Qi* (coughing in case of the Lung, vomiting in case of the Stomach).

Secondly, the Lung is also the most sensitive organ. Wind Excess will attack the Lung before any other organ, but the real enemy of this organ is Dryness. Dryness affects the L when attacking the upper part of the body; on the other hand, it will affect the LI when attacking the lower part of the body. That's why Dryness is in relationship with the meridians Cheou Tai Yin and Cheou Yang Ming. To fight Dryness, we use the points LI1 (Dry and Ting point of the LI), K4 and B17 (Influential point of the Blood, producing liquids and humidifying the Dryness).

The L, placed in the five Elements between Sp and K, will play an important role in the *water metabolism*. Intimately related to the skin, it will disperse part of the fluids as sweat but will cause to descend another part to the Kidney for the formation of urine. Hence, in case of formation of edema, we also must check the functions of the L as well as those of the Sp and K. The L governs the *"external" skin and the body hair*, while "internal" skin or mucosa is dominated by the Spleen. The head hair on the other hand, is under the influence of the Kidney and in a narrow relationship with the presence of Blood (See Chapter on Tchong Mo). We can say that the L commands the skin, sweat, body hair and the Wei Qi. Furthermore, the voice is heard when the original Qi or Zong Qi ascends to the throat. In case of Lung disturbance, we will have disturbances in *phonation*; therefore, the strength of the voice allows one to diagnose a Lung disturbance.

The Lung Qi commands also the *nose*, which is referred to as the "door" of the Lung. It is the passage point of the celestial Qi and the place where the Lung Qi circulates.

The Lung houses the *PRO* (Psychological diseases, See Chapter 14).

Good knowledge of the different physiological symptoms of this organ will lead to an easy understanding and retention of the various possible syndromes involved.

SYNDROMES

WIND INVASION

Since the Qi of the Lung passes through the nose, the Wind excess invades the body through this organ. Wind Excess, known for its changeable symptoms and its association with other Excesses, can either be Wind-Cold or Wind-Heat.

❑ Wind-Cold: the Cold being Yin, has damaged the Yang of the body, decreasing this way the warmth-production. Cold symptoms will predominate:

- Chills
- Cold limbs.
- Sensitivity to cold, patient's fear of the cold.
- Watery nasal discharge. No thirst.
- Edema of the face (the L does not descend the water to the K).
- The pulse will be floating ("conditio sine qua non" for external causes) and slow (Cold).
- Tongue will be pale with white, moist coating.

❑ Wind-Heat: Heat exhausts the body liquids, thus Heat symptoms will predominate:

- Fever and thirst.
- Watery nasal discharge turns yellow and thick.
- Dry cough, sometimes bloody.
- Red face.
- Painful throat and headaches.
- Epistaxis.
- Pulse floating (External condition) and rapid (Heat).
- Tongue: in the beginning, moderately red with a thin, yellow coating. As more liquids are exhausted the tongue becomes redder and drier.

❑ Clinical Examples:

Common cold, influenza, pertussis, acute bronchitis, epistaxis. All of these conditions are a result of Exterior Wind. They may show Cold or Heat syndromes.

❏ Therapy

To extinguish the Wind: GB20, B12, GV16. Wind points have a double function. In the Interior they put the Qi and Xue into movement; in the Exterior, they protect against the Perverse Qi. Looking at two important characteristics of the Wind, putting into movement and the acute, brutal, changeable symptoms it produces, we can understand why we find all these Wind points on Shao Yang (Shao means putting into movement), and Tai Yang (Tai means greatest, highest quantity): GB20, TB17, GB31, B12, SI12 and GV16 (GV is the confluence of all the Yang and hence the most Yang meridian).

To drain Heat out of the body: It is preferable to use points from the level where there is much Qi and Xue; in other words, from the level Yang Ming: LI4, LI11, St44. To drain heat from an organ, it is every effective to puncture the Back Shu point of that organ, B13 in this case.

To relieve Cold symptoms: TB5$^{(t)}$ (facilitates the circulation of stagnated Qi; stagnation is intensified by Cold and improved by Heat).

To relieve the cough: L1$^{(t)}$ (Mo point), L7$^{(t)}$ and CV22$^{(t)}$. These points increase the descending function of the L and will suppress the Rebellious Qi.

To dissolve Phlegm: St40$^{(t)}$ (anti-mucus point), Sp6$^{(t)}$.

HEAT-PHLEGM RETENTION

Whenever the patient shows little resistance (Xu syndrome, too little Wei Qi) or the Excess is very strong (Shi syndrome), the invader will follow the pathway of our key. The Cold turns into Heat, exhausting more and more body fluids and injuring the Yin Qi. The fluids become thick and block the channels, forming Phlegm (water stagnation). The initial dry, bloody cough turns into an abundant, foul purulent sputum. Since this blocks the descending functions of the L, the Qi will ascend (Rebellious Qi) and sputum will be expectorated.

❏ Symptoms

- Fever.
- Shortness of breath.
- Bloody stripes in the sputum.
- Abundant, foul sputum.
- Pulse is rapid and strong (Shi condition), or rapid and weak (Xu condition).
- Tongue: deep red with yellow, greasy coating.

❏ Therapy

- Draining the heat: GV14^{d} (confluence of all the Yang), LI4^{d} and LI11^{d} (points of the level Yang Ming, with a lot of Xue and Qi), L11 (drains the Heat out of the whole body).
- Anti-Phlegm formation: Sp9, Sp6 and St40.
- Descending of the Rebellious Qi, stopping the cough: CV22^{t} and C17^{t}.
- Stop the wheezing: Dingchuann (Extra point, 0.5 cm lateral to GV14).
- Obstruction by Phlegm of the Upper Burner: PC6^{d}, CV 12$^{(t)}$ and CV22$^{(t)}$ (vomiting technique).

❏ Clinical Examples

Chronic bronchitis, bronchial asthma, bronchiectasia, emphysema, cystic fibrosis.

EXHAUSTION OF THE YIN QI OF THE L

Due to a lack of Wei Qi and Qi in general, the disease becomes chronic and damages the most sensitive part of the L, the Yin Qi. This weakness of Yin leads to preponderance of Yang (Heat syndrome of Xu type). The symptoms are Heat and

Excess symptoms, but this is an apparent Yang: dispersing the Yang will only aggravate the patient's condition. Increasing the Yin Qi is the correct solution.

- Symptoms
  - Fever, afternoon fever.
  - Night sweats and low grade fevers in afternoon. Insomnia.
  - Dry cough with bloody sputum (Heat injures the vessels).
  - Dyspnea, lassitude.
  - Warm soles and palms.
  - Weak constitution, hoarse voice.
  - Mouth and pharynx dry, hoarseness.
  - Tongue: dark red, dry with cleavages or yellow coating.
  - Pulse: weak, thready and rapid.
- Clinical Examples
  - Lung tuberculosis.
- Therapy
  - Draining of the Heat: LI4, LI11, GV14.
  - Strengthening the L: L9(t) (heart element), B13/L1 (Yu Mo technique).
  - Coughing Blood B17 (influential point of the Blood), L1 (Mu point).
  - Strengthening of the weakened condition: CV6 (Sea of Qi) and St36, eventually with moxa.

LARGE INTESTINE

The LI receives waste material, sent down by the SI. It absorbs part of the waste material and eliminates the rest as feces. The LI (Yang) is coupled to the L (Yin): disturbances of one organ lead to disturbances of the coupled one: e.g., the formation of Phlegm in an asthmatic patient obstructs the flow of the Qi to the LI, causing constipation. On the other hand, constipation can cause an asthma attack.

Disturbances in the flow of this Qi are caused by overeating, irregular eating and by eating cold and raw food.

SYNDROMES

STAGNATION OF QI

A frequent consequence of eating too much cold and raw food. Cold slows down the flow of the Qi in the LI, leading to its stagnation. The food will stagnate, since the moving force of the Qi has decreased. The Yang is supposed to move the Yin: stagnation of one leads to stagnation of the other. After a while the Cold easily transforms into Heat (formation of Endogenous Heat), injuring the vessels with consequent symptoms).

- Symptoms
  - Diarrhea and abdominal pain (Cold stagnation).
  - Retention of food, leading to distention of the stomach, belching, feeling of fullness, anorexia, nausea, vomiting, pain upon pressure right after meals (fullness of Yin).
  - Mucus in the stool, blood in the stool (Cold transforms into Heat).
  - The tongue picture evolves from a flabby, pale body with white coating (Cold) to a moderately red tongue with yellow coating (Heat).
  - The pulse responds in the same way, going from forceful and deep to fast.
- Clinical Examples
  - Indigestion and diarrhea (Cold), food poisoning, dysentery and appendicitis (Heat-Dampness).
- Therapy:
  - For Cold: CV6, Sea of Qi or Heat, in tonification or moxa.
  - For stagnation of Qi: the Qi is

stagnated at the level Yang-Ming, disrupting the opening of Yang-Ming to the interior: LI11$^{(t)}$, St25$^{(t)}$ and St36$^{(t)}$.

- Vomiting and distention: PC6, CV12 and CV22.

STAGNATION AND FORMATION OF ENDOGENOUS HEAT

As the disease progresses, the Heat becomes more intense, injuring the blood vessels and exhausting the liquids. At the end, the Yin will be extinguished and the patient will show extreme Heat or Yang symptoms (apparent Yang Excess).

- ❑ Symptoms
    - Local inflammation with pain and bright red blood in the stool.
    - Weight loss despite good appetite (Heat in the stomach causes a continuous hungry feeling).
    - Cachexia, abscess formation.
    - Tongue: red body, yellow coating, sticky, evolving to an extreme dry tongue with no fur but cracks.
- ❑ Clinical Syndromes
    - Colitis ulcerosa (very good indication for acupuncture), and Chrohn's disease (granulomatous colitis).
- ❑ Therapy
    - Draining the Heat: B15 (Back Shu point), LI11 and LI4, GV14, L11 (drains the Heat from all over the body), St37 (lower He Sea Point of the LI).
    - Calming the mind: a psychological disturbance seems to be at the onset of the disease, the disease easily triggered off in emotional, fearful patients: H7$^{(s)}$, H3$^{(s)}$ and K3^{t}.
    - Weakness: CV6^{t} and St36^{t}.
    - Stops all diarrhea: new point ZHI XIE (NP 83); one cun under CV6^{t}.

KIDNEY

Very often, deficiency of the K Yang, and even more the K Yin, will be the root of disease. Once we see an older patient in our examining room, we must focus on finding a deficient K Qi. Therefore, knowledge of its physiological characteristics and early recognition of the symptoms will be of great importance.

The Yin-K *stores the essence*, responsible for the growth and the reproductive functions. The Ancestral Qi or Source Qi, inherited from our parents, is localized in this part of the K. The whole *sexual apparatus* (especially the internal sexual organs), is dependent on this Yin K. The Kidney together with the Liver are the most important organs for a normal sexual life. This Ancestral Qi, conserved in the K, is provided by the mother during pregnancy. With any disease, the amount of this Qi will decrease, hence a fullness of the Ancestral Qi is impossible. It is practically impossible to increase the quantity of this Qi by acupuncture (in contrast to the other forms of Qi). One can try with stimulation of the magic triangle: GV4, B23 on both sides.

The Yin-K is also responsible for the *production of bone-marrow* and consequently, for the formation of the brain (Nei Ching: *"The brain is the sea of marrow.")* This marrow production plays an important role in the formation of blood and the bone structure and thus in the relationship of the K with the menstrual cycle, the teeth, bones, etc.

The *Yang* function of the K has also several aspects. It divides the fluids into clear and turbid fluids: the turbid ones are excreted as urine. It is responsible for the warming up of the body: the formation of Endogenous Cold is due to a Deficiency of Yang of the organs. The disease of the "Endogenous Cold" in the Lower Burner is linked to a Deficiency of Yang Qi of the K. The disease of the "Endogenous Cold" in the Middle Burner is most often caused by a deficiency of Yang Qi of the Sp and St. Treatment will be of Sp2 (Fire point),

Sp4 (Luo point), St36, Li13 (Mu point of the Sp), and CV12. The disease of the "Endogenous Cold" in the Upper Burner is especially linked to a Deficiency of the Qi and the L. Treatment is L10 (fire point), L9, CV17 (Influential point of the Qi), GV14 (moxa).

Another function of the K-Yang is to help the Bladder in its function to *hold the urine*. In enuresis nocturna, for example, we tonify the Yang-K. Frequently we see this problem in children going for the first time to school, due to separation anxiety and fear of abandonment (remember, fear is K-related).

The K also *receives the Qi distributed by the L*. According to the Sheng-cycle, this descending Qi must find a good receptor in the K-element. Failure to do so can trigger asthma symptoms; so one must be aware of this possibility when confronted with an asthma patient. The therapy will be entirely different than in a primarily Lung-asthma patient.

The K corresponds with the *ears*. A chronic problem of the ears must be treated by the K. On the contrary, a recent ear-ringing or deafness will be treated by the TB and GB.

The K has a relationship with the adrenals: in TCM, these are not an organ, but their function exists. Their functions and pathology are in connection with the K.

The K houses the *Tche*. (See Chapter 14)

SYNDROMES

DECREASE OF QI OF THE K

Numerous factors decrease the K-Qi during our lifetime. Sexual excesses and masturbation ("affairs of the bedroom") can easily exhaust this Qi. In homeopathy, this is called "*Never well since loss of fluids.*" It is written in the *Su Nu King* (the ancient Chinese book of sexuality, a common marriage present and wrongfully considered in the Occidental world as a soft-porno book), that a technique for increasing the Qi of the K in a male is for him to give a female as many orgasms as possible in order to capture the Yang liberated by the female, while at the same time he must avoid having an orgasm himself (so that he may not lose his Ancestral Qi fixed on the spermatic Qi).

Another cause of K Qi decrease is old age or aging in general. It is well known in Western medicine that nearly everybody past the age of forty shows signs of arthrosis deformans, different in severity from one person to another. To acupuncturists, this is clear since the bones are related to the K, and the more we spend our K-Qi, the worse our degree of arthrosis can be. Of course, we have to mention the cold climate and the emotion fear, also related to the K and aggravating factors in this disease if present.

- ❏ Symptoms:
  - Nocturnal enuresis and incontinence: the K is in a Biao-Li connection with the Bladder; the B, being a Fu organ, has a storage function. When the K Qi decreases, the B loses its capacity to retain urine.
  - Asthma, dyspnea and wheezing: the K not receiving the Qi from the L is responsible for this secondary asthma, in contrast to the primary form due to deficient Yin-L.
  - Pulse will be slow and deep, the tongue pale and enlarged with white, thin coating.
- ❏ Clinical Syndromes:
  - Enuresis nocturna, incontinence, irregular menses, dreamless variety of spermatorrhea.
- ❏ Therapy:
  - B 23, GB 25: Yu-Mo technique.
  - Sp 6: intersection of the three leg Yin channels.

DECREASE OF YANG OF THE K:

According to the key, decrease of Qi quickly leads to decrease in Yang Qi.

- ❏ Symptoms:
  - Sensitivity to cold, cold limbs: the Yang-K is responsible for provid-

ing warmth to the body and together with Tchong-Mo, for keeping the temperature of the body. The K-Yang feeds the Sp-Yang, which assures the optimum temperature for the four limbs.

- Backache with sensitivity to cold.
- Edema: the K does not split the fluids between turbid and clear. According to the Su Wen: "*The Kidneys are the door to the Stomach*". The doors being closed, the liquids coming from the St cannot be evacuated; they reach the flesh and skin causing edema. It is very important to note that according to TCM, the L also has functions of circulation, elimination and spreading of the water: in case of edema of the superior part of the body, one has to treat the Lungs, e.g., edema of Quincke. The L is the superior source of water, the K the inferior one.
- Impotence, oligospermia, ejaculation praecox: deficiency of the Yang root of the K is often the source of impotence and priapism. On the other hand, the Yang K in fullness will stimulate the sexual desire or libido.
- Pulse: slow and deep (Xu Cold syndrome).
- Tongue: pale, white moist coating.

❑ Therapy

- CV9 and Sp9: both are anti-edema points, tonification sometimes causes strong diuresis.
- Strengthening of the Yang Qi: either the combination of K3, GV4 and B23 left or K2 (fire point), CV4 and CV6 (where the Yuan Qi and the Yang Qi are produced and where they leave the body).
- Sp 6: has the advantage of strengthening the Li Qi too, in case of impotence, since it is a confluent point for the three Yin foot channels.

DECREASE OF YIN OF THE K:

Due to a lack of resistance (Xu syndrome) or a strong pernicious factor (Shi syndrome), the disease progresses deeper, injuring the most precious part of the K, the Yin. Xu of K-Yin will lead to Xu of Li-Yin (Sheng-cycle), causing a disruption in the Yin/Yang unity of the Li. The Yang of the Li will ascend after forming Endogenous Heat and Interior Wind. This pathogenesis is important to remember when we see a patient with signs of Li-Yin deficiency. To restore this Li-Yin, we have to increase the K-Yin.

❑ Symptoms

- Poor memory and reasoning impairment due to poor formation and supporting of the brain.
- Backache without sensitivity to Cold.
- Hearing impairment, tinnitus, dizziness, headaches.
- Prospermia, and sterility. It is important here to emphasize the effectiveness of acupuncture in the treatment of sexual disorders.

Therefore, different terms with their corresponding disease are mentioned.

- *Jingguan* or spermatic barrier: this barrier is controlled by the K-Yang: the sperm will be ejaculated at the optimal moment. Xu of this K-Yang will lead to spermatorrhea, ejaculatio praecox and nocturnal emissions.
- *Jingshi* or spermatic room: the spermatic Qi or Essence are stores in this room, controlled by the K-Yin (who says storage, says Yin-organ!). Too little storage will lead to sterility. Not only the quantity

will be important, but also the quality of what is stored in this room (corresponds to the normal configuration and mobility of the sperm in Western Medicine).

- *Erection:* this implies movement of muscles and hence involvement of the Li, but erection is also commanded by the K-Yang. Xu of the Qi of the latter leads to impotence, incomplete erections.
- *Libido*: in TCM, the libido is ruled by the K-Yang, deficiency leads to lack of libido and frigidity in women.
- Arthritic complaints.
- Blurred vision.
- Pulse rapid and thin.
- Tongue: red, contracted, yellow coating.

❑ Clinical Syndromes:

- Prostatitis, hypertension, epilepsy, neurasthenia,Meniere's disease, glaucoma, and arthritis.

❑ Therapy:

- GB20, GV16 and Li2: to extinguish the Interior Wind and drain the Li Fire.
- Li3, B18, L14 and GV14: to drain the Heat.
- B23(t) on the right, Sp6 and CV4: to tonify the K-Yin.

RELATION OF THE KIDNEY TO THE OTHER ORGANS:

With the H:

❑ Physiology:

- The Yang or Fire of the H descends to the K to equilibrate with the water of the K (Yin).
- The Yin of the K ascends to the H to feed the Yin of the H to avoid the escape of its Yang.

❑ Pathology:

- If the Qi of the H does not ascend, the water of the K ascends to the H, causing edema and palpitations.
- Xu of the Yin of the K will create an imbalance in the H Yin-Yang, hence insomnia, nervositas (the H-Yang escapes).
- If both organs are disturbed, we observe insomnia, palpitations, nervositas, nocturnal emission of sperm, fatigue in the back.

With the Liver:

❑ Physiology:

- The Yin of the K feeds the Yin of the Li (Sheng cycle) but the essence of the K needs also the blood of the Li.

❑ Pathology:

- Xu of Yin of the K creates a Xu of the Li-Yin, with escape of the Li-Yang: vertigo, irregularities in the menstrual cycle, warm palms and soles, headaches, poor memory and stroke.
- Xu of Blood of the Li causes a deficient K-Yin: insomnia, low-grade fever, pollyuria, nocturnal spermatic emissions, fatigue in the back.

With the Lung:

❑ Physiology:

- The L sends water down to the K.
- The Yin of the K ascends to the L to participate in the water metabolism.

❑ Pathology:

- Xu of Yin of the K; the Yin does not ascend to the L, hence an escape of the L-Yang; dyspnoe upon effort, fever in the evening, spermatorrhea, nocturnal perspiration.

- If the L-Yin is Empty, then this Yin does not descend to the K, causing an escape of the K-Yang: cough aggravated at night and fever in the evening.

With the Spleen:

- ❑ Physiology:
  - The Essence is stored in the K and is strengthened by the essence of the food (Ancestral Qi is completed by the Acquired Qi).
  - The K-Yang feeds the Sp-Yang.
- ❑ Pathology:
  - Xu of Yang of the K causes Xu of Yang of the Sp, causing morning diarrhea, anorexia.
  - Vice-versa, emptiness of the Sp. causes either Yin K deficiency or Yang K deficiency, with their corresponding symptoms.

CLINICAL EXAMPLE XU K-YIN:

Mrs. Kathleen N., 29 years old, suffered for six months from progressive fatigue without apparent cause. She was a flight stewardess, with the irregular schedule typical for many airline employees. Another complaint was the daily occurrence of night sweats. Due to these complaints, Mrs. N. has not been able to work on a regular basis. At the first visit, I saw a slender-looking woman, anxious, somewhat fearful and nervous.

Conclusion One:

The night sweats were the first important indication of what was going on with this patient: there was an overall deficient Yin Qi. The cause was not difficult to find. The patient admitted eating very little and irregularly, because of the obligations of her work.

Further inquiry revealed the following:

- Cold limbs and immediate postpandrial fullness: fullness of Yin central with non-distribution to the periphery.
- Low grade fever for one month: apparent Yang excess due to Yin deficiency.
- Concentration and memory disturbances: deficient Blood or Yin the upper part of the body.
- Vertigo, especially when changing position.
- Appetite: poor and irregular.
- Thirst: especially for cold drinks.
- Stool: constipation for 2 months, def. Yin, burning up the liquids.
- Sleep: nightmares, palpitations; the K-Yin does not feed the H-Yin, creating an imbalance in the Yin-Yang of the H.
- Chest: normal, no needle feeling (excludes Yin Wei Mo).
- Smoking: increased in the previous months: creates internal Heat; no alcohol.
- Previous history: arthritis complaints and lower back pains, no cystitis. This signifies a deficient K-Yin; no other diseases.
- Family history: mother had arthritis. A deficient K-terrain was created from the beginning of her life.

Conclusion Two:

All symptoms indicate a deficient K-Yin, hence presence of Yang or Fire symptoms. There is a block of the Yin central with non-distribution to the periphery. The menstrual cycle was always disturbed: long cycles, coming too early with profuse bleeding, increasing the Xu Yin.

- ❑ Tongue
  - Narrow body: def. Qi.
  - Red with cracks, especially in the Middle and Lower Burner: drying up of the liquids, presence of Heat in the body.
  - Very little fur.
- ❑ Palpation
  - Mo points: GB25; very sensitive; Li14 sensitive.
  - Back-Shu points: B23; bilateral: sensitive.
  - Pulse: ratio p/r=5/1 acceleration. Left stronger than right. Weak K pulse.
- ❑ Therapy:
  - GB25, Li14: to increase the K-and Li Yin.
  - CV4 and 6: with moxa, to increase the original Qi.
  - Sp6, St36, CV12: to unblock the Middle Burner.
  - B23, B17: to regulate the K Qi and increase the Yin in general.
  - PC7: Iu and Shu-point, to disperse this Yin.

Results:

Right after the treatment, something strange happened. I had just left this patient and she was paying her bill, when suddenly she had an overwhelming feeling of relief and started to cry. She had to sit down, and I had a revealing conversation with her. She felt that this was the first time in months that she could open her feelings to the exterior world. Apparently, she had much responsibility on the plane, kept all her problems to herself, with a great deal of frustration and anger, creating Interior Fire, causing even more Yin-deficiency. In a way she was caught in a vicious circle and unable to break out of it. So far no doctor had found anything special (except the usual "psychosomatic story"). The patient recovered beautifully in as little as three visits, over two weeks. The tongue picture had already changed after the first treatment: no cracks were seen anymore.

BLADDER

The bladder *stores the urine* and *discharges* it from the body with the help of the Yang of the Kidney. In other words, there is a possibility of "opening" disturbances and "closing" disturbances of the Bladder. The former is illustrated by a spasm of the B, the latter by a feeble B, causing incontinence. The K and B are in a Biao-Li connection and hence have an important influence on each other. Disturbances in one organ inevitably cause a dysfunction in the coupled one.

SYNDROMES

DAMP-HEAT ATTACK

The combination of Damp and Heat is extremely pathological for most of the Fu organs, (B, GB, SI, LI, etc.). Damp-Heat will block the Qi of the B, disturbing the storage function; frequent and urgent urination are the consequences. It is very important to remember that dysuria is not only due to an energetic disturbance in the B. Often Damp-Heat of the SI passes into the B causing dysuria. This is easy to understand when we remember that in the Chinese Clock, the SI, is followed by the Bladder, connected by SI18 and B1. The Heat, injuring the vessels, is responsible for hematuria, pyuria and formation of stones (the latter when the Damp-Heat persists for a certain time). The pulse will be fast and deep, the tongue is red and yellow-coated.

- ❑ Clinical Syndromes:
  - Cystitis, renal colic, and prostatitis
- ❑ Therapy:
  - B23 and B28: to drain the Heat from the B and the K.
  - CV4 and Sp6: to facilitate the function of the Lower Burner. No moxa is used, only needles!

LIVER

One of the most important functions of the Li is the *storage of blood* (the Sp produces it, the H circulates it). When an increased amount of blood is required (such as in strenuous muscular activity or during menstruation), the Li must be able to provide the blood supply to the body. It is the organ that contains the greatest amount of blood: in TCM, movements, eyesight, standing up, etc., all need blood supply and hence are under the influence of Li.

The Yang part of the Li is responsible for the maintenance of the *flow of Qi* throughout the body. Anger, frustration and irritability will lead to stagnation of Qi of the Li and affect this organ. At the same time, it will also affect the free flow of Qi to the other organs, especially the stomach (Ko-cycle). This will lead to stagnation and formation of "rebellious Qi" of the Stomach, and the patient will exhibit symptoms of nausea, vomiting, dyspepsia, oppression, and diarrhea.

The Yin part of the Li, in addition to storage of the blood, will *nourish the tendons and muscles*. Ample Li-Yin is necessary for good muscular functioning. Disturbances of the volume of the muscles, or in other words "the flesh", are in the domain of the Sp: e.g., consequences of polio with atrophy are treated by points of the Sp. But disturbances of the muscular functions and movements, such as dyskinesia, akinesia, spasms, cramps, etc., are treated by puncturing points of the Li.

Different organs have an impact on the functions of the eyes (H, etc.) but the Li especially will contribute to ocular functions. The Li has an important "eye-branch", going down the cheek and encircling the mouth: "the *eyes are the openings of the Li.*"

The Li, in a Biao-Li connection with the GB, helps this organ in storing and *excreting the bile*.

The Qi of the Li contributes to the *defense against the exterior*: the Qi of the Li empties itself into the Lungs via the internal circulation and takes away the Qi of the Lower Burner.

SYNDROMES

DECREASE AND STAGNATION OF THE LI QI

Anger, frustration and irritability will stagnate the Qi in the Li. Stagnation of Li Qi leads to Fire, consuming the Li-Yin. Hence, the Li-Yin will not be in harmony with its Yang: "the hepatic Yang is released and will ascend." (One of the consequences is hypertension.)

- ❑ Symptoms
  - Pain in the right upper quadrant and discomfort in the chest (stagnation of Qi always means pain "at the place of stagnation.")
  - Symptoms due to Endogenous Fire and ascending Li Yang: insomnia, red eyes, irritability, headache, and bitter taste in the mouth.
  - Hematemesis and epistaxis: due to extreme Interior Heat formation, injuring the vessels and aggravated by smoking and alcohol intake.
  - Pulse is wiry and fast, tongue will be red and yellow-coated.
- ❑ Clinical Symptoms
  - Hypertension, stomach ache, stroke, and psychosis.
- ❑ Therapy:
  - GB20, Li3: extinguishes Exterior Wind conditions; another two points are Li2 and GV20.
  - GV14, LI4 and LI11: drains Heat, calms the mind. Li14, Li8 and Li5: activates the circulation of the Li Qi .

EXTREME ENDOGENOUS HEAT FORMATION

Invasion of Exterior Heat will increase the amount of Endogenous Heat. This will exhaust the Yin, transforming the fluids into phlegm which blocks the channels. In its extreme form, the Li Fire Ascending Yang attacks the Yin of the H (after penetrating the protecting shield of the PC) and phlegm will block the heart channels.

❑ Symptoms

- Derangement of the mind, with logorrhea, weeping without reason, excitability and hysteria.
- Extreme irritability, anger, vertigo, and red eyes.
- Malfunctioning of the muscles and tendons with convulsions, opisthotonos and coma.
- Pulse: rapid and wiry.
- Tongue: ranges from bright red, dry, with yellow, sticky coating to a deep red color with sores (the latter indicates invasion of the Heat in the Heart).

❑ Clinical Syndromes

- Hypertension, stroke, and hysteria.

❑ Therapy

- "Interior Wind": Li2, GB20.
- Draining Heat: LI4, LI11, GV14.
- Calming the mind: H7, H3 and St36.

DECREASE OF LI YIN

There is a separation between the Yin and the Yang of the Li: the Yang ascends, characterized by anger and irritability. Vice versa, too much anger will decrease the Li-Yin. The symptoms in this syndrome are symptoms of excess: red face, vertigo, and redness in conjunctivae. In reality we have a deficiency of Yin: this is called the *"apparent"* Yang. It is very important to differentiate between the apparent Yin or Yang and a true Yin or Yang Excess. Failure to recognize this leads to progression in the course of the disease with aggravation of the symptoms.

❑ How do we recognize these symptoms? (Table 1)

Other symptoms of Li-Yin Deficiency

- Malnourishment of tendons and muscles with spasms.
- Dry eyes.
- Prolonged menstrual cycle.

❑ Therapy

- B18, Li3 and Li8: tonify the Liver or Li 14. (Mu point).
- B17: influential point of the Blood.
- B23, K3 and Sp6: indirect tonification; to increase the Li-Yin, we have to crease the K-Yin.

Table 1

EMPTINESS of Li Ying	**EXCESS of Li Yang**
Fever	Fever
Vertigo	Vertigo
Ringing in the ears	Ringing in the ears
Red face	Red face
Pulse: deep, slow, feeble	Pulse: rapid, strong, wiry
It is a chronic disturbance	It is a recent disturbance
The above symptoms are constant	The above symptoms are intermittent (they correspond to the release of the Li Yang: this happens in waves).
Therapy is tonification (LI14, Li8 and Li3)	Therapy is dispersion (B18, Li2 or season dispersion point)

GALL BLADDER

The main function of the GB is the *storage and excretion of the bile* to help the digestion. As mentioned above, the liver, in a Biao-Li relationship with the gall bladder, plays an important role here. We have seen that the liver stores the blood and regulates the circulation of the Qi. When the Li is "full or filled", the arriving Qi will be transferred to the GB: this organ is the helper or adjunct of the Li.

The GB is the organ that makes *decisions*: the Li can be compared to a general in the army who thinks about the strategy of the coming battle. The GB, on the other hand, is the chief of staff, responsible for the action. In case of emptiness of Qi of the GB, the chief of staff cannot help the general to make a decision; hence, we will have an army that is confused, hesitant, fearful, unconfident and incapable of fighting. Another characteristic attributed to the GB is *courage*. Xu of Qi of the GB leads to cowardice, Excess of Qi on the other hand to irritability, *stubbornness and dissatisfaction* with everything and everybody. It is evident that very important psychological characteristics are related to the GB. Therefore, when we see a patient who complains that he has a hard time making decisions in important matters, is fearful of starting a new job or taking an examination (anticipation anxiety), the Li and at the same time the GB will be tonified. In order to have an army that can take action, both the general and the chief of staff have to function well as one entity.

SYNDROMES

ACCUMULATION OF DAMP-HEAT IN THE GB

As with many Fu-organs, Dampness-Heat is the main cause of disturbance. It leads to a stagnation of the Qi in the GB, with an overflow of the bile. This pathology is often linked to a digestive problem: either irregular meals, too fat or rich, or, in other words, spicy foods. Associated with a sedentary lifestyle, this excess of calories creates an accumulation of Dampness-Heat.

- ❑ Symptoms:
  - Pain in the sides, especially on the right side, radiating to the shoulder: stagnation of the Qi leads to eventual formation of gallstones, causing pain, following the trajectory of the meridian.
  - Bitter taste in the mouth, anorexia: normally, the Qi in the GB circulates freely. Blocking of the GB will disturb this movement. The Qi can ascend to the mouth and the patient notes a bitter taste, or this Qi can circulate in the whole body, causing jaundice. Finally, this Qi can enter the Stomach (Ko-cycle), disturbing its function, with anorexia as a consequence.
  - Alternating chills and fever: the alternating occurrence of the symptoms shows penetration of Excess in the Chao Yang level. The latter is one of our levels of defense against the Excesses, protecting the more important Yin: the Exterior protects the Interior.
  - Pulse is rapid, deep and slippery.
  - Tongue is moderately red with greasy coating.
- ❑ Clinical Syndromes:
  - Cholecystitis, and gallstones.
- ❑ Therapy
  - Heat in the GB: GB24 (Mu point), B19 (Yu point), GB34 and TB6 (the latter acts on the level Chao Yang, GB being Cheou or Tsou Chao Yang).
  - Vomiting, to calm the St: St36, Sp4.
  - Distention in the abdomen: PC6.

EMPTINESS OF QI:

Decrease of Qi of the GB is mostly caused by emotional problems: either by suppressing one's feelings (emotional and verbal abuse leading to indignation) or by receiving repetitive strict orders, allowing no opportunity for personal initiative. It can also be the opposite, as the example below describes.

I remember a case of a female patient whose mother died when she was eleven years old. She was forced into the role of the mother at too young an age, obliged to make decisions at a time when normally she could have followed her mother as the primary example. Hence, the GB's Qi decreased considerably in the following years of her life, changing totally the personality of this poor woman. At the age of 25, at the time of consultation, she was a frightened, indecisive person much to the surprise of her relatives who had known her always as this courageous little girl, capable of doing anything.

- ❑ Symptoms
  - Vertigo, insomnia and especially problems of falling asleep.
  - Vision disturbances: diplopia, myopia, night blindness.
  - Pulse: wiry but small, reflecting the emptiness.
  - Fearfulness: indecision and lack of courage.
- ❑ Treatment
  - Direct action on GB-Li through Yu-Mo technique: B18 and B19 with Li14 and GB24.
  - Heart points for the psychological symptoms: H3 and H9, H7, and B15.
  - Mo-point of the Lower Burner: CV5.

HEART

This is the most important organ: it is the *Emperor*, commanding and controlling the other organs. The heart plays an important role in the *blood circulation*, together with the liver and the spleen. The heart commands the vessels: it disperses the blood in the vessels everywhere in the body to assure the nutrition in the organism.

Another main function of the Heart is the *housing of the Shenn or the vital activity*. It is the totality of the mental activities. One must first consider a disorder of the Heart in treating a mental disorder. Daily neuroses are treated by points of the Heart meridian, circulation and heart disorders are treated by points of the Pericardium-channel.

The *tongue* is the opening of the heart. The heart meridian has a branch connected with the root of the tongue. Especially the tip of the tongue will reflect the state of the heart. At the same time, it will command the *speech*.

The heart commands the *perspiration*. The H directs and guides the Blood, hence it guides also the liquids. Practically we can say that abundant perspiration in the day reflects a Xu of Qi, or since the L is the master of the Qi, a disturbance in the Lung. Nocturnal perspiration is caused by an Emptiness of Yin or disturbance in the Heart or Kidney.

DECREASE OF QI OF THE H:

In the first stage of heart disease, the pumping action of the Blood decreases, leading to a decrease in the Yang Qi of the heart.

- ❑ Symptoms
  - Xu of Yang leads to a decrease in the warming up of the body, the patient feels chilly, and is sensitive to Cold.
  - Shortness of breath and palpitations.
  - Nocturnal perspiration.
  - Oppression in the chest.
  - Pale face, anorexia, and lassitude.
  - Pulse is weak and thready or arrhythmia.
  - Tongue is distended, pale with a white moist coating.
- ❑ Clinical Syndromes
  - Angina pectoris, and heart failure.
- ❑ Treatment:
  - Strengthening of the H: PC6 and PC5.
  - Edema: Sp9 and CV9.
  - Anorexia: St36, CV12.

- Lassitude: CV6 and CV4 with moxa.

Recently acupuncturists in Shanghai have proven the great benefit of acupuncture in cardiology, especially in the coronary pathology and rhythm disturbances.

- ❑ Angina pectoris: dispersion of the following three points, St36, Sp4 and PC7. The needles are kept in for 15′ to 20′. The analgesic effect is demonstrated at the moment of treatment and even long afterwards. One treatment every other day for one month.

In general, an improvement in health is observed and permits to suppress the vasodilators. A certain number of patients need some treatments after the initial program. During the crisis, CV17 is also a useful point. The effectiveness of these points are indicated by ECG: we see an increase of the systolic volume and increase in the amplitude of the ventricular movement, whereas no reaction is seen in a normal individual.

- ❑ Extra-systoles: St36 and PC4 in dispersion for 20′. The results are swift and mostly, need no further treatment.

XU OF YIN OR EMPTINESS OF BLOOD OF THE HEART

In the next stage, the Yin is deficient and can lead to a stagnation of Blood. Xu of Yin leads to preponderance of Yang of the Heart.

- ❑ Symptoms
  - Insomnia with excessive dreaming and palpitations upon awakening.
  - Poor memory, vertigo, and headache.
  - Excessive perspiration
  - Pale face, and oppression in the chest.
  - Cyanosis of lips and nails due to stagnation of Blood.
  - Hypothermia.
  - Pulse is very rapid and thready.
  - Tongue is red with yellow coating (deficiency); dark, purplish in case of stagnation.
- ❑ Clinical Syndromes
  - Heart failure, insomnia, anemia, and hyper function of the thyroid.
- ❑ Therapy
  - Primary therapy: B14, B15, B17, Sp10 (the latter two points are the source of Blood or Yin).
  - Calms the mind: H7, PC6.
  - Accelerates the Yin: Chao means acceleration: we find the point back on Shao Yin of the Foot, starting point of the Yin: K6[t].
  - Drains Fire from the Heart: PC5[d].

OBSTRUCTION OF THE CHANNELS OF THE HEART

In the most advanced stage of this disease, the depressed Qi may turn into Endogenous Fire, stirring up the Wind and disturbing the mind. In extreme forms, there will be formation of Phlegm-Fire, obstructing the channels of the Heart, leading to a derangement of the mind (see the key).

- ❑ Symptoms reflect extreme Heat
  - Bitter taste in the mouth, insomnia.
  - Hysteria, incoherent speech.
  - Depression possible leading to coma.
  - Pulse is rapid, submerged and long.
  - Tongue is deep red with sores, yellow-coated, greasy in case of phlegm formation.
- ❑ Clinical syndrome
  - Insomnia, and hysteria.

- Therapy in this stage
  - Calms the mind: H7, PC6 (clears the H-orifice).
  - Drains Heat: PC5, L14, and LI11.
  - Elimination of Phlegm: Sp6, Sp9, Li13, St40.

PERICARDIUM

The Pericardium is the main *protection of the Heart*. It is the first protection shield for the heart against the Six Excesses and Seven Emotions. Among them, Heat and Joy are the most important ones. The syndromes of the pericardium can be compared to those of the Heart. It is important to note that we use the points of the PC to treat *heart diseases*.

THE TRIPLE BURNER (SANJIAO)

The Triple Burner is not an organ, but a function. Syndromes of the TB will be related to the organs in the respective Burners. The Triple Burner is divided into three parts:

- The Upper Burner, situated at the level of the heart, contains H and L, and is responsible for the distribution of the Qi, Blood and Water.
- The Middle Burner, situated at the level of the stomach, contains Sp and St and is charged with the transformation and transportation of the food and liquids.
- The Lower Burner, situated at the level of the Bladder, is composed of the Small and Large Intestine, Kidney, Liver, and Bladder and is responsible for elimination of toxins.

We can say that a certain Burner is affected when all the organs in that Burner are disturbed: e.g., the Upper Burner is disturbed when we find symptoms of disturbance of the L and H. This can be the case in progressed heart deficiency associated with lung edema.

Needless to say, a disturbance of a Burner is always a very serious problem which will require from the acupuncturist much skill and patience.

SMALL INTESTINE

The SI plays an important role in *digestion* and *transportation*. It receives waste material sent down by the stomach, absorbs part of it and sends the rest to the colon. It is the pure part that is absorbed, enters the body and will be part of the circulation. The impure part is re absorbed in the SI or B and eliminated.

Another important function of the SI is the *elimination of water*. If we have in the clinic a problem of water elimination, then SI should be considered in our treatment plan The SI is linked to the umbilicus at the level of CV9. This point has the Chinese name Shui Fen or *"separation of the water"*. In other words, it is the place where the impure liquid is split from the pure. This point CV9 can be tonified in any retention of water.

ACCUMULATION OF HEAT

This syndrome is caused by absorption of too fat and rich food or by an emotional shock (fear, anger). We are not surprised that the origin of this problem is often found at the level of the heart. The Heat is the biggest enemy of the heart, but this organ is well protected by the pericardium. The Heat attacking the heart will be diverted to the SI, coupled in a Biao-Li connection with this organ.

- Symptoms
  - Diarrhea: the water is not re-absorbed at the level of the SI and enters in the LI.
  - Aphtosis, rectal tenesms.
  - Non-digested food in the stool: can also be a sign of disturbance in the stomach.

- Cystitis: the Heat from the SI can go to the B; the Bladder follows the SI in the Chinese Clock and has an internal connection with this organ.
- Pain in the penis or meatus externus: the Heat descends from the B.
- Thirst: the Heat dries up the liquids.

❏ Clinical Syndrome

- Cystitis.

❏ Therapy

- Eliminates the Heat at the level of all organs Tsang and Fu: L11.
- Eliminates the Heat in the B: B28.
- CV3, Mo point of the B.
- Aphtosis: CV24, LI4 and LI11, Sp6 and Sp5, B21, the last three points in case the origin is in the Sp; H7, PC7 and 6, B15 if the origin is in the H.

ATTACK OF THE PERVERSE QI COLD

The syndrome occurs when there is an extreme attack of External Cold, often associated to Dampness. It is clear that the Excess can only have its negative effect when the patient is already in a deficient state (decreased Vital Energy).

❏ Symptoms:

- Diarrhea, undigested food in stool: the Cold invades the SI and hinders the elimination.
- Pain in the lower abdomen: according to the Eight conditions, it will be an Emptiness of Yang; the pain diminishes with pressure and Heat.
- Clear, abundant urine: the water is not absorbed and enters in the bladder.

❏ Clinical Syndromes:

- Chronic diarrhea and enteritis.

❏ Therapy:

- CV8: moxa or indirect moxibustion with salt.
- CV9: moxa.
- To warm up the body, one must increase the K-Yang: K3 or K6.
- Stops all diarrhea: new point ZHI XIE (NP83), one cun under CV 6.

SPLEEN

The main function of the Spleen is its *transportation* and *transformation* of the blood and energy. The food in the Stomach is split in an impure and pure fraction, the latter going to the Spleen. The Sp-St entity is considered as the root of life. Its disturbances will be reflected in the functions of all the other organs. The Sp is the main organ in the digestion and a balanced function provides good appetite, normal stools and adequate digestion.

The Sp is also responsible for the *uplifting of the tissues*, the maintenance of muscle strength: the Sp is building up the muscle volume; in other words, the inert of Yin state. The movement of our body due to the muscle actions are under the control of the Liver. Disturbances of the Spleen function cause muscle atrophy: to increase the muscle volume, one has to tonify the Spleen.

The Sp *produces blood and keeps it inside the vessels*. Weakness of the Sp will cause presence of blood outside of the vessels, translated into all kinds of bleeding such as epistaxis and menorrhagia.

Another important function is its role in the *water metabolism*. This can be manifested at different levels. At the intestines, causing diarrhea, at the bladder, causing anuria and at the subcutaneous level, producing edema.

The *mouth* is the origin of the spleen and permits the communication with the Exterior. In TCM, the mouth consists also of the lips, teeth, palate except the tongue which belongs to the Heart

The Sp houses the *I* (See Chapter 14 on Psychological Diseases).

DECREASE OF QI OF THE SP

Numerous are the causes of deficiency of the Sp Qi. External causes, especially Dampness, and internal causes, food and emotions (worry, obsessive compulsive behavior). Humidity or Dampness is the biggest enemy of the Sp. Distinction must be made between exogenous and endogenous Dampness. Exogenous Dampness is characteristic for the Late Summer and comes from the humid climate, especially in that season. The Endogenous Dampness is due to a deficient function of the Sp: it can no longer distribute the organic liquids to the whole organism. Three principles direct the treatment of Dampness in TCM. Induce sweating: LI4-K7; facilitate the urinary elimination, K7, Sp6, Sp9; and tonify the Sp, Sp4, B29, and St36.

I remember the case of an obese female patient, who during the consultation showed all the symptoms of a deficient Sp (see below). Eager to lose weight and plagued by a peri-arthritis humero scapularis (Fullness of Yin), she mentioned that her daily diet consisted of salads. To her surprise, but not to mine, she did not lose any weight. Indeed one internal cause that has decreasing affect on the Sp Qi, is the intake of cold and raw foods. Intrigued by the acute obesity six months before the consultation, I asked her if she had traveled at that time in country where the climate was extremely humid. Her answer was positive. She had been more than a month in Indonesia, known for its humidity; the PHS had also started at that moment. Strengthening the Sp and eliminating the Dampness cleared her problems

A second internal factor, decreasing this Qi is one of the Seven Emotions, Pensiveness. It is typical for the students in their examination periods or people who do not alternate their intellectual jobs with physical exercise. Lack of movement with their sedentary lifestyle will have a severe impact on their Sp Qi. Numerous are those people who exhibit belching, abdominal distention, and gas formation. It is also remarkable that these people have an obsession for things and events which happened in the past (in contrast with "Lung People", who are obsessed with the future.).

❑ Symptoms:

Lassitude: the Sp, together with the St, is the main organ of the Middle Burner in which will occur the first splitting of the food into pure and impure Qi. If the Qi of the Sp is weak, this dividing and formation of Qi will not happen smoothly, and a decrease in the production of the Qi is a consequence. During exercise or strenuous activity, the Qi and Blood are not sufficiently produced hence the lassitude.

Anorexia is also experienced. Since the transformation and the transportation of food is insufficient, the Middle Burner is easily full, causing a feeling of distention in the Stomach and reducing the appetite.

Prolapsed uterus, prolapsed rectum: the Spleen sustains the muscles and uplifts the tissues. The decrease in Qi will weaken this function, leading to a state of relaxation of the different muscles, especially in the lower Burner.

Hemorrhages, uterine bleeding (especially meno-menorragy), abnormal bleeding at another site. The Sp is too weak to control the blood in the vessels. Simultaneously, there is less production, leading to anemia and a shortened menstrual cycle.

❑ Clinical Symptoms

- Chronic diarrhea, indigestion, and menstrual problems (particularly abnormal uterine bleeding).

❑ Therapy:

- Tonify the Sp: B20, Sp6, Sp4, CV12, St21.
- Increasing the appetite: CV12, St36, Sp6 or Sp4.
- Prolapsus uteri, recti: B20, Sp6, Sp4, CV12, St21, GV20.

EMPTINESS OF SP-YANG

This is only an aggravated situation of the previous syndrome. This syndrome coincides with a deficient K-Yang. The K-Yang feeds the H-Yang which in turn feeds the Sp-Yang (Sheng-cycle).

- ❑ Symptoms:
  - Cold limbs, sensitivity to cold: the K-Yang is responsible for warming up functions of the body.
  - Anorexia, vomiting, chronic diarrhea, and post-pandrial abdominal distention.
  - Asthenia.
  - Deep and weak pulse, tongue will be pink and covered with a thin coating.
- ❑ Clinical Syndromes
  - Chronic gastritis and enteritis, cirrhosis, leucorrhea.
- ❑ Therapy
  - Sp6, Sp9, St36, B20, Li13.

INVASION OF COLD-DAMP

An invasion of Cold-Damp is likely to occur by the body's intake of a lot of raw or cold food. The cold blocks the Qi in the channels and causes a stagnation in these pathways. Hence, all the functions of the Sp will be blocked too.

- ❑ Symptoms:
  - Nausea, vomiting.
  - Sticky feeling in the mouth.
  - Feeling of heaviness in the head (as if there were a bag on the head) and the whole body.
  - Mucus in the stool.
  - Leucorrhea.
- ❑ Clinical Syndromes
  - Chronic gastritis and enteritis, leucorrhea.
- ❑ Therapy:
  - Three principles direct the treatment of Dampness in TCM.
  - The "anti-mucus" point: St40 will eliminate and liquefy the mucus.

ATTACK OF HEAT-DAMPNESS

With time, the intake of raw and cold food can turn into Heat.

- ❑ Symptoms
  - Icteric face, icteric sclerae, anorexia.
  - Nausea, vomiting, fatigue.
  - Fever, small amounts of urine, deep-yellow colored.
  - Itching, constipation.
- ❑ Clinical Syndromes
  - Hepatitis: it is an accumulation of Heat-Dampness, originated in the Sp. This Heat-Dampness will go to the GB. Cholecystitis, and pancreatitis.
- ❑ Therapy
  - Disperse the Sp: Sp2, Sp3, Sp4.
  - Disperse or drain the Heat: L11 (drains Heat from the whole body), GV14 (confluence of all the Yang, drains effectively the Heat).
  - Traditional "Hepatitis" point: GV9.
  - Drain Heat from the Li-GB: B18 and 19.

STOMACH

Since the Stomach is in a Biao-Li connection with the Spleen, it is obvious that the functions of the St will match those of the Sp. The Stomach is the organ that *receives* the solid and liquid food stuff. All the food goes first through the St, hence in case of anorexia, we may presume that there is a St-problem. It is not only a point of passage of the food, but an *active center* where the splitting into pure Qi (going to the Sp) and impure Qi happens.

In light of the above characteristics, we are not surprised that the St is called in ancient literature: "*the Mother of all organs.*" A problem of the St (think St-Sp entity) has a consequence on all the other organs. Hence the immense importance the TCM links to the appetite: "*When the patient keeps his appetite, then the prognosis of the disease is not bad.*"

XU OF THE YIN OF THE ST

Causes are multiple. The Xu of Yin of the St can be part of a Xu of Yin in the whole body, as is the case in a post-febrile disease where the intense Heat has dried up or burned up the liquids or the Yin, especially in case of a long term sub-febrile disease with unknown cause. The Xu of Yin can, of course, also be a direct consequence of a loss of Yin or liquids: chronic or excessive vomiting, excessive diarrhea or dehydration, post-operative bleeding and excessive sexual activity.

- Symptoms
  - Anorexia, dry lips: Xu of Yin leads to an imbalance between Yin and Yang; the Yang escapes and ascends to the upper part of the body (normal tendency of the Yang), where we find this Heat symptom.
  - Abdominal distention right after the meals: the patient cannot digest properly; the moment he eats, a block occurs.
  - Hiccough, nausea.
  - Tongue is dry and red with little or no fur, another sign of the ascending Yang.
  - Pulse is weak and rapid.
- Clinical Syndromes
  - Indigestion, chronic gastritis, and diabetes.
- Treatment
  - Increase the Yin and liquids in general: B17, Sp10, Sp6.
  - Strengthen the Middle Burner: CV12, St36.
  - Distention, nausea: PC6, CV13, CV22.

ACCUMULATION OF HEAT

Again, we have exterior and interior causes. We can have an attack of the Perverse Qi Heat during a spell of extreme Summer-Heat, or it can afflict people who live in a Cold-climate, when they travel to the desert or arrive in the Heat-Dampness of Florida, for instance. Food and emotions are another possible cause: too much sugar, too much hot and spicy food, pensiveness and worry.

- Symptoms
  - Bulimia, gingivitis, excessive thirst.
  - Bad odor in the mouth.
  - Toothache.
  - Dry stools.
  - Tongue is red and dry, rapid pulse.
- Clinical Syndromes
  - Gingivitis, diabetes, and stomach ulcer.
- Treatment
  - Eliminate the Heat at the level of Yang Ming: LI4 and 11, St44.
  - Drain the Yang or Heat: St36, 37, 38, the Lower He Sea points of the St, LI and SI.
  - Strengthen the Middle Burner: CV12 and Sp21.

The Cold-Damp, turning into Fire, and the accumulation of Heat will trigger the formation of Phlegm, causing an obstruction and accumulation of Dampness in the Sp-St entity. The symptoms will be an extreme version of the previous ones, and the same therapy will be essential, except for the elimination of Phlegm and Dampness.

CONCLUSION

The theory of the Zang and Fu shows the important impact of the Exterior and Interior Factors. Climate, psychological and food factors are more and more accepted, even by Western medicine, as the roots of all disease.

I read a remarkable story about a patient suffering from leukemia. As is known in any terminal disease, he went through the stages of denial, anger, depression and when he entered the acceptance stage, he had an astonishing insight in his disease. He said: "Although I lead what could be considered, according to our norms, a healthy life, (he went into detail about his physical fitness program and his superb diet) I failed in an important aspect of my life. I could never regain peace of mind; there was too much anger in my body, too many unresolved psychological problems still hanging around, a raging fire that consumed my Vital Energy."

It is my strong belief that Western Medicine should take the previous factors into greater consideration when looking for the causes of many mysterious diseases. It is also clear to me that what the Chinese Masters have advocated for 5,000 years should be looked at more carefully by Western Medicine in order to arrive at the only true medicine: preventive medicine. In ancient China, a Doctor was held responsible for the death of his patients, because it was his job to keep his patients fit through his skills in preventive medicine. Every time one of his patients died, he was obliged to light a lantern in his garden: darkness in the garden of the doctor of that time meant great healing power.

7

Differentiation of Syndromes According to the Eight Principles

Upon seeing a patient in our office, our first concern must be to make a differentiation according to the Eight Principles: we have to recognize what is going on with the Yin and Yang Qi. Is there a fullness of Yin or Yang in the upper part of the body? In the lower part? Or is it more a deficiency? Is the Yin not ascending properly? Is the Yang not descending properly, therefore causing a block at a certain level? All these questions have to be answered properly before we ask anything else and certainly before we do something.

It has surprised me that students on their final exams were not able to make this easy diagnosis. Most of the students know that there are eight principles, but for some unknown reason they inquire only about two or four of them, resulting in a wrong and incomplete diagnosis. In those circumstances, what then can we expect from the therapy!

It cannot be stressed enough that this must be our first diagnostic step and hence, our first therapeutic step. Many practitioners will only influence the *local* Yin-Yang balance on the first visit of their patient. The result is often a *temporary* disappearance of symptoms. Do not consider this law of Eight Elements as a secondary approach, as I have seen many times. It corresponds to the primary law of acupuncture, the equilibrium of the Yin and the Yang.

THE EIGHT PRINCIPLES

The Eight Principles, or rules are formed by four pairs:

YIN—YANG
FULLNESS (SHI)—EMPTINESS (XU)
COLD—HEAT
EXTERIOR—INTERIOR

The most important ones are Yang and Yin, since the three other pairs can be classified within the previous pair:

Yang: Shi, heat, exterior, Qi
Yin: Xu, cold, interior, Blood

YANG-YIN

Yang-Yin indicates the type of condition and the overall qualitative aspect of Energy in order to differentiate between the patient and the symptoms. One has only existence because of the other: the night is only Yin by comparing it to the day, Yang. In this section particular attention will be paid to the symptom of pain and how it is experienced by the "Yang person" as opposed to the "Yin person".

But how do we recognize these different personalities? Never forget that our diagnosis, or should we say our source of information, starts at the moment our patient walks into our consultation room. His attitude, way of walking, introducing himself and shaking hands, backed up by a good inquiry, will provide valuable information. Needless to point out, what an advantage the former "house" doctor had by following his patients from birth, by delivering them, being involved in their diseases and emotional lives all along. Now that this is obsolete, a keen observation and inquiry about the patient's interests, social activities, previous diseases, family diseases, etc., must supply enough elements to classify our patients in Yang-Yin and its gradations. The first base of diagnostic is the determination of the Yin-Yang equilibrium of our patient.

YANG Person (+)	YIN Person (–)
· Sleeps little, eats a lot	· Sleeps a lot, eats little
· Dry mouth	· A lot of saliva formation
· Slender, active	· Calm
· Improvement by cold	· Improvement by heat
· Needs sugar	· Needs salt
· Short and rare menses	· Frequent and long menses
· Mediterranean type	· Nordic type
· Urinates little	· Urinates much
· Perspires much	· Perspires little
· Baldness, beard growth	· Scant facial hair, no baldness at young age
· Virility	· Little virility
· Talks and laughs a great deal	· Talks slowly and quietly
· Joyful personality	· Depressed personality
· Black hair	· Blond hair
· Is always at ease	· Timid
· Dynamic	· Lymphatic
· Warm limbs	· Cold limbs

This list is infinite. More important is to stress the fact that *nobody* is 100% Yin or Yang. We have to determine if there is an important disequilibrium in our patient: we will have then a person presenting himself with an excess in one or the other form. This diagnostic can be easily confirmed by the palpation of the pulses. The Yang type is subjected to superficial, burning, painful and febrile illnesses, easy to cure. The Yin type will demonstrate conditions of stasis, and chronic illnesses which are more difficult to cure. Keep in mind that the *Yin harms the Yang and the Yang harms the Yin*, or a Yin illness harms the Yang of the person, a Yang condition the Yin of the person. Consequently, a Yin person can easily neutralize a Yang condition, the Yang conditions "drowns" in the excessive Yin. On the other hand, that same Yin person will not have enough Yang to neutralize a Yin illness and therefore, a Yin person often has a Yin malady. With the same reasoning, a Yang patient can easily neutralize a Yin disease, but not a Yang one. Do not use moxa when a person is hot.

Once we have established the diagnostic of the Yin-Yang in general, we must determine if there is a *local* Yin-Yang disequilibrium. If this is not the case and the patient consults for a general disease without any particular location, then our first therapeutic gesture will be the *restoration of the Yin-Yang equilibrium in general.*

How is this done? Excess of Yang in general: GV19, GV14, CV12 and GV4 in dispersion. With an Excess of Yin in general, we could disperse the Yin, but our therapeutic gesture will be more rapid by acting on the Yang (more mobile): St36, CV12, GV19 and LI14 in tonification (the Yang fights the Yin).

However, in most cases patients will come with local complaints and the most frequent one that brings them to the doctor is pain. It is most important that the acupuncturist be able to differentiate the Yin from the Yang pain.

Differentiation of Pain:

YANG Pain (+)	YIN Pain (–)
· Recent.	· Chronic
· Intermittent.	· Continuous.
· Maximum during the daytime hours.	· Maximum during the night time hours.
· Erratic.	· Fixed in location.
· Movement worsens the pain.	· Movement and warmth alleviate the pain.
· Rest and cold lessen it.	· Cold and rest worsen it.
· Electrical.	· Itching.
· Superficial.	· Deep.
· Local heat and redness in the area of the pain.	· Cold in the local area of the pain, ankylosis, atrophy

DO WE TREAT THIS LOCAL YIN-YANG DISEQUILIBRIUM?

A special technique uses the Wonder Meridians (Extra Meridians) or, in other words, we act on their opening points. We know the Wonder Meridians can be considered as rivers, ready to absorb the local Yin or Yang Excess in the body. As we can see, they are an important defense mechanism in our organism, preventing the overflow in our body of Yin or Yang Qi.

- ❑ Yang Chiao Mo or Keo absorbs the Excess of Yang of the R or L side.
- ❑ Yang Wei Mo or Keo absorbs the Excess of Yang of the upper or lower part.
- ❑ CV or Jenn Mo or Keo absorbs the Excess of Yang of the front of the body.
- ❑ Tchong Mo or Keo absorbs the Excess of the *interior* of the body.

What is the therapeutic rule?

"To decrease the local Yin or Yang Excess, we disperse the opening point of the Wonder Meridian of the disturbed region."

EXAMPLES

- Excess of Yin in upper part of the body: Yin Wei Mo, PC6(d).
- Excess of Yang in upper part of body: Yang Wei Mo, TB5(d).
- Excess of Yang in lower part of the body and only on the R side: Yang Wei Mo and Yang Keo, TB5(t) (tonification: we bring the excess of the lower part to the upper part) and B62(d)
- Excess of Yin at the anterior body: CV, L7(d).
- Excess of Yin at the left and in the upper part: PC6(d) and K6(d).

OPENING POINTS WONDER MERIDIANS

GV: SI3 CV: L7	Yin Wei Mo: PC6	Yang Wei Mo: TB5
Tchong Mo: Sp4	Dai Mo: GB41	Yang Keo: B62
	Yin Keo: K 6	

At this point, the most common mistakes are made. Acupuncturists have listed the patient's local complaint and focus their attention only on the local complaint, forgetting that we have here a disturbance of Qi in the whole body. This is also a common mistake in Western medicine, where the doctor treats the disease or diseased part, not the whole person! For instance, the patient complains of a painful knee. The doctor determines that it is a Yang pain and disperses the Excess Yang locally with the previous technique. Great will be his surprise when he will only have a very temporary improvement, requiring repetitive treatment.

We have to *combine* what we found in the previous step: the findings of the Yin-Yang person with the local Yin-Yang Excess.

There Are Four Different Modalities

A Yang pain in a Yang person.
A Yang pain in a Yin person.
A Yin pain in a Yin person.
A Yin pain in the Yang person.

a. A Yang pain in a Yang person

Example: a meniscus lesion in a young, sportive person.

This means that there is an overall present Yang Excess. The only logical therapeutic gesture is to disperse this Yang in the whole body: GV14 and TB5 for the upper part, CV12 and GV4 for the middle and St36 for the lower part of the body.

b. A Yang pain in a Yin person

Example: a Yang knee pain in a Yin person.

This means that most of the Yang of this patient is located in one place: his knee. In other words, in this patient there will be a Xu of Yang everywhere in the Body except in the lower part of the Body. Therapy: strengthen the Yang in the upper and middle part of the body, TB5, GV20, CV12, GV4, and disperse the Yang in the lower extremity, St36.

c. A Yin pain in a Yin person

Example: Toothache in a depressive, old patient. Rather than dispersing the overall present Yin, we tonify the overall missing Yang: TB5, L14, CV12, GV4, St36.

d. A Yin pain in a Yang person

Example: toothache in a sportive, young person.

This means that most of the Yin of this person is located in the upper part of his body; therefore, we must strengthen the Yin in the middle and lower part of his body, CV6 and Sp6.

Only by bringing the Yin and Yang as a whole in balance can we be assured of a long-lasting effect. Do not fall into the trap of looking only at the local problem and forget that you have a whole person before you and not just a leg or a knee. This notion Yin-Yang can also be used in the diagnostic of the patient. The old texts tell us that *"if in a malady **all** the signs are either Yang or Yin, death is certain!"* I. e., the classical Shao Yin syndrome or "emptiness of Cold" in which the patient has a feeling of cold in the whole body, cold limbs, the patient fears cold, diarrhea with undigested food and a thin, small and feeble pulse, the prognosis is severe. But if this same person has warm limbs, which translates in having a certain quantity of Yang energy, then a cure is possible. The Yin-Yang law is the first and most important law in acupuncture and their unity is expressed as follows:

> *"When the Blood and Qi circulate in harmony, the body is in good health."*
> *"When the Qi is deficient, the Blood slows down."*
> *"When the Qi is deficient, the Blood stagnates."*

FULLNESS (SHI) - EMPTINESS (XU)

The second pair indicates the *quantitative* aspect of the Qi. Also, it reveals to us whether the resistance of the person is strong or weak and whether the intensity of the Excesses is predominant or not. The syndrome of emptiness manifests itself through a decrease in the patient's general resistance. The syndrome of fullness manifests itself when the Excesses are particularly strong.

All the ancient texts proclaim that one must treat a patient according to the Xu or the Shi. The Nei Tching says: *"Fullness is abundance of Qi"* and *"Emptiness is not having the essential Qi."* The diagnosis of emptiness and fullness is easy to make:

> *"All emptiness improves through pressure." Applying pressure to a painful area adds energy and will improve emptiness of Qi.*
> *"All fullness worsens when pressure is applied." We are adding Qi by the pressure when there is already too much Qi*

It is a mistake to believe that the applied pressure must be strong. The pressure of a belt will be enough to worsen a post-prandial fullness. A post-prandial fullness, directly after a meal, is a Yin fullness, since food is Yin. If the fullness starts two hours after the meal, it is a Yang fullness, since by this time the Yin food has been transferred to energy or Yang.

Clinical signs of fullness are (Su Ouenn, Chapter 19): full pulse, hot skin, constipation, distended abdomen, difficult urination and no perspiration. Signs of emptiness are: asthenia, weight loss, diarrhea, incontinence, vomiting, spermatorrhea, and asthma.

In diagnosing symptoms of fullness-emptiness, some important questions need an answer:

- How do we recognize the Xu of Shi of a Meridian and what is the therapy?
- Is the Emperor strong in its season?
- Is the Son-organ energetic?
- Is the Mother-organ weak?
- How do we diagnose the quantity and quality of the Qi?
- How do we diagnose the Shi and Xu of an organ?

HOW DO WE RECOGNIZE THE XU OR SHI OF A MERIDIAN AND WHAT IS THE THERAPY?

The Shi or Xu of a meridian can be gauged by applying pressure to the Source point. Pressure on the source point can demonstrate the fullness or emptiness the patient is experiencing.

> *"When the meridian is empty, the Source point and the season tonification point need to be strengthened."*

The use of seasonal points is already described in the ancient literature and is not at all a modern finding, as some people may believe. How do we find the seasonal tonification points? It should be remembered that the Ting points of the Fu organs start in the Autumn, while those of the Tsang organs start in the Spring. The second rule to remember is that to *disperse* an organ, we use the Son-point. To *tonify* we use the Mother-point. Some examples will clarify this matter.

The seasonal tonification points of the Li are: Li8 in the Spring, Li1 in the Summer, Li2 in the Long Summer, Li3 in the Autumn and Li4 in the Winter.

> *"When the meridian is full, the Source point and its seasonal dispersion point should be drained."*

For example, the seasonal dispersion point (Son-points) of the Li are: Li2 in the Spring, Li3 in the Summer, Li4 in the Long summer, Li8 in the Autumn, and in the Winter, Li1.

The list of all the seasonal points can be found at the end of this Chapter. In applying this important rule, the practitioner needs a small calendar, showing the changes of the seasons in order to adjust the tonification and dispersion seasonal points. There are four periods of seventy-three days and four periods of eighteen days (the fifth season, referred to as "Long Summer"). The calendar is only valuable if the climate corresponds well to the season: e.g., if it is still cold on the twenty-fifth of February, then the Spring points should not be used, but rather the points of the fifth season. Another exception is an unusual meteorological change in an otherwise normal season: e.g., a cold humid day in the middle of the Summer needs, beside the usual Summer points, special protective points, the Penn Points as discussed in Chapter 4).

In summary, it can be said that the season points are much more important than the normal tonification or dispersion points. As mentioned before, Li 8 can be tonification point (in the Spring) as well as dispersion point (in the Fall). hence the disappointment some practitioners encounter when they do not follow this important therapeutic rule.

Is the Emperor Strong in its Season?

The Emperor is the organ belonging to the current season:
Spring: Li   Summer: H   Long Summer: Sp
Fall: L   Winter: K

It is normal that an organ will show fullness in its own season. It is not only normal but mandatory. The Emperor must be strong enough to create the normal balance in the Five Elements cycle. For comparison, this strength can be expressed in "percentages" (e.g., in Figure 33 the current season is Spring).

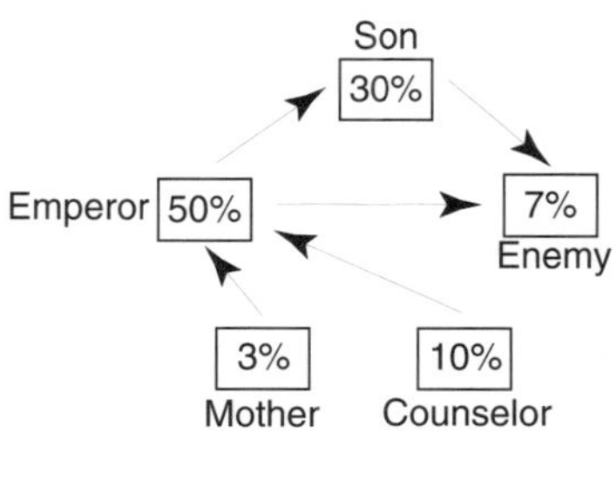

Figure 33

HOW DO WE DIAGNOSE THE FULLNESS (EXCESS) OR EMPTINESS (DEFICIENCY) OF AN ORGAN?

One diagnostic step is to take the pulses (See Chapter on Pulses). Another step is to question the patient as to the effects of the Five Elements. The following table will aid the practitioner in asking proper questions, in order to diagnose the patient's disorder in terms of Xu or Shi of the seasonally dominant organ.

SPRING (LIVER AND GALL BLADDER)

FULLNESS (Shi)	EMPTINESS (Xu)
Tears in eyes	Dry eyes, bad vision
Tired from walking	Energized by walking
Dislikes taste of lamb	Likes lamb
Dislikes sour taste	Craves sour taste
Improves with sugar intake	Aggravated by sugar intake
Irritable disposition	Calm disposition
Condition aggravated in spring	Condition improves in spring
Muscle spasms	Weak muscles
Avoids the wind	Likes the wind
Likes sweet, perfumed odors	Likes sour odors
Nail breaking	White nails

SUMMER (H-PC-SI-TB)

FULLNESS (Shi)	EMPTINESS (Xu)
Dislikes bitter taste	Likes bitter taste
Calmed by pungent odors	Aggravated by pungent odors
Very excited, laughing	Depressed
Aggravated in summer	Improves in summer
Hypertension	Hypotension
Dislikes the taste of poultry	Likes poultry
Dislikes burning odor	Likes burning odor
Red face	Pale face
Avoids heat	Seeks heat

LONG SUMMER (Sp-St)

FULLNESS (SHI)	EMPTINESS (XU)
Dislikes sweet taste	Likes sweet taste
Worries a lot	Worries rarely
Excessive salivation	Scant salivation
Aggravated by long summer	Improves in long summer
Prefers to remain standing	Likes to sit down
Dislikes beef	Likes beef
Avoids dampness	Seeks dampness
Herpes simplex on lips	Pale, dry lips

AUTUMN (L-Li)

FULLNESS (SHI)	EMPTINESS (Xu)
Dislikes pungent odors	Likes pungent odors
Depressed	Seldom depressed
Highly energetic	Lethargic
Aggravated in autumn	Improves in autumn
Dislikes to recline	Likes to recline
Dislikes rice	Likes rice
Avoids dryness	Seeks dryness
Abundant body hair	Scant body hair

WINTER (B-K)

FULLNESS (SHI)	EMPTINESS (XU)
Dislikes salty taste	Likes salty taste
High state of anxiety	Little anxiety
Frequent urination	Scant urination
Aggravated in winter	Improves in winter
Prefers not to stand	Likes to stand
Dislikes pork	Likes pork
Avoids cold	Seeks cold
Abundant head hair	Bald

The Emperor in the Spring is the Liver, hence, feeling a Shi pulse of the Liver at this time is normal. To disperse at this point is a severe error. If the patient was not very sick at the moment of the visit, we can be sure that he will be afterward.

The Son-element, the Heart, receiving Qi from the strong Mother (Li), should already be strong, waiting to take over the position of the Liver in the next season. The Spleen, on the contrary, is at this time the defeated enemy, having very little energy (7%).

The Lung, being the counselor of the Emperor,

must show a certain strength in order to give advice and control the Emperor. The Kidney, Mother of the Emperor in the Spring, has just given all its Qi to the Liver, the Son, and is therefore relatively weak (3%). In this way, our patient is well-balanced.

WHAT HAPPENS IF ANOTHER ELEMENT BECOMES EXCESSIVE (SHI OF QI)?

For example, suppose the Spleen is strong in the Spring instead of the Liver. Two organs are in danger: first, the Liver, because the Liver normally has an "overacting relationship" (Ko-cycle) with the Spleen. The Sp will counteract the Liver's function. The second organ in danger is the Kidney. The Sp, which under normal circumstances is controlling the K, will decrease the K Qi too much and hence will weaken the K in this season. A clinical example will clarify this important relationship and will give us at the same time the answers to the questions: Is the Son-element energetic and is the Mother-organ weak?

Clinical Example:
Patient Mark D., 25 years old, consulted in the winter time with Herpes simplex labialis. The pain was sharp, intermittent, and the blister appeared three days before the visit. The patient was sportive, outgoing and always smiling.

The first step is to differentiate according to the Eight Conditions. This is a Yang person (sportive, outgoing, smiling) with a Yang pain (intermittent, sharp, superficial and exterior lesions).

Therapy
LI4-GV20-GB20 (as the blister is caused by Wind-Heat, GB20 disperses Heat and Exterior conditions and eliminates Wind), CV12 and St36, all in dispersion. The employment of the latter two points is a step towards equalizing the Yang-Yin in the patient's body as a whole.

The next step is to focus on the blister formation on the lips. Lips are within the domain of the Sp, and the symptoms indicate an Excess of this organ. Since the season is Winter, the K is the Emperor while the Sp is the counselor and is normally moderately strong (10%). However, the symptoms indicate that the Sp is in excess here, and thus the counselor has become a threat to the Emperor (Sp is too strong for the K). The Li will also be threatened by this Sp excess (the Li is relatively strong in this season, 30%), by the Sp counteracting the action of the Li. Tonify the K and the Li in accordance with the seasonal balance and sedate the Sp. Season tonification point of the Li and the K: Li4$^{(t)}$ and K7$^{(t)}$. Season dispersion point of the Sp: Sp1$^{(s)}$.

This Emptiness and Fullness can pertain to the IONG Qi, the ANCESTRAL Qi, the WEI Qi, the ESSENTIAL Qi (IONG + WEI Qi) and the GLOBAL Qi (IONG + WEI = ANCESTRAL) as well as to the BLOOD. These different possibilities are discussed below with their symptoms and therapy.

EMPTINESS OF QI AND BLOOD

Emptiness of Wei Qi
The skin will lack warmth and flexibility, the hair is brittle and falls easily out, the skin pores are dilated with increased perspiration, recurrent attacks by Pernicious Energies (i.e., recurrent colds), and often we can find in this patient disturbances in the Lower Burner (because the Li and K are responsible for the production of Wei Qi). These are expressed as prolaps uteri, rectal and vaginal prolaps, hernia, etc.

Treatment will consist of: TB3^{t}, B67^{t}, L9^{t}, St36^{t}, CV5^{t} and CV7^{t}.

Emptiness of Iong Qi
Causality is a deficiency of Qi of the Middle Burner or a deficiency of the Heart Yin Qi (H is the mother of the Sp!). Symptoms are maldigestion, anorexia, nausea, vomiting of bile, bloating, constipation, stomach ache and insomnia.

Treatment is CV12^{t}, CV7^{t}, St36^{t}, St41^{t} and CV23^{t}. H7 and H9^{t} and CV14^{t} in case of Xu H Yin Qi. Symptoms in this case will be palpitations, cardiac pain, radiating to the back, nightmares, anxiety, nocturnal perspiration and deep, thin, small pulse.

Another causality is a Xu of the 3 YIN (Deficiency of the Yin root of the Kidneys!). Symptoms are back pains, weak back, cold limbs, red tongue, spermatorrhea, constipation with hard and dry stools, oliguria, tinnitus, vertigo, deafness, and fear. If the condition is unchecked, symptoms of Xu Yin of the Li, H, Sp and L will appear in this order.

Treatment is K1, 3, and 7[t], and GB25[t] (Mo point of K).

Emptiness of the Ancestral Qi

Vertigo, tinnitus, psychasthenia, forgetfulness, and pain in the bones and spine.

Treatment is GV4, K2, B23 bilateral, CV4, and CV6.

Emptiness of Essential Qi

Symptoms are fatigue, lack of stamina, short respiration, weak voice, does not like to talk or move, profuse perspiration.

Treatment is CV10, 12 and 13, St42, Sp2 and TB5.

Emptiness of Global Qi

Severe asthenia, losing weight rapidly, profound depression, perspiration day and night, chronic diarrhea and spermatorrhea, vomiting, incontinence (loss of fluids), oppression in chest with short respiration, deep pulse but very small and weak.

Treatment CV10, 12, and 13, St36, St41, GV4, K2, CV4, 6 and 7, H9 and B43.

Emptiness of Blood

Causalities are deficient nutrition, excessive bleeding and a severe disease in evolution. Symptoms are pale lips and face, nocturnal perspiration, dry skin, heart pain, insomnia, melancholy, anger, and weak and small pulse.

Treatment is to tonify the Liver and the Heart: Li3, Li8, H7 and H9.

FULLNESS OF QI AND BLOOD

Fullness of Qi

A Fullness of Qi is mostly caused by *heat*, either of exterior origin (Perverse Qi) or interior origin (the YANG heat in the interior does not circulate towards the exterior, which is its normal course). The heat can be associated with dampness. The mechanism of a fullness can take different "faces": Perverse Qi, stagnation, obstruction and compression of the body Qi.

The clinical picture shows oppression, indigestion, shoulder blades drawn backwards, abdominal distention, constipation or diarrhea, acid vomiting, and a full, hard, superficial pulse.

Treatment is dispersion of the heat. Su Ouenn has 4 points of dispersion of the PERVERSE "YANG": LI1, St12, B12, St27.

Fullness of Blood

Is caused by a stagnation of Blood. It can be GLOBAL, as in certain hypertensions. Treatment will be LI11, St36, Li2, Sp6, PC6, PC9, and B17. The Fullness of Blood can be LOCAL, with stagnation of blood in the muscles (fever and chills, cold sweat) or stagnation of blood in the Primary meridians or secondary meridians (pain and contractures).

EXTERIOR-INTERIOR

This pair has two meanings. It expresses the *superficial* or *deep* location, the *central* or *peripheral*, the *interior* or *exterior* location. On the other hand, knowledge of these syndromes will lend important information regarding the *prognosis* of a disease. A favorable prognosis is a disease coming from the interior, but progressing to the exterior. The reverse condition indicates an unfavorable prognosis. An external disease evolves from the Yang towards the Yin and will follow the reverse way in its cure. An internal disease starts from the center and will express itself at the exterior. This law in acupuncture is also well-known in Homeopathy where it is one of HERING's Laws.

- ❑ There are different systems of reference to express Exterior-Interior.
- The first one is the *anatomical* one, identical to Western medicine.
- The second system of reference is according to the *layers of the body*

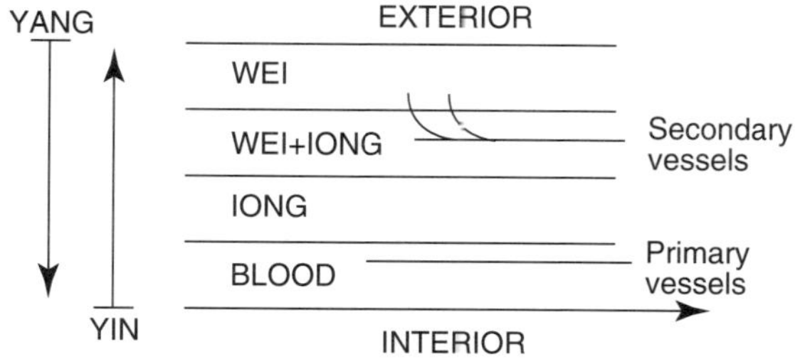

- The third system of reference are the *energetic levels.*

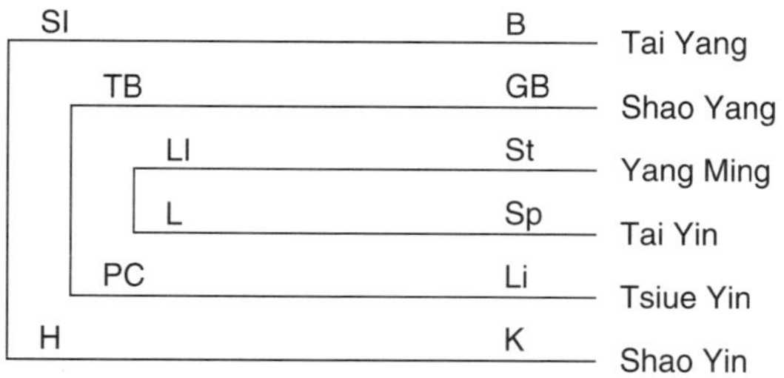

- The fourth system of reference is the *Yin-Yang of the Interior/Exterior.*

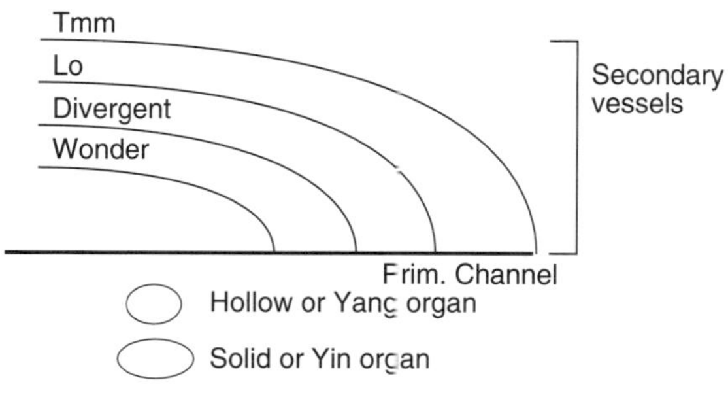

At the surface, the meridians= YANG
In the depth: the organs= YIN
The secondary vessels= YANG of the YANG
The primary vessels= YIN of the YANG
The hollow organs= YANG of the YIN
The solid organs= YIN of the YIN

Other possible locations of the disease:

Anterior=YIN	Posterior=YANG
Right=YIN	Left=YANG
High=YANG	Low=YIN

CAUSES OF THE DISEASE

The etiology is intimately connected with the location of the disease, because the symptomatology varies according to the "power of penetration" of the pathogenic agent, and the quality of the pathogen. The latter can be an external perverse Qi, or an internal digestive problem or internal mental problem. The Interior or Exterior are in emptiness and allow the penetration of pathogenic agents which can be of internal or external origin.

External causes

Depending on the strength of the pathogenic agent and on the Vital Qi of the patient, the perverse Qi's of cosmic origin (heat, dampness, dryness, fong, cold) will penetrate more or less into the body.

If the superficial Wei Qi is very little weakened, the penetration will be halted quickly. The attack will not penetrate deeper than the Tmm. Treatment is often not necessary, Nature or the body has enough resources to resist the attack.

A greater deficiency of the Wei Qi will allow a deeper penetration through the Ting and Iu point, going to the Ho point and from there, through the Divergent vessels, into the organs. Of course, the Primary vessels, can protect the Interior through several defense mechanisms. The perverse Qi can be diverted to muscles and bones in the King point, or it can be absorbed by the Wonder meridians, Divergent meridians or Lo vessels. The Wonder meridians have no direct connection with the organs, but the Divergent and Lo vessels pass through the organs. Therefore, attack of perverse Qi in these vessels is of no big importance and does not lead to severe consequences. (Figure 34)

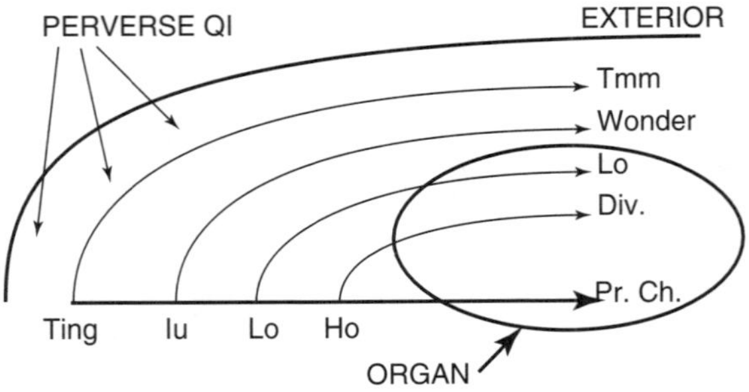

Figure 34

Internal Causes

Digestive causes

Foods are metabolized at the level of the Middle Burner. From this mass, which will be transformed into Yong Qi, the stomach will extract and send to the taste system, the different tastes. This system under the control of the spleen, will direct each taste to its organ. There is an absolute specificity:

Pungent goes to the L.
Salt goes to the K.
Sour goes to the Li.
Bitter goes to the H.
Sweet goes to the Sp.

A certain quantity of all these tastes is necessary for a good functioning of the organs.

This notion is important in the diagnostic of emptiness and fullness. We must know that the taste, which is Yin in comparison with the Qi, makes up the Yang of the food of which the matter is Yin. The tastes themselves are separated in Yang (bitter, pungent and sour) and Yin (sweet and salt). All excesses of taste can create an imbalance. The taste Yin will increase the Yin polarity of its receptive organ, the taste Yang the Yang polarity. I.e., the salty Yin taste will increase the Yin root of the kidney, the bitter Yang taste the Yang root of the heart.

How is a pathology created? Either through *chronic* intoxication or abuse of certain foods, creating an imbalance at the level of the organ, like sweets in hypoglycemia, then in diabetes. Or when the organ was already in imbalance and a certain amount *acutely* of the taste brought into the body will cause an acute pathology of Fullness, like a liver crisis after too many sour foods.

Mental/Emotional causes

According to the Chinese, all pathology can be explained through psychological causes dating from infancy. It is evident that a disturbance at the level of the Ancestral Qi will favor the onset of such pathology. Emotions are also necessary for the well-functioning of the organs. We know that:

Happiness stimulates the H.
Meditation stimulates the Sp.
Sadness stimulates the L.
Fear stimulates the K.
Anger stimulates the Li.

We need a little of all these emotions to function well in life. However an *excessive emotion* will cause:

- a transitory fullness of the organ (a couple of hours)
- a secondary emptiness
- because of this emptiness, an attack of the same emotion reoccurs; e.i., recurrent fears cause a state of continuous fear evolving into real phobias.
- this emotional "stress" leads to an obstruction of the energetic circulation of the organ involved. The energy is blocked *in* the organ. We will have then symptoms of emptiness at the level of the Primary channel with "apparent" fullness through obstruction at the level of the organ.

EXTERIOR CHARACTERISTICS	**INTERIOR CHARACTERISTICS**
Fever and chills, headache, rhinorrhea, articular pains the limbs, floating pulse, superficial location, sensation of cold, tongue with white coating, rapid onset, quick evolution of disease	Diseases of Seven Emotions, syndromes of the organs, in deep and strong pulse, fever without chills or chills without fever.

WHAT FALLS IN THE DOMAIN OF THE EXTERIOR?

- The Tmm or Tching Kan .
- The skin.
- Ear, nose and throat.
- Acceleration of the Exterior (See Chapter on Tchong Mo).

· Is it a deep disease, expressing itself at the Exterior?

The same rules and laws as in homeopathy are applying here. We are curing the patient if symptoms go from the interior to the exterior. Favorable signs of exteriorization are, pains at the level of the meridians, joint pains, appearance of rashes, discharges, warts, cysts, and polyps. The body brings the disturbance to a safe place of the body (skin, mucosae, articulations): the worst thing we can do is interfere with this natural healing reaction of the body, as so often is done in Western medicine through cortisone creams, vaginal suppositories or creams, cutting, burning or lasering. This is nothing but *suppression* of symptoms, going against the course of healing resulting in much more severe organic disease. A typical example is the "curing" of eczema in child, followed by asthma!

· Is it a disease of the Exterior going into the depth? This is a bad prognosis or a result of a wrong treatment described above. Instead of superficial signs, signs of pathology of organs will appear. Another sign of interiorization is the onset of mental/emotional signs or an aggravation of these symptoms. On the contrary, if we effect in the patient a "sense of well-being" even before the physical symptoms start disappearing, our treatment was effective and should be continued.

WHAT FALLS IN THE DOMAIN OF THE INTERIOR?

- The organs.
- The deep meridians or Tching Pié.
- The Upper Burner: Wei Qi.
- The Middle Burner: Iong Qi.
- The Lower Burner: Ancestral Qi.

Examples of Exterior Diseases (Biao):

- Dermatoses, discharges, warts, cysts and polyps.
- Diseases of the sensory organs.
- Diseases of the ligaments, muscles, hair, and nails.
- Capillary diseases.

Examples of Interior Diseases (Li):

- All the deep organs.
- Peritoneum.
- Deep nervous system.
- Deep articulations.
- Deep vessels.
- Mental/Emotional diseases.

COLD-HEAT

The fundamental axis in men is the SHAO YIN axis, which is Kidneys-Heart, or Cold-Heat, or Water-Fire. This is very precarious balance in men, hence the abundant and severe pathology we find at this level. Hence, the preponderance of these specific energies: people are chilly or hot.

Cold and Heat have two meanings:

A quantitative action

Cold: aggravates Fullness of Yin.
aggravates Emptiness of Yang.
Heat: aggravates Fullness of Yang.
aggravates Emptiness of Yin.
Cold: improves an Emptiness of Yin.
aggravates a Fullness of Yang.
Heat: improves an Emptiness of Yang.
improves a Fullness of Yin.

A dynamic action

- Cold aggravates any stagnation, Yin or Yang.
- Heat improves any stagnation, Yin or Yang.

The symptoms of stagnation are discussed further. This dynamic action explains why in TCM, cold means also slowing down or lagging: e.g., oligomenorrhea, or menstrual cycle too late. On the other hand, heat means acceleration: polymenorrhea, or a menstrual cycle too early.

CLINICAL MANIFESTATIONS OF COLD AND HEAT SYNDROME

COLD SYNDROME	HEAT SYNDROME
The patient avoids the cold, has diarrhea, cold limbs, likes hot drinks, has a pale face, white caoting on the tongue, polyuria, somnolentia, silent and slow pulse. Dull pains, paresthesias and formication.	The patient likes cold drinks, has a fever, hot limbs, thirsty, has a red face, tongue dry, red in color with crevices and yellow fur, dry mouth, oliguria, insomnia, fast pulse, constipation, exterior redness and heat

Of course, things are not always that simple. Heat or Cold can be located in the higher or lower part of the body.

- COLD in upper part of the body leads to oppression, indigestion and vomiting.
- COLD in lower part of the body is reflected by constipation with hard, dry stools, hernia, abdominal pain and ice cold limbs.
- HEAT in upper part of the body translates in red, teary eyes, headaches, toothache, and inflamed throat.
- HEAT in lower part of the body is shown in lumbago, edema of lower extremities, constipation and cystitis.

All this is schematical but a combination of all of the above is possible. There is even worse. The Sou Ouenn, Chapter 5, says: *"When Cold is in Fullness and reaches its maximum, it will transform into Heat. When Heat reaches its maximum, it will transform into Cold."* At this point, there is a transformation of "True Cold in apparent or false Heat" and "True Heat into false Cold."

Hot Disease Transforming into Cold: "True Heat-False Cold"

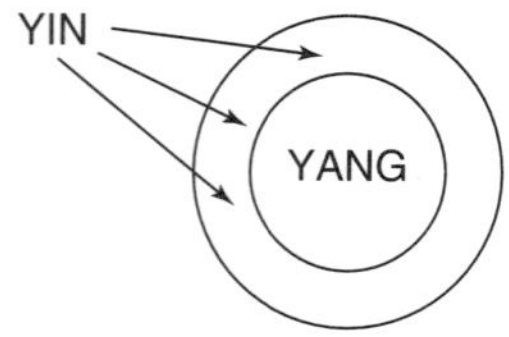

The Heat is in Fullness in the interior of the body, is enclosed and compressed by the Yin. The Yang cannot circulate to the exterior and the limbs: the face is pale and the four limbs are ice cold. These cold symptoms are accompanied by symptoms of "True Heat:"

Strong thirst, dry mouth, lips and throat; bad breath, constipation, hard stools, distended abdomen, oliguria, tongue is yellow-black and painful, the pulse is deep and strong (Yang condition in the interior).

Treatment of this severe condition consists in chasing the heat from the interior to the exterior through:

- *Treatment of Yang Ming*: St25 (Mo point of LI, tonifies the Yin of Yang Ming and directs it to the interior), St27 (one of the 4 dispersion points of the perverse Yang according to the Sou Ouenn), LI11 and 1, St40 and 43 (Treating the obstruction and circulation of Yang Ming, St42 brings Yin or Cold.
- *Urgent treatment*: Evacuation of the Heat (Yang) at the points of concentration of Yang, GV20, GV14 and GV9 (where the Yang arrives).

Cold Disease Transforming into Heat: "True Cold into False Heat"

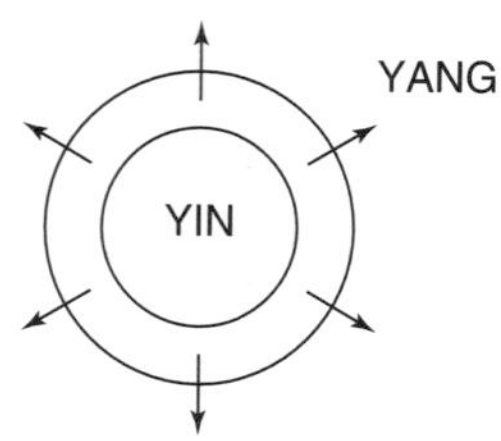

This is the opposite picture as the previous one: the Yin is concentrated in the interior in such a matter that the Yin and Yang cannot communicate with each other. The Yang will follow its natural tendency of escaping especially to the *upper* part of the body, causing the following symptoms:

Dry mouth, painful throat, epistaxis, red face, red, teary eyes, insomnia, restlessness, palpitations and constipation. These "false Heat symptoms" can mask the symptoms of Fullness of Cold such as, cold sweat, cold limbs, feeble voice, asthenia, abdominal distention, clear, pale urination, diarrhea alternating with constipation, supple and swollen tongue with black coating (is a sign of destruction of the fire by the water element) and small, deep and feeble pulse. This disease picture is caused by the *great fullness of the Cold of the Yin kidneys*, dominating the Heart (Fire) and counteracting the Spleen (Earth). The Perverse Qi Cold could penetrate to the level of Shao Yin or Kidney.

Treatment consists of B23 (MOXA, will make the Heat penetrate directly in the Kidney-organ), GV4 (Ming Menn, tonification point of the Ancestral Qi), K10 (dispersion of the Cold, point Ho), K3 and 7 (tonification of the K through its meridian) and L9 (tonification point of L, the L is the "mother" of the K!).

SUMMARY:

The notion of EIGHT CONDITIONS (not six or four) is easy to understand and to apply in the practice. Nothing has to be learned by heart, but only understood and meditated upon to be useful.

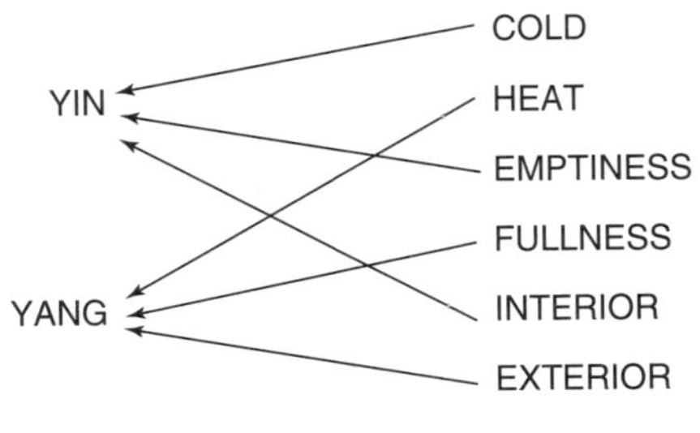

CLINICAL EXAMPLE

Pt, R., 45 years old, was sent to me by another acupuncturist. The reason for referral was the onset of erection disturbances after acupuncture treatment for a pain in his right hand. The pain started 7 years ago after he fell with his hand on a piece of glass. The pain was located in the palm radiating in the direction of PC. After each treatment of acupuncture, the patient had temporary relief, but a repeated treatment was necessary each month. After several months, the patient noted erection problems, something he never experienced before. The acupuncturist as well as the patient feared that this was a direct consequence of his treatments.

The first time I saw the patient, he avoided carefully giving me his right hand. It was obvious that there was still a great sensitivity in his palm. In other words, according to the Eight Conditions, there was a fullness, since pressure aggravated the pain. This was not a stagnation, as pressure does not influence a stagnation.

Fullness of Yin or Yang?

This was undoubtfully a Yin pain:

- Seven years of existence, continuous, dull.
- Patient himself mentioned that cold was aggravating; deep pain, sometimes during the night.
- On the right or Yin side: a Fullness of Yin manifested itself by preference on the right side.

The patient was a jovial, outgoing person, had an active life. He had no trouble talking about his sexual life; no swearing, liked cold drinks, and liked to be in company.

All this indicated that we had here a *Yin Fullness in a Yang person*. This means that all the Yin of this patient went to the right hand, leaving the rest of the body (middle and lower part) in deficiency of Yin.

What was done before? How did the erection problem occur?

The first acupuncturist concluded correctly that his patient had a Fullness of Yin in the right hand but made an often made mistake: he dispersed only points of the Yin meridians: PC 6 and PC7. This was wrong for several reasons. To fight an excess of Yin, it is easier to increase the Yang, since the Yang is more mobile, hence will give faster results.

- He did not take into consideration the whole person and therefore did not increase the Yin in the middle and lower part of the body. This is a common mistake, and we can say that this acupuncturist acted as if only the hand of his patient came on a visit. This is practicing according to Western medicine methods, neglecting our Laws and Principles of Acupuncture or to treat the patient as a whole.
- The acupuncturist forgot the dual function of the PC: it has not only a circulatory function but is also the meridian of the sexual functions; by dispersing PC, he dispersed or decreased the sexual functions of his patient. This was undoubtedly a sequence of errors in the judgment of point choice but at the same time, it shows the strength of an acupuncture treatment.

How did the erection problem get resolved?

There are several possibilities:

1. According to the Eight Rules:
   - CV4(t): increase the Yin of the middle part.
   - Sp6(t): increase the Yin of the lower part.
   - LI4(t) and TB5(t): increase the Yang in the R hand.
2. According to the Tsang-Fu:
   - The erection depends on Tsiue Yin and on the K Yang: CV4 and Sp6, crossroads of the three foot Yin meridians will do the job. K3, B23 and GV4 will increase the K-Yang.
3. The *Miu-technique* (Su Ouenn, Chapter 63)

   "The Ting point and the Lo point are tonified on the opposite side, together with the Lo point of the meridian in the law "Midday-Midnight." In this case, this means: PC9(t) and PC5(t) together with St 40(t), all on the left side.

The latter technique has two advantages:

- We don't have to puncture the painful hand.
- The PC meridian or sexual meridian is tonified, which is favorable for his hand and sexual problem. A few treatments corrected the patient's problems (five treatments, once a week).

WHAT IF THE LOCAL SYMPTOM DOES NOT RESPOND TO THE EIGHT CONDITIONS?

Various disturbances are possible.

STAGNATION OF QI, YANG OR YIN.
Most acupuncturists can apply the Eight Rules, but are totally puzzled when they discover a local Yang symptom, which to their great despair, improves with Heat. How do we distinguish this stagnation from an Excess, Yin or Yang? *The pressure, applied locally will neither aggravate nor improve the pain;* Another important characteristic of stagnation is that any stagnation, Yin or Yang, *improves with Heat, massage and movement*, rest and Cold will worsen any stagnation.

The above characteristics will provide the symptoms for a Yin and Yang stagnation.

Yang Stagnation:

- Yang pain: sharp, intermittent, superficial.

- Pressure is ineffective.
- Heat, massage and movement improves.
- Cold and rest aggravate.

Therapy: Shao Yang means "putting into movement of the Yang." We find the points to improve our stagnation of Yang on the Cheou (Tsou) Shao Yang for the upper extremities and on Tsou or Zu Shao Yang for the Lower extremities: TB1 and TB8 for the upper, GB39 for the lower part.

Yin Stagnation:

- Yin pain: dull, continuous, deep.
- Pressure is ineffective.
- Heat, massage and movement improve.
- Rest and Cold aggravate.

Therapy: Shao Yin means the putting into movement of the Yin: we find the points to improve the stagnation of the Yin on the Cheou Shao Yin (H1) for the upper extremities and on Tsou Shao Yin (K1, K6) for the lower extremities.

DISTURBANCE DUE TO A MECHANICAL TROUBLE

a. A block of a vertebra is a contra-indication for acupuncture. After correction by a chiropractor, acupuncture will be used to correct the energetic disequilibrium that has allowed this block.

b. A disturbing focus at a distance
   - A scar
   - Sinusitis
   - Dental focus (caries, cyst)
   - Appendicitis
   - Chronic Cholecystitis
   - Infectious amygdalitis

Any of the above-mentioned foci can cause a local symptom at a distance. Neural therapy, a technique existing of injection of Impletol, will eliminate a lot of these problems.

c. Tumors and fractures are other causes of mechanical trouble.

EXTERNAL DISEASE

There will be either involvement of the Six Excesses or a de synchronization of the patient with the macrocosm.

a. The involvement of the Six Excesses is stated in the Nei King:

"Wind-Cold, Dryness, Heat, Summer Heat and Dampness cannot harm an individual if there is not already an existing deficiency within the body."

Treatment will consist of a number of steps:

- Increasing the Wei Qi: St36(t), L9(t), B67(t) and TB3(t).
- Treatment of the local Emptiness.
- Use of protection points or the Penn points (See Chapter4).
- If the local symptom is sensitive to weather changes, then Yang Wei Mo is involved: TB 5, command or opening-point of this Extra-meridian is punctured.

b. The External disease due to a de synchronization of the microcosm of the patient with the macrocosm is a different story. In this case, we have a disturbance of one of the Five movements: movement of the Wood, Fire, Earth, Metal or Water. There is no involvement of a Pernicious factor (Excess). A clinical example will clarify this situation.

Pt. S., 53 years old, consults for a shoulder pain. It started four days ago, without apparent cause and not improved by pain medication or infiltrations. The pain is located in the zone Yang, but difficult to pinpoint. There is no sensitivity to pressure, Cold, Heat and exterior weather conditions. The pain is aggravated by every movement.

Further questioning of the patient provides the following information:

- *In 1976, he had a similar attack of tennis-elbow, located on Cheou Tai Yang, with spontaneous appearance and disappearance. At the same time, he had the strange perception of feeling his stomach and intestines.*

- *There was a needle feeling in the heart area*
- *Tendency to soft stools*
- *Olfactory hallucinations*

ANALYSIS:
It is clear that the symptom does not respond to the Eight Rules. This eliminates a disturbance of internal origin. The spontaneous appearance of the tennis-elbow on Cheou Tai Yang indicates a disturbance with Exterior origin, due to a de synchronization between the patient and his macrocosm at the level of the Five Movements.

CONCLUSION:
We have a patient with a shoulder pain, from External origin, located on Cheou Tai Yang. Hence, the primary disturbance is located at the level of the movement of the Fire with involvement of the movement of the metal:

The Fire is in emptiness.

- *Pain on Cheou Tai Yang*
- *Precordial needling*
- *Soft stools*
- *Sensation of feeling the intestines*

The Metal is in fullness.

- *Olfactory hallucinations*

Because the movement of the Fire is in emptiness, each time that we have an emptiness of a stem or branch of the Fire at the level of the macrocosm, the patient's situation will be aggravated. By the same token, each time we have a fullness of a stem or branch of the Water in the macrocosm, the patient will be aggravated again. The same situation happens in case of fullness of the movement of the Metal. This explains the spontaneous appearance and disappearance of the symptoms. In general, we can say that in case of an acute pain, not responding to the Eight Conditions, the origin is most likely external.

TREATMENT:
The Miu-technique (Chapter 63, Su Wenn): H9 and H5 at the left side in tonification. We couple the previous treatment with the Midday-Midnight Rule: Li5 at the R side.

INTERNAL DISEASE: SEVEN EMOTIONS

The impact of the Seven Emotions on each organ is described in Chapter 14. The impact of the movement of the Yin gives us four possibilities:

a. *Non-Exteriorization of the Yin from the center to the periphery.* This causes Fullness of Yin in the center with oppression in the chest, dyspnea, palpitations. Therapy: Li13.
b. *The Yin does not enter from the periphery in the center*: stagnation of Yin at the shoulder. Therapy L2[(t)].
c. *Non-exteriorization of the Yang from the center to the periphery causes:* Fullness of Yang in the center with poor digestion, abdominal distention, and pain in the stomach upon pressure. CV12[(t)].
d. *Non-Interiorization of the Yang from the periphery to the center* causes stagnation of Yang in

the periphery. TB1[(t)] and TB8[(t)].

APPENDIX: SEASONAL POINTS OF THE MERIDIANS

SEASONAL DISPERSION POINTS

	SPRING	SUMMER	LONG SUMMER	FALL	WINTER
H	8	7	4	3	9
PC	8	7	5	3	9
K	10	9	8	5	11
Sp	2	3	5	9	1
Li	2	3	4	8	1
L	10	9	8	5	11
LI	5	11	1	2	3
SI	5	8	1	2	3
TB	7	10	1	2	3
St	41	36	45	44	43
GB	38	34	44	43	41
B	60	40	67	66	65

SEASON TONIFICATION POINTS

	SPRING	SUMMER	LONG SUMMER	FALL	WINTER
H	3	9	8	7	4
PC	3	9	8	7	5
L	5	11	10	9	8
K	10	1	2	3	7
Sp	9	1	2	3	5
Li	8	1	2	3	4
LI	2	3	5	11	1
SI	2	4	5	7	1
TB	2	3	7	10	1
St	44	43	41	36	45
GB	43	41	38	34	44
B	66	65	60	40	67

The Moment to Puncture 8

INTRODUCTION

Chronobiology is an idea that gains more and more acceptance by practitioners of TCM. This is not surprising: every acupuncturist knows that a particular therapeutic act works better at some hours of the day than at others. In fact, according to the Chinese, we see this statement reversed. It is not the medication, herb or therapeutic gesture that works better at a certain moment. It is the fact that the disturbed organ is more sensitive at that particular moment of the day! Energy cycles are formed by the rhythm of years, days and hours, and periodically, an organ is at its maximum or minimum of energy. The Chinese always believed that these cycles depend on Heaven and Earth. Men positioned between these elements are influenced by them and are affected by the power of these magnetic fields.

It is mentioned in the Sun Wenn and the Ling Throu that certain factors have to be taken into consideration before treating a patient. These books mention the seasons, lunar, phases, days and hours during which we should or should not puncture the patient. In view of the busy schedule of some acupuncturist, or simply the ignorance of most doctors regarding these important rules, it seems strange that they still achieve positive results. This indicates the existence of a certain "Auto-Regulatory" system of our body. Certain points, for example, having no action at the moment they are punctured, produce the desired effect later; and it is precisely at those moments that the action of the point has its maximum effect.

In spite of all this, there is no doubt that the results will be longer lasting and better for the acupuncturist who takes the greatest number of factors into account. Therefore, we all should strive to follow as closely as possible the various important energy cycles. In practice, the simplest factors to consider are:

- **Phases of the Moon.**
- **Position of the Sun.**
- **Seasons.**
- **Hours of the Day.**
- **Stems and Branches of the Chinese Astronomy.**

LUNAR PHASES

The movements of the Qi and Blood in relation to the moon are well described in the Sun Wenn. During the phase of the *new moon,* we will find very little Wei Qi in the meridians. It is prudent to avoid puncturing a patient because the treatment will be futile.

When the moon is *waxing,* the Qi and Xue become more abundant and circulate better. This will be the moment to tonify our patient.

At *full moon,* the Qi and Xue are abundant and, therefore, Excesses will manifest themselves. This will be the moment to disperse our patient.

When the moon is *waning,* the meridians empty their Qi and Xue. Tonification at this time will slow down this natural cycle and thus will be inefficient. Again, dispersion is indicated.

We also should remember that the moon is the symbol of the Yin, governing the cycle of the woman. It is very important to consult a lunar calendar before regulating the menstrual cycle.

POSITION OF THE SUN

The Qi and Xue follow the movements of the Sun. In the *morning,* when the sun is rising, the Yang Qi is growing. This will be the moment for tonification of the Qi (Yang) and dispersion of the Xue (Yin).

In the *afternoon,* the Yang Qi decreases, while the Yin increases. Therefore, this will be the ideal time of the day to tonify the Yin Qi and disperse the Yang Qi.

The Su Wenn indicates also that in the *winter,* when cold weather predominates, the Qi will go to the Interior and the circulation of the Blood will slow down. We stimulate the circulation of the Blood through moxa or needles, puncturing deep to reach the Qi. On the other hand, in the *summer,* when warm weather prevails, the Qi will circulate in the superficial layers, and the flow of Blood is not hampered. In this case, we will not puncture deeply, in order to avoid injury of the organs. Also, moxa will be contra-indicated.

SEASONS

According to the Five Movements, each season is more ore less indicated for our patients. According to the "Energy Disequilibriums, "we have to take advantage of the proper season to bring our patient into equilibrium.

From *February to May,* we have to watch closely patients with hepatobiliary diseases, eye diseases, tendon and muscle disease, etc. All of these are a translation of an imbalance at the level of the Wood.

From *May to August,* disturbances in the movement of the Fire are common. This will be translated into heart disease, tongue and saliva disturbances, diarrhea, cystitis, etc.

From *August to November,* disturbances of the Metal are common. This is a very sensitive period for asthma, skin diseases, depression, sinusitis, etc.

According to the seasons, the depth of the puncturing will change. We puncture very superficially in the summer, since the Qi flows in the Yang or superficial layers. To reach the deeply hidden Qi in the winter, we puncture deeply, while in the fall and spring we reach the middle layers.

HOURS OF THE DAY

A general rule says that *"In case of an empty energy syndrome, whatever the nature of the emptiness, tonification of the Mother organ is indicated (See cycle of Five Elements)."* For instance, from 3-5 a.m. Cheou Tai Yin has its maximum Energy. During these hours, Sp2, tonification point of the Mother organ of the Lung, is indicated to correct the deficient syndrome. From 5-7 a.m., on the other hand correction of the emptiness is achieved by the puncturing of St41, tonification point of the Mother organ during this period. As we can see, this rule has nothing to do with the Deficient Organ but is applied to correct the empty state of Qi.

In case of a *full energy syndrome,* whatever the nature of the fullness, *the dispersion point of the Son organ is indicated.* For example, from 1-3 p.m., energetic hour of the Small Intestine, we use St45, the dispersion point of the St.

Using this rule in order to know how to tonify and disperse an organ is one side of the coin. We can also use this system in the opposite sense. For instance, we want to disperse the Gall Bladder. The GB is the Son of the Bladder which has its maximum Qi during the hours 3-5 p.m.. Therefore, GB38 in dispersion will be more effective during the hours 3-5 p.m., than at any other given moment.

STEMS AND BRANCHES OF THE CHINESE ASTRONOMY

The Stems and Branches are described in Chapter 6 of the Su Wenn. It is not my intention here to elaborate on all the different aspects of Stems and Branches, and Knots and Roots, since this would go beyond the goal of this book to be practical, rather than theoretical. Too many times, I have listened to lengthy explanations of this important aspect in TCM, only to feel very frustrated afterwards, since I did not see any practical application. Therefore, I want to illustrate this phenomenon with an actual case history.

EXAMPLE

We see our patient on the 11th of January, 1983. The moment of consultation is 12 o'clock. Before we can elaborate on this example. Here are some charts we must use:

Chart of the years and months:

				Leap years
* '80	9	January	0	1
'81	15	February	31	32
'82	20	March	59	0
'83	25	April	30	31
* '84	30	May	0	1
'85	36	June	31	32
'86	41	July	1	2
'87	46	August	32	33
* '88	51	September	3	4
'89	57	October	33	34
'90	2	November	4	5
'91	7	December	34	35

***NOTE**: Leap Year

To find the new figure for the next year, we add five to the previous number; e.g., going from '83 to '84, we go from 25 to 30. For the leap year we add six from 30 to 36 in '85. If the sun is more than sixty, we deduct sixty and the remainder will be our new figure (from 57 to 2 in '90).

Chart of the Chinese days:

1	2	3	4	5	6	7	8	9	10
Chia	I	Ping	Ting	Chen	Chi	Keng	Hsin	Jen	Kuei
Tzu	Chou	Ying	Mao	Chen	Szu	Wu	Wei	Shen	Yu
11	12	13	14	15	16	17	18	19	20
Chia	I	Ping	Ting	Wu	Chi	Keng	Hain	Jen	Kuei
Hsu	Hai	Tzu	Chou	Ying	Mao	Chen	Szu	Wu	Wei
21	22	23	24	25	26	27	28	29	30
Chi	I	Ping	Ting	Wu	Chi	Keng	Hsin	Jen	Kuei
Shen	Yu	Hsu	Hai	Tzu	Chou	Ying	Mao	Chen	Szu
31	32	33	34	35	36	37	38	39	40
Chia	I	Ping	Ting	Wu	Chi	Keng	Hsin	Jen	Kuei
Wu	Wei	Shen	Yu	Hsu	Hai	Tzu	Chou	Ying	Mao
41	42	43	44	45	46	47	48	49	50
Chia	I	Ping	Ting	Wu	Chi	Keng	Hsin	Jen	Kuei
Chen	Szu	Wu	Wei	Shen	Yu	Hsu	Hai	Tzu	Chou
51	52	53	54	55	56	57	58	59	60
Chia	I	Ping	Ting	Wu	Chi	Keng	Hsin	Jen	Kuei
Ying	Mao	Chen	Szu	Wu	Wei	Shen	Yu	Hsu	Hai

Chart of the hours of the day:

Tsu	23-01	Wu	11-13
Chou	01-03	Wei	13-15
Ying	03-05	Shen	15-17
Mao	05-07	Yu	17-19
Chen	07-09	Hsu	19-21
Szu	09-11	Hai	21-23

OPENING POINTS ON THE DIFFERENT DAYS:

On the days Chia-Chi

Hours	Opening points day Chia	Opening points day Chi
Chia-Tzu		GB 38
I - Chou	Li 2	
Ping-Ying		SI 8
Ting-Mao	H 7 K 3 PC 7	
Wu Chen		TB 6
Chi-Szu	Sp 5	Sp 1
Keng Wu		
Hsin Wei	L 5	L 10
Jen Chen		
Kuei-Yu	PC 9	K 3 Sp 9
Chia-Hsu	GB 44	
I - Hai		Li 4

On the days I and Keng:

Hours	Days I	Days Keng
Ping-Tzu	SI 2	
Ting-Chou		H 3
Wu-Ying	St 43 GB 40	
Chi-Mao		PC 5
Keng-Chen	LI 5	LI 1
Hsin Szu		
Jen-Wu	B 40	B 66
Kuei-Wei		
Chia-Shen	TB 2	GB 41 LI 4
I- Yu	Li 1	
Ping-Hsu		SI 5
Ting-Hai	H 8	

On the days Ping and Hsin

Hours	Day Ping	Day Hsin
Wu-Tzu		St 36
Chi-Chou	Sp 3 Li 3	
Keng-Ying		TB 10
Hsin-Mao	L 8	L 4
Jen-Chen		
Kuei-Szu	K 10	K 2
Chia Wu		
I - Wei	PC 8	Li 3 L 9
PingShen	SI 1	
Ting-Yu		H 4
Wu-Hsu	St 44	
Chi-Hai		Sp 9

On the days Ting and Jen

Hours	Day Ting	Day Jen
Keng-Tzu	LI 3 SI 4	
Hsin-Chou		PC 3
Jen-Ying	B 60	B 67
Kuei-Mao		
Chia-Chen	GB 34	GB 43
I - SZU		
Ping-Wu	TB 3	SI 3 B 64 TB 4
Ting-Wei	H 9	
Wu-Shen		St 41
Chi-Yu	Sp 3	
Keng-Hsu		LI 4
Hsin-Hai	H 7 L 9	

On the days Wu and Kuei

Hours	Day Wu	Day Kuei
Jen-Tzu		TB 1
Kuei-Chu	K 7	
Chia Ying		
I- Mao	L 8	
Ping-Chen		
Ting-Szu	PC 7	
Wu-Wu	St 45	
Chi-Wei		
Keng-Shen	LI 2	
Hsin-Yu		
Yen-Hsu	B 65 St 42	
Kuei-Hai		K 1

We return to our example. The date of consultation was January 11, 1983. We apply Chart A:

- Year '83: 25
- Month of January: 0
- Day: 11

The total is 36 (25+0+11).

The second step is the application of Chart B: the Chinese day under the figure 36 is Chi Hai. The moment of consultation was at noon. Looking at Chart C, this corresponds with the hour Wu.

In summary, we have day *Chi, hour Wu.* The opening point for this particular patient is found in Chart D 1: TB6.

Some important aspects must be mentioned. The opening point will be punctured bilateral, neither in tonification nor in dispersion but in regulation. It will always be the first point to puncture and can be used in combination with other points or alone. This technique will be especially useful if we are dealing with a difficult case, where all kinds of other therapeutic steps have failed. Mostly, we puncture only this point at that moment!

RESTRICTIONS

Restrictions in regards to puncturing the patient are mentioned in the Nei King and Ling Shu.

Restrictions in case of pregnancy can be found in Chapter 16. Lunar phases have to be taken into consideration in gynecological disease and, as mentioned before, we do not puncture in case of a New Moon.

Nei King (Chapter 9) also advises not to puncture a patient who:

- is intoxicated.
- is exhausted (Yin and Yang energy empty).
- is fearful
- is nervous.
- has just eaten, or is now hungry.
- has just returned from a long trip.
- is angry.
- after sexual intercourse

Also don't puncture on the moment that the Perverse Qi is in full force, since the Qi in the body will be empty at this point.

There is another restriction, indicated in Chapter 51 of the Ling Shu:

- During the first three months of the year, the Qi of man being predominant at the left lower limb, we must not puncture the Yang of this region during these months.
- During the fourth, fifth and sixth months the Qi of man being predominant at the right lower limb, we do not puncture the Yang of this region during these months.
- During the seventh, eighth and ninth months, the Qi of the man being predominant at the right lower limb, we do not puncture the Yin of this region during these months.
- During the tenth, eleventh and twelfth months, the Qi of man being predominant at the left lower limb, we do not puncture the Yin of this region during these months.

Nei King (Chapter 38): *"When the patient is robust or obese, puncture deeper than for a thin one, and let the needle stay longer in. When a patient is muscular and fat, and the tissue is resistant, keep the needle less longer in and puncture less deep. When one puncture children, puncture with a small needle, superficially, and for a short time. Do not puncture more than once a day in this case."*

There are moments that the acupuncturist cannot disperse (Nei King, Chapter 61): *"When there is a severe bleeding, or an abundant perspiration, or after a severe diarrhea or after delivery when there was abundant bleeding."* All these circumstances correspond to the "loss of fluids," so well-known as pathology in Homeopathy.

Also, according to an ancient work of Dr. Tsou Lienn, one should avoid puncturing when, *"A point is located on a vein or artery, on a scar"* (puncture just next to it unless the scar is too large, then choose another point).

ACCIDENTS DURING THE SESSION

The patient can fall in syncope during a treatment (in a very sensitive patient or the Perverse Qi can be too much stimulated). Leave the needle in place and let the patient lay down, feet up. If the punctured point was on the upper part of the body, puncture St36. If the point was on the lower part, puncture LI4. In general, in case of syncope, whatever the location of the point, stimulate the following points: St36, LI4, GV20 and L11.

To avoid such incidents, always explain the patient what you are going to do before the session. If it is the first visit, don't let the patient sit on a chair, lie him down! Always puncture the points located on the Yang side of the extremities first, since the sensitivity is less on that side. Don't puncture someone if you don't know anatomy. In pregnancy, after 5 months, don't puncture points below the umbilicus. From the first pregnancy month, don't puncture points above the umbilicus.

And of course, there are always points that should never be punctured nor getting moxa applied. Refer to modern day charts for this aspect.

Tchong Mo 9

CHARACTERISTICS

Tchong Mo is one of the "Eight Extras", vessels which have particular functions in the organism. They intervene at the moment that the Primary Channels are not able to properly handle the Excess (Shi) of Qi, and in this way, help to regulate the Qi in the channels again. They also help bring Qi into the main channels in case of Deficiency (Xu).

Tchong Mo shares some other characteristics with the other Extras. The Extras do not have their own points except for the Governing Vessel and Conception Vessel. Rather, they incorporate points from the regular channels and are connected with them through special points: the confluent points or opening points. They are generally not punctured in the beginning stages of treatment, but usually only when other treatments have failed. There is Qi running through these Extras in both directions, except for GV and CV which are uni-directional. Other characteristics are mentioned in Chapter 4.

Why are there only eight Extras and not more or fewer? The reason is that in three-dimensional space, an object can be described in eight different ways.

Anterior-Posterior.

Interior-Exterior.

Right-Left.

Superior-Inferior.

Each of the Eight Extras will correspond with one of these directions:

Anterior/Posterior:	**CV-GV**
Interior/Exterior:	**Tchong Mo-Tai Mo**
Right/Left:	**Yin Tchiao Mo-Yang Tchiao Mo**
Superior/Inferior:	**Yang Wei Mo-Yin Wei Mo**

Each of these Eight Extras has corresponding pathological manifestations. If the patient describes these symptoms, the corresponding confluent point may be punctured. The specific syndromes are described in Chapter 4.

ORIGIN, BRANCHES AND FUNCTIONS OF TCHONG MO

Tchong Mo originates in the kidneys and even more specifically, the adrenals. Together with CV and GV, Tchong Mo descends to the genitals and splits into two branches: an anterior branch and a posterior branch. The anterior branch follows CV to CV 4, where it connects with the kidney meridian at K11. In its ascending trajectory, it goes from K11 through K21, passes through K27, CV23, and emerges around the lips. At K11, there is also a descending branch going to St30 and down the inner side of the thigh. The posterior branch goes to GV1 and ascends from there, following the vertebral column to GV16. Hence, it is also responsible for the growth of the hair on the head. If the posterior branch of the Tchong Mo has enough energy, there will be sufficient hair growth. With *excessive sexual activity,* there may be a Xu of Qi in the posterior branch, which may lead to baldness, although hair may be growing elsewhere.

Tchong Mo is classically seen to have a relationship with the blood as explained in the following chapter in Ling Tchrou:

> *"Tchong Mo and CV begin in the woman at the uterus; from there, they climb on the right side of the abdomen, pass to the throat, then outline the mouth. When the Qi and Xue of the Tchong Mo meridian are in equilibrium, the temperature of the body is normal and the hair grows normally. But in the woman, Tchong Mo has more Qi than blood; it is because of this disequilibrium that women do not have beards. This lack of blood is due to the menses, which cause women to lose blood regularly."*

One also reads about beard growth:

> *"If the blood and the Qi are strong in the upper part of the body, the beard is abundant. If there is more blood than Qi, then there is little beard growth. If the Qi and the blood are deficient , one is beardless and has a lot of wrinkles."*

Tchong Mo also classically relates to the Five Organs and Six Bowels (Ling Tchrou, Chapter 28):

> *"Tchong Mo is the Sea of the Five Organs and of the Six Bowels."* This means that they receive their energy from it. This meridian climbs toward the upper part of the body, and on its way it moistens the diverse organs. Toward the lower part, Tchong Mo flows into the capillaries of the Shao Yin, in the region of St 30. It runs along the internal surface of the thigh and the calf and passes to the internal malleous, where it is integrated into the Shao Yin meridian. It moistens the three Yin meridians, passes again to the ankle and then goes to the big toe.

The normal circulation of the Wei Qi in the couple Du Mo-Tchong Mo starts in GV16. From there it descend along the spine and GV to end in GV1. The Wei Qi descends in the opposite direction of the Ancestral Qi running in this meridian. The Wei Qi descends very slowly: it takes 21 days to finish this tract. From GV16 on (the 22nd day), the Wei Qi will follow a part of Tchong Mo. CV1-CV4-K11-CV23 is the tract followed to finish at GV16. This route takes 9 days to be finished. The perverse Qi will attack the GV-Tchong Mo couple in GV16. This point is called Fong Fou or the "Palace of the Fong" or the Wind. Penetration of Wind in this point will cause fever and stiffness in the spine. Once this Fong arrives in Tchong Mo, secondary symptoms such as abdominal distention, diarrhea and digestive disturbances will appear with a sensation of heat in the body.

The ancient books describe that Tchong Mo and Yin Keo have their proper Qi, called, "Ancestral," originating from the kidney. This Qi circulate in and out of the meridians, at the same time with the Yong and Wei Qi. Its role is twofold: regularization of the temperature of the body and transportation of the organic liquids to the intercellular spaces. Tchong Mo has numerous side branches which connect with the Tmm, especially at the level of the chest and abdomen. No wonder Tchong Mo is called the sea of the meridians and secondary vessels.

DIAGNOSIS OF DISEASE OF TCHONG MO

Tchong Mo is the *"Master of the Internal World"*. In the Ling Tchrou it is stated: *"If Tchong Mo is affected, the exterior Qi will be accelerated."* Since Tai Mo is responsible for the connection with the external world, this phrase can be translated in:

"If Tchong Mo is in Deficiency, Tai Mo is in Excess."

In case of disease of Tchong Mo, it can be seen that:

- The disease is internal or organic.
- There is an acceleration of the Exterior Qi.
- Tchong Mo is affected only in serious cases and not in simple ones such as diarrhea.
- The acceleration of the exterior has to correspond with the area of the diseased organ. Only then is Tchong Mo involved. For example, in a patient with a stomach ulcer, if there was pruritus along the area of the St meridian. Tchong Mo would not be involved if the pruritus was present along the region of the Gall Bladder meridian.

EXAMPLES OF DISTURBANCE OF TCHONG MO

- Adrenal deficiency.
- Anorexia nervosa, obesity, viral hepatitis, parasitosis, and abdominal pain.
- Edema, pruritis, conjunctivitis, olfactory hallucinations intolerance to light and noise, and tinnitus.
- Hyperesthesia, chills, brachycardia, and palpitations.
- Dysuria, nocturnal enuresis, and thirst.

The above symptoms relate also to the acceleration of the exterior or excess of Tai Mo.

THERAPY

Sp 4 — activates Tchong Mo (confluent point). This will be the first point to puncture. According to the involved Burner, other points will be activated.

- Lower Burner (Women):
  - K11
  - CV3 (connection and reunion point of Ying and Yang)
  - CV4
  - CV6
  - All of these points must be tonified and heated with moxa
- Lower Burner (Men):
  - St30(t)
  - GV4(t)
  - CV5(t)
- Middle Burner
  - St30(t)
  - CV12(t)
  - CV15(t)
  - St36(t)
- Upper Burner:
  - CV14(t)
  - CV21(t)
- Barrier points:
  - between the lower TB - middle TB = PC6(d)
  - between the middle TB and upper TB = CV4(d)
- For distention before menstruation:
  - CV4(d)

Moxibustion 10

INTRODUCTION AND HISTORY

In ancient times, when people referred to acupuncture, they always used the expression "Chen chiu" or "Zhen Jiu Fa." This means nothing else than "Method of needles and extended fire", indicating the close connection between acupuncture and moxibustion. But there are distinct differences between these two approaches. Acupuncture treats the energy disequilibrium through implantation of needles on the different points of the meridians. Moxibustion, sometimes neglected, treats essentially the chronic disease through direct or indirect application of moxa. Experience also indicates that acupuncture produces faster results, while moxibustion has more long-lasting effects. The word moxibustion is derived from the Japanese word "Mogusa", meaning "Herb to burn". Moxa is also called, KAO which means fire. Moxa is from Japanese origin, while Kao is the real Chinese term. Even today, moxibustion is extensively practiced by the Chinese population, even more so than acupuncture.

The Book of Internal Medicine, the *Nei King*, written between 700 and 300 BC., states that moxibustion was born in North China, known for its long and severe winters. The population consisted principally of Nomads, who through their migrations brought Moxa to the rest of the country.

Many Chinese doctors wrote about moxibustion, even as early as 2700 BC. During the Han Dynasty (-206 to -220 BC.), one of the most famous surgeons was Hua Tuo, specialist in acupuncture, moxibustion, nutrition and Chinese pharmacopoeia. He was especially known for the invention of an anesthetic agent, Ma Fo San, to suppress pain during an operation. He cured a famous army general of his headaches and vertigo, but declined to work for the general full time. That led to his imprisonment at the age of 97: ingratitude existed even at that time!

In the Sui-Tang Dynasty (seventh century), the emperor Huang Di edited a famous book *"Etiology and Symptoms of Disease"*. In this book one could find treatment of goiters by acupuncture and treatment of infantile convulsions through moxibustion. One of his most famous students was Sun Si Miao, who was a master in classical literature at the age of twenty. He started his studies in medicine at that time and traveled through all the Cantons of China, collecting popular prescriptions. He compiled them in his famous book *"A Thousand Golden Prescriptions."*

During the Ming Dynasty (1368-1344 AD.), Wang Chi was one of the best-known doctors. He wrote *"Questions and Answers on Acupuncture,"* consisting of three books. The first two described acupuncture, the third Moxibustion only.

After 1912, Jie Yi Bin Wei wrote *"Principles of Moxibustion"*. Working with a moxa stick, he stimulated the empty meridians through moxibustion of the Lo points.

ARTEMISIA VULGARIS

The plant used for moxibustion is Artemisia Vulgaris, a variety of the chrysants, which grows wild in numerous countries including the U.S.A. The plant has a stem of 40 to 120 cm in height and irregular leaves, green on one side and silver on the other. On top of the plant are flowers, violet or brown in color, according to the species.

Pharmacological the plant has significant characteristics: bitter, warm and sharp. This indicates its Yang nature, allowing it to cure any Yang Deficiencies. Only the flowers and the leaves are used. They are dried for a long time (as long as three years), preferably in the sun. When the moxa is too recent and still humid, the patient feels a strong burning pain. Then they are grounded as finely as possible. The longer the drying time, the more beneficial the effects of the moxa!

Recent analysis has indicated the chemical richness of moxa: protein, sodium, potassium, calcium, iron, aluminum, magnesium, Adenine, Choline, several acids and Vitamins A, B, C and D. Other research programs have indicated that moxa is the only combustible without flame that can provide a temperature of 670 degrees C! Electrical devices invented to replace moxa have never been able to match its quality and healing power. Moxa has some qualities that cannot be replaced, hence its use is highly recommended in many patients.

The size of the Kao depends on for who it is intended. For instance, in children we use very small kaos (like a rice grain). They are also used in sensitive patients. For adults, we have the size of a halve dade. This strong stimulation causes an increase of white and red blood cells. Sometimes, one can put a slice of ginger or garlic between the skin and the Kao. Or we put the moxa on the implanted needle which will transmit the heat deep in the tissues.

INDICATIONS AND EFFECTS OF MOXIBUSTION

INDICATIONS

Moxibustion is especially indicated in chronic diseases and Yang Deficiency syndromes. Examples are malaria, tuberculosis, impotence, prolapsus, fatigue, apoplexy, cholera, continuous perspiration, etc.

More general indications can be found in the Ling Tchrou: *"In any case where acupuncture is inhibited, moxa is indicated."* If both the Yin and Yang meridians are empty, we will do only moxibustion. Moxibustion can also disperse the Qi in case it is accumulated in the meridians. The Nei King (chapter 51), mentions also that it is better to apply moxa on the Back-Shu points rather than needles. Moxa has a tonifying action when it consumes itself; the dispersion action is obtained when we blow on the Moxa to activate its combustion.

Some important points regarding moxibustion are listed below. Small cones are preferred on the limbs and the head, while larger ones are applied on the abdomen.

- In case of Fong symptoms, moxibustion is done on GV20 and GB20.
- In edema, CV9 is indicated, while LI4 is preferred for the head and eyes.
- For the lower extremities, we have GB30, while LI15 and LI11 are indicated for the upper extremities.
- On the points L11 (disperses the Heat in the body), CV25 and K1, very few moxas are applied.
- On the points CV12, St36, LI11 and 15, we apply as many as a hundred moxa cones.

EFFECTS OF MOXA

It is important to remember that needling can be forbidden in case of extreme fatigue. There is a lack of Energy to work with and patients will be prone to syncope. In those cases moxibustion is the logical therapeutic step.

The effects of Moxibustion improves the patient in four ways:

- Dispersion of the pain.
- Strengthening of the Yang Qi.
- Improvement of the circulation of Qi and Xue.
- Prevention of disease.

Dispersion of the pain
The main characteristic of moxa is the Heat (670 degrees C). Next to trauma, Cold and Dampness are the most frequent causes of pain. Fighting the Cold with Heat is the most logical step: the patient has a sensation of pleasant warmth and a noticeable decrease of pain when the heat penetrates the skin, muscles and meridians.

Strengthening of the Yang Qi
Yang is the cornerstone of life. Its good function provides good health. In case of deficiency, the Yin is abundant and produces shock if not corrected, which is easily done by moxa.

Improvement of the circulation of Qi and Xue
According to TCM, the source of disease is the disequilibrium between Energy and Blood: *"The Yang protects, the Yin feeds."* In case of deficiency of Yang, the Yin stagnates (the Yang moves the Yin) and cannot fulfill its nourishing function. The heat (moxa) resolves any stagnation and improves the circulation of the Blood.

Prevention of disease and maintenance of good health
In China, acupuncturists and patients always considered moxibustion as an excellent way of maintaining health. One of those Golden Rules is to apply moxa on CV4 (source of original Qi), CV6 ("Sea of Qi") and CV4 (strengthens the original Yang and the Kidney Qi). Another popular prescription is Moxibustion of St36 and LI10.

METHODS OF APPLICATION

GENERAL RULES
It is recommended to place the patient in a comfortable position to avoid irritation of the eyes by the fumes of the Moxa. In case different parts of the body need to be stimulated, a certain order should be followed:

- First moxa on the head.
- Then the back, before the front of the body.
- The upper extremities before the lower ones.
- The left side before the right side.

The daily climate factors should also be considered.

- In warm weather, the empty syndromes can be stimulated by using a point of tonification plus a point of the Yin that will have a cooling effect. The only exception to the latter is when the patient already shows symptoms of Yin Excess (See Eight Conditions).
- In cold weather, the internal Yin syndromes will be dispersed and warmed up.

METHODS OF APPLICATION

They can be classified in two groups: direct moxibustion or cauterization, and the indirect or heating.

Direct Moxibustion

We apply a certain amount of moxa directly on the skin. The moxa will have the shape of a cone whose base will be attached to the skin through a greasy substance (almond oil). Treatment will consist of applying a certain number of cones on the same point. This number varies according to the type of affection, the physical condition of the patient, and the area to treat. Very rarely, especially in Europe and the U.S.A., the moxa will be burnt until it forms a blister and subsequently a scar. More popular is the method where the moxa cone is removed with tweezers the moment the skin feels hot. This is the non-scarring moxibustion, since application of moxa causes only redness (temporary) of the skin.

Indirect Moxibustion

We heat the points from a distance or through various materials.

a. Cigar form

The Moxa is rolled in the form of a cigar, surrounded by rice paper. It has a length of twenty-one centimeters and is lit on one side. It is held at a distance of one *cun* of the meridian point that we want to stimulate. Three different methods are described.

(1) Stable, prolonged heating

The cigar is held at a fixed distance from the skin until a redness of the skin is obtained. The patient can also indicate if the heat becomes too intense or unpleasant. This method is applied for general fatigue, abdominal pain and diarrhea.

(2) Intermittent heating

The burning end of the cigar is lifted up and down in order to bring a stronger stimulation. We bring the moxa closer to the skin than in the first method; therefore, we have to be more careful to avoid a blister. This method is indicated in case of paralysis and syncope.

(3) Circular heating

This permits us to heat an area that exceeds the meridian point. In a rapid circulation we can bring the cigar closer to the skin; in a slower movement we will obtain a fast heating of the area. This method is used for skin diseases, but is also applied for Xu syndromes. After puncturing the meridian point, we heat the zone around the needle. The reactions of the patients can be different during this moxibustion: in case of extensive emptiness, we can heat for a long time, because the heat is quickly absorbed. In China, a whole cigar can be used to heat one or two points for about forty minutes. On the contrary, if the patient has an unpleasant feeling after a few minutes, we should stop the moxibustion, since the stimulation is either sufficient or there is no Emptiness of Yang.

b. Moxa on needle

This is the perfect union of acupuncture and moxibustion. This method is especially indicated when the needles have to be inserted for a long time, such as Xu or Cold syndromes. The needle is implanted at the required depth, then moxa is put on the handle of the needle and burnt.

c. Moxa on salt

The salt is put in the umbilicus on CV8. The best salt is natural sea salt, containing multiple minerals. On the salt we put a big cone of moxa and let the patient indicate the tolerable heat effect. This form of moxibustion is indicated for vomiting, diarrhea, apoplexy, hemorrhage and Emptiness of Yang Qi.

d. Moxa on ginger

Fresh ginger is cut in slices of two millimeters in thickness. We perforate the slices with a needle to allow the heat to diffuse. The slice is put on the treated area, with a large cone in the center of the ginger slice. Once the heat becomes too intense we remove the slice with a tweezer, then put it again on the treated zone after a few minutes. The special "hot" quality of the ginger is frequently used in the treatment of vomiting, diarrhea, abdominal pain and other gastro-intestinal disorders. Pei diseases due to Cold and Dampness are also excellent indicates.

e. Moxa on needle and ginger

This is a combination of the two previous methods: we put some moxa around the handle of the needle and perforate a slice of ginger on the treated area. Arthritis is an excellent indication.

f. Moxa on garlic

We cut the same slices as in the ginger method, but the cones of moxa used are considerably smaller. The garlic has some excellent anti-infectious and anti-inflammatory characteristics, successfully used in cases of pulmonary tuberculosis, furoncels, abscesses and insect stings.

THERAPEUTIC EXAMPLES

STROKE

Causes:

- External Fong.
- Excessive Heart Fire, deficient Water Kidney.
- Liver Fire Yang, stirring up the Interior Wind.
- Attack due to a deficiency of Yang Qi.

Only the last cause is an indication of moxa.

Symptoms (of Xu Yang Qi):

- Cold limbs: the Qi does not reach the extremities.
- Cold perspiration: deficient Qi.
- Vertigo: emptiness of Qi in the brain.
- Tongue: white, damp coating.

Treatment:

Moxibustion is applied on the following points:

- CV4: source of original Qi.
- CV6: increase the Qi of the Inferior Burner
- K1: causes the Fire to descend.
- St36: circulates the Qi in the lower and upper body.
- Sp6: regulates the Blood.

To increase the Yang Qi, we add the following points:

- B23: tonifies the Fire.
- K3: golden needle or moxa.
- GV4: Ming Men, tonifies the original Qi of the Kidneys.

ABDOMINAL PAIN

Pathogenesis:

An accumulation of Cold is caused by an external Cold attack, especially when the Earth element is already in emptiness. The same symptoms appear when excessive quantities of cold food are absorbed, even more so in the Winter when the Yang of the body fights the Excessive Yin. As a consequence, the Spleen does not transform the food, the Qi stagnates and pain appears. Alleviation is obtained by Heat and warm food.

Treatment:

- St36: treats the Earth Element.
- CV6: tonifies the central Qi and fights the Cold.
- CV11: harmonizes the St/Sp.
- B20: strengthens the Earth Element.

The former points are done in tonification while the following will be done with moxa:

- CV4: Mu point of the Small Intestine.
- CV8: this point is treated with salt or ginger and will increase the Middle Qi and disperse the Cold.

PROLAPSUS UTERI

Pathogenesis:

Due to excessive fatigue after delivery or multiple pregnancies, the uterus prolapses through the vagina, since the Sp and K Qi are in emptiness. This is accentuated in standing position, while the supine position reduces it.

Treatment:

Moxa on:

- CV4.
- GV20: increase the Yang Qi, reduces the ptosis.

Heated needle:

- Sp 6: tonifies the Sp Qi, regulates the Blood.
- B20 increases the central Qi.
- B23: nourishes the Kidney.

LATE MENSTRUAL CYCLE

Pathogenesis:

At the origin of this syndrome are ingestion of cold and raw food and a concentration of cold on the Lower Burner.

Symptoms:

Pale face, sensitivity to cold, depressive, sleepy and pale, small amounts of blood, as well as pale tongue and a thin coating.

Treatment:

- CV6: heats the Lower Burner.
- Sp10: equilibrates the Original Qi and strengthens the Blood.
- Sp6: increases the three Yin channels and the Blood.

EDEMA IN A YIN KNEE

Pathogenesis:

Due to acute trauma, the articulation of the knee is red, swollen and painful. This is a Yang knee and moxa is prohibited at this stage. We puncture in dispersion St36, St35, GB34, Sp9 and Li8. If the traumatized knee is too painful to puncture, the technique "Piqûre a l'Opposé" is indicated (See Chapter 4). Failure to treat this acute knee leads to a stagnation of Blood and the symptoms become Yin: redness and the warm feeling disappear, the edema is pronounced, and the pain becomes constant and dull.

Treatment:

In tonification:

- GB34, Influential point of the ligaments and the tendons.
- St34.

Hot needle:

- Sp9: eliminates the Dampness.
- St35: "The eyes of the Dragon", treats the articular affections of the knee.
- GV3: treats the lower limbs and increases the Yang in that area.

- B23: strengthens the K Qi, master of the bones.
- St36: balances the St/Sp.
- Sp5: eliminates the Dampness and is indicated in case of diffuse articular pains.

FATIGUE

Pathogenesis

Either we have a temporary deficiency or a chronic deficiency of Yang Qi. The former is due to grief, worry and excessive labor, the latter caused by sexual excesses or alcohol abuses.

Symptoms

They are preponderantly Yin in both cases: chills, looks for a warm environment, tired with every effort, loose stools, pale face and feeble pulse.

Treatment.

- St36: strengthens the central Qi.
- K1: calms the mind.
- CV4: tonifies the Original Qi.
- B23: tonifies the Yang Qi of the Kidneys.
- B13: increases the Lung Qi, master of the Qi.

LONGEVITY

Since ancient times, the Chinese tried to conquer and master the physical and spiritual aspects of life in order to come into harmony with nature. With the help of martial arts, music and especially preventive medicine, they tried to preserve all their capabilities until old age. We are talking here about "a real art of long life", or better expressed as "road of immortality."

Moxibustion on the following points is applied to achieve this goal:

Principal points are CV4 and St36; auxiliary points are CV12, CV8, B13 (master of the Qi), B17 (master of the Blood) and B23. Three to seven moxa cones are used on each point, and this is once a week.

CONTRA-INDICATIONS OF MOXIBUSTION

GENERALITIES

Moxibustion is prohibited on areas where the meridians are superficial or in dangerous zones: eyes, nose, area of the heart, penis, vulva, mouth, etc. Except for some situations, moxa is not applied in pregnancy nor during the menstrual cycle: we would induce too much Yang for these excessive Yin states. Acute situations or excitations do not call for moxa: extreme hunger, thirst, right after meals, or after a violent emotion. In Chapter 9 of the *Ling Throu* it is mentioned: *"Moxibustion is never done in case of Fullness of the St 9 pulse"*, or in other words, in case of fullness of the exterior (See Chapter 5).

FORBIDDEN POINTS

The points are mentioned according to their meridians.

- L: L8 and 10
- LI: LI19
- St: St1, 4, 8 and 17
- Sp: Sp7, 16 and 20
- H: H8 and 9
- SI: SI9 and 18
- B: B1, 6 and 62
- K: K2
- PC: PC5, 8 and 9
- TB: TB1, 4, 6, 16 and 18
- GB: GB2 and 3
- Li: Li2
- CV: CV5, 14 and 23
- GV: GB15, 16, 25, and 27, 28

In any event, we have to use our common sense

and knowledge of TCM. In case of pregnancy we can use moxa for fatigue or lower back pain, but points of the abdomen will always be forbidden! Experience dictates also that we use moxa sparingly on all the systems of the Yang Qi in the body: Li, H and Tchong Mo, and the Fire points of the meridians.

CONTRA-INDICATIONS FOR THE PRACTITIONER

This is a warning for the acupuncturist who can be exposed chronically to the fumes of the moxa. Quite often, we see rhinorrhea, epistaxis and conjunctivitis. Good aeration in the treatment room easily avoids these risks. This is a better solution than the one that some of our colleagues prefer: not doing any moxibustion at all! The value of moxa is too great for us to withhold this excellent technique from our patients!

11 Dialectic of the Acupuncture Points

INTRODUCTION

When we talk about the significance of the acupuncture points, the terms Tai, Shao, and Ming or Chiueh have to be explained thoroughly. It was during my teaching days that I was confronted with heated discussions among my students about the exact sequence of these terms. Before attending my class, they learned from several teachers various combinations, which caused total confusion among the students. Consequently, none of them knew anything about the practical value of these different acupuncture levels.

So, who was right — the one who claimed it was "Tai Yang, Shao Yang and Yang Ming", or the one who saw the sequence more as "Tai Yang, Yang Ming and Shao Yang"? I hate to disappoint anyone; in fact, they both could be correct or both incorrect! It is just a matter of what we are talking about. As we will see, there are four different classifications for these Six Levels. They are classified according to:

Intensity or Strength
Transformation or Mutation
Space or Exterior/Interior
Movement

For clarification, an example with the YIN QI in general is given, followed by their practical application in the Group Lo points of the Kidney meridian.

THE THREE YIN LEVELS

The first classification is according to the *intensity* of the Yin Qi in these levels. They are found in the Energetic Medicine, so well explained in the books of Dr. Maurice Mussat, an eminent acupuncturist-physician in France. When we put the different levels on a circle with their corresponding trigram (Figure 35), we see that:

- Tai Yin is the greatest Yin, closest to the Sea of Yin or CV (Jen Mo).
- Shao Yin is the middle Yin and weaker.

- Chiueh Yin is the weakest Yin, far from the original Yin source (CV).

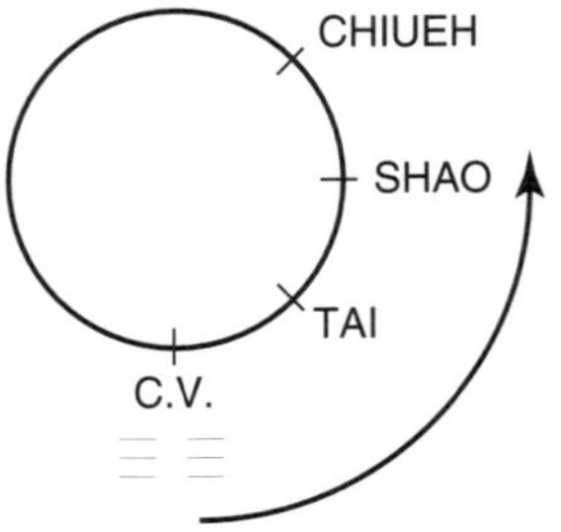

Figure 35

Further explanation of trigrams is beyond the scope of this work and not relevant for this chapter.

The second classification of this Yin Qi is according to the *transformations and mutations* of the Yin. Now our sequence will be "Shao Yin—Chiueh Yin—Tai Yin", since Shao Yin is the deepest Yin level or last defense barrier of our body before the Perverse Qi will penetrate into the organs.

Thirdly, the Yin can be considered in *space*. As is expressed in the Six Levels or the Great Meridians (Chapter 4, Par. VI), Tai Yin and Tai Yang have their opening to the Exterior, Shao Yin and Yang Ming open to the Interior, while Chiueh Yin and Shao Yang are the hinges of the Yin and Yang, respectively, opening to the Interior and the Exterior. The sequence of the Yin is going from the Exterior to the Interior, Tai Yin—Chiueh Yin—Shao Yin.

To summarize, we take an example of the Yin, Chiueh Yin. This Yin is the smallest Yin, the second stage of transformation and mutation, the hinge of the Yin in space, and the end of the movement of the Yin in time.

DIALECTIC OF THE GROUP LO POINTS

The Group Lo points are cited in the classical works of acupuncture and are the following:

- **TB 8 or Cheou Shao Yang: three Upper Yang.**
- **GB 39 or Tsou Shao Yang: three Lower Yang.**
- **PC 5 or Cheou Chiueh Yin: three Upper Yin.**
- **Sp 6 or Tsou Tai Yin: three Lower Yin.**

They all have Lo functions: they regulate the relations Yin/Yang of the type Right/Left, Interior/Exterior, Front/Back and Up/Down. These Group Lo points will be analyzed, one by one, according to the four previous classifications.

SP6 OR 6 TSOU TAI YIN

Its principal name is San Yin Jiao:

- San: three, three times.
- Yin: Inn.
- Jiao: exchanging, linking of relations or crossing.

Thus, this ideogram groups the ideas of great Yin, organization, support and fusion of the three Yin. Indeed, Sp6 governs the Yin of the lower part of the body. This point will unblock the accumulations of the Yin in this area and bring this form of Qi up to the trunk and the head. By the same token, Sp6 is the linking point of the three leg Yin channels.

Why Tai Yin and not a point of Shao or Chiueh Yin? We divide the human body into three parts: head and upper extremities are heaven; trunk is linked to man; and the lower extremities are earth. According to the intensity of the Yin, earth is Yin when compared to heaven, and lesser Yin when we compare it to man. Figure 36 shows that:

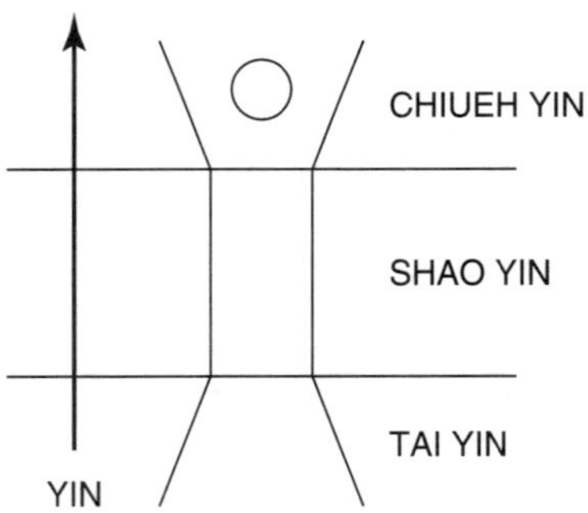

Figure 36

- The lower extremities are the greatest Yin, which corresponds to Tai. (See beginning of this chapter).
- The trunk is the middle Yin or Shao

Yin.

- The head and upper extremities are the smallest Yin, since they are the farthest removed from the original Yin; hence this area is Chiueh Yin.

To summarize, the point with its functions described in Figure 35 is found on the meridian with the same name, Tai Yin, and it is Tsou (lower part of the body) Tai Yin or Spleen.

PC5 OR CHEOU CHIUEH YIN

The principal name is Jian Shi:

- Jian: in the middle.
- Shi: guides, governs or serves.

According to this ideogram, PC5 leads and guides the Yin of the superior part of the body. There is an idea of movement, an expression of dynamism and quantity. Indeed, Figure 36 demonstrates that the Yin of the superior part of the body is quantitatively the smallest Yin or Chiueh Yin. But this is only one aspect of PC5. As mentioned in this chapter, Chiueh Yin is the end of the movement Yin, while Shao Yin puts the Yin into movement and Tai Yin accelerates this same Yin. Therefore, the final Yin in intensity and movement is found on Chiueh Yin, necessarily on Cheou (upper extremities). What point of this meridian fulfills these characteristics? Only one Antique Su point has this function: PC5.

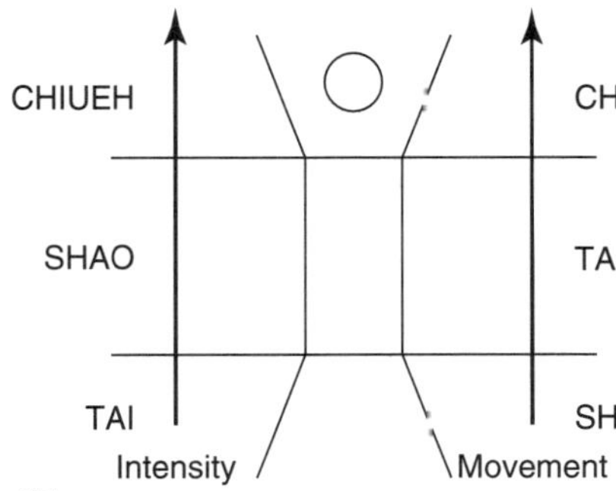

Figure 37

OTB8 OR CHEOU SHAO YANG

The principal name is San Yang Luo:

- San: three.
- Yang: of the couple Yang/Yin.
- Luo: ideogram of the points and meridians Lo.

In this name we find a notion of three Yang, exterior/interior relationship (Lo), and communication. This point is situated on Shao Yang, on the upper extremities, because it rules the putting into movement of the Yang in the superior part of the body. Normally the Yang descends from the upper part of the body to the lower part, as opposed to the Yin, which ascends from the lower extremities to the head. Therefore, the Yang is put into movement in the upper part of the body and is called Shao Yang; the middle of the movement is Tai Yang; and the end of the Yang is Yang Ming, at the lower extremities. (Figure 38)

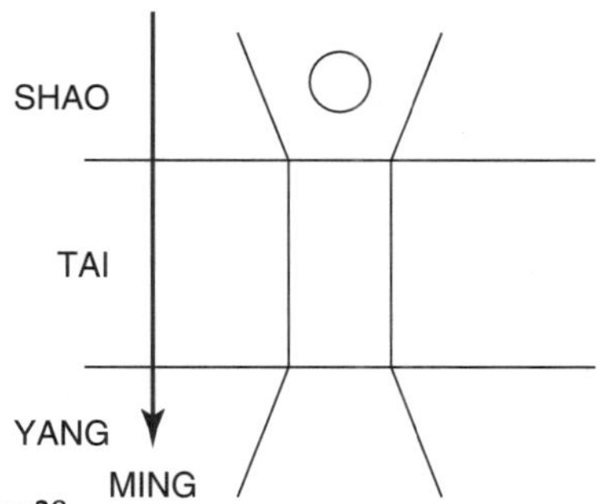

Figure 38

What are the indications of this point? All the indications involve the notion of movement:

- Aphony (cannot speak).
- Immobility.
- Somnolence.

The indication of this dynamic point is putting into movement the Yang of the upper extremities; hence, the point is punctured in any stagnation of Yang in the upper part of the body.

GB39 OR TSOU SHAO YANG

The principal name is Xuan Zhong:

- Xuan: separated, at the end.
- Zhong: clock, alarm clock.

Here is an idea of "far", "at the extreme end". The point is situated on Shao Yang of the lower extremities (Tsou). This can only be for a reason of Exterior/Interior or *spatial* relationship:

- It cannot be for a reason of intensity, because the Yang is the smallest in the lower part of the body and is called Yang Ming.
- It cannot be for a reason of putting into movement of the Yang, because this occurs in the upper part of the body and is called Cheou Shao Yang.

Shao Yang is the hinge of the Yang and assures the free movement of the Yang in the Interior. Indications of this point find their origin in the translation of its symptoms:

- There is a Fullness of Yang superficially, expressed by symptoms such as fear, anger, apoplexy, epistaxis, tightness of the chest, and itching of the skin.
- Shao Yang does not move the Yin. Therefore, symptoms of stagnation of deep Yin appear with thick blood and paraplegia.

Summarizing, this point circulates the Yang in the superficial part of the body and causes the Yang to descend, in order to circulate the deep Yin (Figure 39).

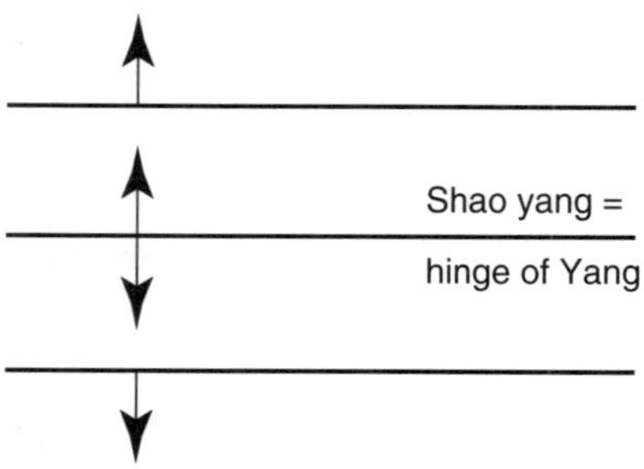

Figure 39

DIALECTIC OF THE TSOU SHAO YIN POINTS OR KIDNEY POINTS

As stated in Paragraph II of this chapter, we can look at the points of the Kidney meridian from four different angles:

- Their intensity,
- Their mutations,
- Space, and
- Time.

According to the *intensity*, we consider Shao Yin as the middle Yin:

Tai Yin —	Shao Yin ———	Chiueh Yin
Great Yin	Middle	Final or smallest Yin
***	**	*

In its *mutations*, going from matter of Qi, Shao Yin is the beginning of the mutation:

Shao Yin —Chiueh Yin ——— Tai Yin

In *space*, Shao Yin is the closing of the Yin to the Interior. (Figure 40)

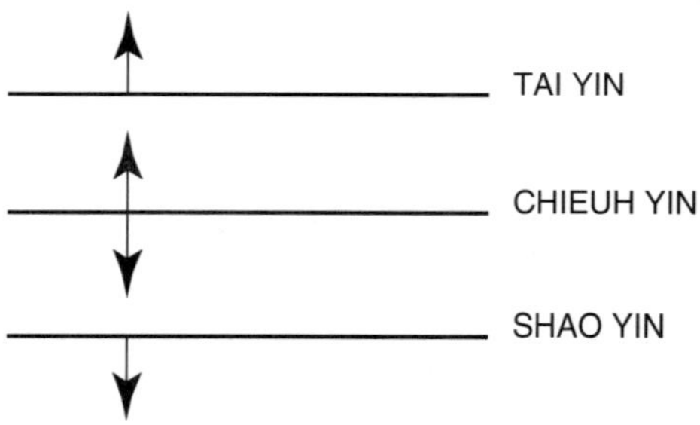

Figure 40

In *time* Shao Yin is the putting into movement of the Yin.

We will consider now the points of Shao Yin according to these previous criteria.

INTENSITY OR MIDDLE YIN (Figure 40)

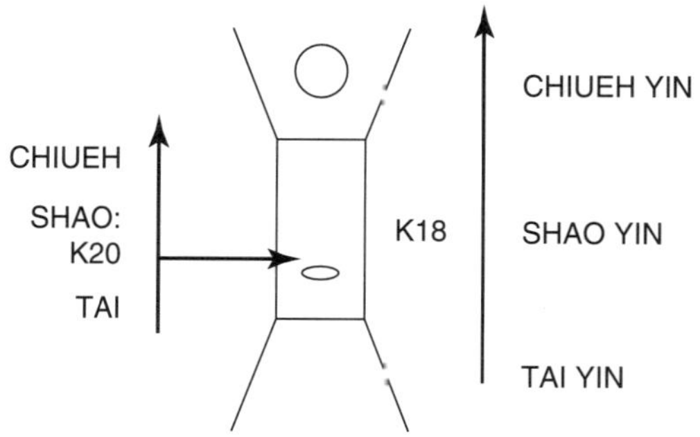

Figure 41

Two points correspond to this criterion:

· On a *global* plane, or at the level of the whole body, the trunk is Shao Yin with a relation to the lower extremities and the head. K 18 facilitates the passage of the Yin of the trunk to the head. Hence, its indications of fullness of the Yin of the trunk with emptiness of Yin in the superior part of the body: oppression, the superior part of the body: oppression, dyspnea, slow digestion with abdominal distention two hours after meals, constipation and painful menstrual cycle. All these symptoms are aggravated by pressure.

· On a *local* plane, or at the level of the trunk, the epigastrium is Shao Yin compared with the pelvis and thorax. The point K20 facilitates the passage of the epigastric Yin to the thorax. Puncturing this point is indicated in case of fullness of Yin in the epigastrium with emptiness of Yin in the thorax: palpitations, slow digestion, epigastric cramps and vomiting aggravated by pressure and meals.

BEGINNING OF THE MUTATIONS.

Three points rule the first stage of a mutation: *K9, K11 and K24*. Let us consider these points separately.

· K9 governs the mutations during conception. It was the "Father of Acupuncture" in Europe himself, Soulié de Morant, who claimed that puncturing this point during pregnancy "creates a child with a nice color, immune to diseases, and healthy in body and mind." We also notice that this point is the Xi point of Yin Wei Mo.

· K11 rules the putting into movement of the food mutations. The point is indicated in case of digestive dysfunction with cachexia, fatigue and weakness.

· K24 dominates the spiritual mutations and is punctured in case of mental fatigue and absence of ideas.

IN SPACE

Shao Yin is the closing of the Yin to the Interior. (Figure 42)

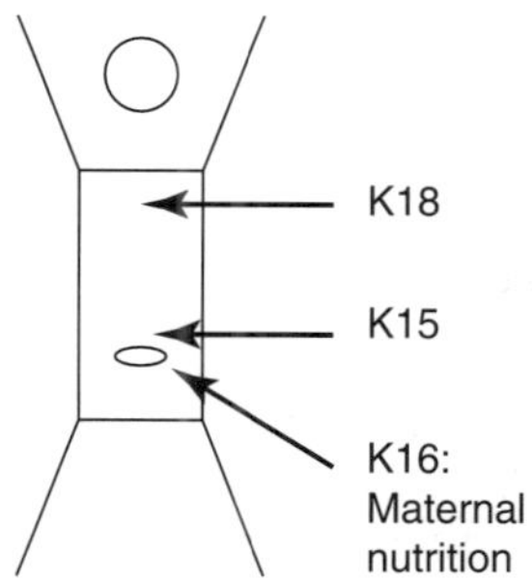

Figure 42

Three points correspond to this criterion: K15, K26 and K16.

· K15 is the closing of the Yin to the abdomen; it is indicated in abdominal Yin Emptiness through non-interiorization. Genital Yang inflammation, burning sensation in the abdomen, and diarrhea or constipation are commonly noted and improve under pressure (emptiness!).

· K26 is the closing of the Yin to the thorax, punctured in case of Emptiness of the Yin in the thorax. Symptoms are anger, congestion in the head (superficial Fullness of Yin), palpitations, dyspnea and cough (Emptiness of Yin in the thorax).

· K16 is the closing of the nourishing maternal Yin the fetus. It is indicated in case of recurrent abortions due to a malformation of the fetus, or due to maternal malnutrition or affective malnutrition. We note here a lack of warmth, hence a symptomatology type Cold: gastric spasms and diarrhea aggravated by exterior Cold or food.

IN TIME

Shao Yin is the putting into movement. (Figure 43) Four points rule this activity: K8, K19 and K12.

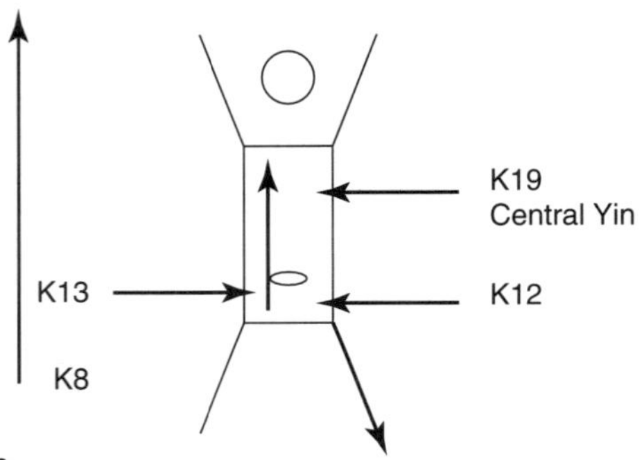

Figure 43

· K8 puts into movement the Yin of the lower part of the body and is punctured in stagnation of the Yin in the lower extremities, with Heat in the pelvis through the non-ascending of the Yin.

· K13 moves the pelvic Yin, therefore is punctured in stagnations of Yin the pelvis. Symptoms are spastic pains, backaches aggravated by cold and alleviated by heat, massage and movement.

· K19 puts the Yin into movement at the level of the trunk; it is the central Yin that is not distributed to the periphery. This point is indicated in stagnations of the central Yin, dominated by epigastric contractions and slow digestion, alleviated by warmth, massage and movement.

· K 12 puts into movement the genital Yin and is therefore punctured in case of difficult erection, sterility and genital congestion due to stagnation of Yin.

CASE HISTORY

Mrs. Jane, 55 years old, consults for "an ophthalmic" migraine on the left side. The recurring headache has existed for three years and irradicates to the thyroid and the naso-labial groove. One week ago, the situation became more complicated with the sudden appearance of a peri-orbital edema and the sensation that the eye was being pushed forward, without noticeable pain. Then three days ago, sharp pains appeared around the thyroid, especially in the evening. During the night, the pain disappears and sleep is not disturbed. The characteristics of the pain are important: less pain during the summer, aggravated by the pressure of glasses, aggravated by the movement of the eyes and improved by the application of a heated towel.

Analysis 1

According to the Eight Conditions:

- Sharp pain indicates a Yang state.
- Improvement by pressure indicates an emptiness. But pressure, or rather rubbing, by the glasses aggravates, while we would expect improvement since rubbing activates the circulation and offers more Qi.
- There is no aggravation with dampness, cold or wind, indicating that the disease is of Internal origin.
- The pain is improved by heat. Any Yang pain improved by heat must be a stagnation of Yang; but the pain is aggravated by massage whereas it should be improved.

Conclusion: the pain does not respond well to the Eight Conditions. What we must do is make a distinction between the pain peri-orbital and the eye pain itself.

1. The eye pain

   The pain is sharp (Yang), improves upon local pressure and heat, but is aggravated with eye movements. It is a Yang pain due to emptiness of the intra-cranial Yin (Xu Yang syndrome). Movement aggravates, since it uses Qi that is already exhausted.

2. The peri-orbital pain.

   Around the eye, there is pain and edema. The latter is a sign of stagnation. Heat improves any stagnation and therefore, in the summer (maximum Yang or Yang of the Yang), the pain is alleviated.

Inquiry.

- Social history:

  Father died of throat cancer at the age of 72; mother died at 69 of generalized Ca; familial problems and emotional disappointment in the marriage; patient is an introvert and does not share her problems with anybody.

- Personal history:

  For some years gastritis, with frequent vomiting and burning, contributed to her familial psychological problems (blockage at the level of the Stomach).

  Migraine, due to an Emptiness of Yin (lightheadedness, pressure on the eyeballs improves).

  Periodic pain in the ears, present since the onset of the headaches, confirms that we have an endocranial problem.

  Memory disturbances, especially since the headaches began, due to a lack of Yin or Blood in head.

  Menopause at 45, since the death of her husband, causing some hot flushes with perspiration. One normal pregnancy.

  For the rest, the history is negative and provides no special clue to her "migraine".

Analysis 2.

There is no trouble in the limbs or trunk that could explain the endocranial Yin. There is a blockage at the level of the St. which has been resolved for one year. This blocking was important, since it was at the level of the solar plexus, which is the center of the human being. From here the Yin and the Yang are distributed from the center to the periphery.

On the psychological level we find some important disturbances: amenorrhea when her husband died and loneliness, which causes an interiorization. There is a relation between this loneliness and the fact that the Yin does not ascend to the head (which is the normal movement of the Yin). The Yin is blocked in the Interior and cannot exteriorize.

At the level of the Five Elements, the center corresponds to the solar plexus. It is the center of man, distributing the Yang through CV12 and the Yin through Li13. With this knowledge, we try to find the cause of emptiness of Yin in the superior part of the body. There are two possibilities.

- Central blocking of the Yin caused by loneliness.
- A non-exteriorization of the Yin to the Yang.

For the second option, we cannot find an argument, since there is no symptomatology found in the inquiry, explaining a disturbance of a Yin or Fu organ (what we would expect in that case). There are also no symptoms of a non-passage of the Yin to the Yang in this patient: no troubles at the trunk and extremities, no cold feet, heavy legs or menstrual disturbances, indicating a stagnation of the Yin the pelvic area.

Conclusion: we find a central blocking of the Yin due to a psychological cause: loneliness creating an intra-cranial emptiness of Yin!

Therapy:

1) Treatment of the root: Li13 disperses the central Yin to the periphery; we strengthen the action of this point with Li3, Shu point or transporting point that helps to feed the Yin.
2) Cause the Yin to ascend to the head: once the central Yin is put into movement, we bring it to the head with a Sky-Window point. (See Paragraph VI on the Sky-Window points). SI17 makes the Yin ascend to the head and supplies the head with the Yin from the center.
3) Stagnation of Yang in the head: we need to put the Yang into movement. As explained in this chapter, this is accomplished by a point of Shao Yang or Cheou Shao Yang (head). This point is TB23.

The patient's problem was resolved in three treatments and no follow-up was necessary.

THE SKY-WINDOW POINTS

INTRODUCTION

In order to deal with a patient's problem, we must be able to skillfully adjust the Yin and Yang Energies in his body. An excess Yin condition in the lower portion of the body leads to a deficiency of Yin in the upper part with an excess Yang.

Symptoms will be heat in the head, with headaches, red eyes and anger. Excess Yin below will give cold symptoms, with varicose veins, cold feet, menstrual disturbances and leg cramps in the night.

To correct the condition we must bring the Yang to the lower portion of the body which will move the Yin, while we also will bring the Yin to the head. All the points involved in these movements are mentioned in this chapter. However, there is one important class of points extremely effective in this therapy, the Sky-Window points. From classical material (Ling Shu, Chapter 21), we first encounter a class of points located at or near the neck. These are **TB16, St9, LI8, B10 and L3.**

Through many years of clinical experience in Europe, it has been found that these Sky-Window points (so-named because they are grouped around the point TB16, Tien Yu, which roughly translates as *"Celestial Window"*) and other additional points, have an important energetic action. They may be used to open the channels in the neck area, thereby allowing the ascent or descent of their Yin or Yang. We will discuss the action of these different Sky-Window points, as well as other strong energetic points.

ACTION OF THE SKY-WINDOW POINTS

The Celestial-Window points, connecting the Earth-Qi to the Sky-Qi, all have connections with the Tching Pie or Divergent channels.

❑ **B10**

This point is indicated in case of Fullness of Yang in the upper part of the body. It makes the Yang descend from the head to the thorax. It will do wonders in case of headaches localized along the Bladder meridian. The sharp, intermittent headache, alleviated by Cold, will disappear instantly by opening B10.

❑ **St9**

This point has the opposite action of the previous one: it will be indicated in case of deficiency of Yang in the head. St9 makes the Yang ascend to the upper part of the body.

❑ **SI17**

This point has a similar action to St9. Instead of the Yang, it will make the Yin ascend to the head. Other points, such as K6 and PC5, will bring the Yin up to make it available in the neck area.

❑ **TB16**

All the other points are grouped around this Sky-Window point. It is especially indicated for deafness and loss of visual acuity.

❑ **LI18**

Dispels the Wind, relieves pain and is also indicated in case of aphasia.

❑ **L3**

Indicated in epistaxis and bleeding from the mouth.

OTHER POINTS FOR MOVING THE YIN AND YANG

Movement of the Yin

- Acceleration of the Yin: Yin Tsiao Mo and Shao Yin; we puncture K1, K6 and Sp6.
- Exteriorization of the Yin from the center to the periphery, causing a Fullness of Yin in the chest and Emptiness of the Yin in the head: L2.
- Stagnation of Yin in the pelvic area: CV4 will mobilize the Blood. B53 commands the "envelope" of the uterus. CV6 in tonification has the same action as CV4 in this case.
- Movement of the Yin at the level of the head: SI17 and GV22 will make the Yin ascend, while PC1 will make the Yin descend.
- Stagnation of Yin in the upper part is helped by H1.

Movement of the Yang

- Acceleration of the Yang, with points of Yang Tsiao Mo and Shao Yang: TB1, TB8, GB39, GB43 and B62.
- Exteriorization of the Yang to the center of the periphery, causing a Fullness of Yang central and Emptiness of the Yang in the periphery: CV12.
- Stagnation of the Yang in the pelvic area: GB28 and B32.
- Movement of the Yang at the level of the head: B10 and St9, mentioned in Paragraph II.
- Fullness of the Yang in the upper part of the body: St37 in tonification.
- Emptiness of Yang in the upper part of the body: St39 in dispersion.
- Emptiness of Yang in the lower back: GV4 and GV3.
- Stagnation of Yang in the upper part: TB1 and 8.
- Stagnation of Yang in the lower part: GB39.

BARRIER POINTS

GENERAL REMARKS

Pain, in Chinese Medicine, is translated as an obstruction or a disturbance in the Qi-circulation. Through the limbs, a person can communicate with the surrounding world: the extremities are places where there is a shifting of Energy from the exterior to the interior, and vice-versa. The "barriers" discussed in this chapter are the large joints in the body, the "articulations" that the Qi has to overcome. These articulations are under the command of certain important points: the *"barrier points"*. Puncturing these points will influence the inflow or outflow of Qi. These points can be compared to valves which can be opened or closed to allow free flow of the Qi (either Yang or Yin). The direction of the flow will be from the extremities toward the body, or vice-versa (Figure 44).

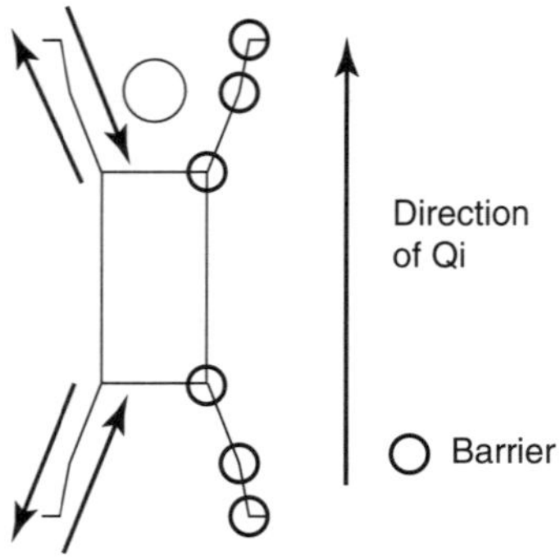

Figure 44

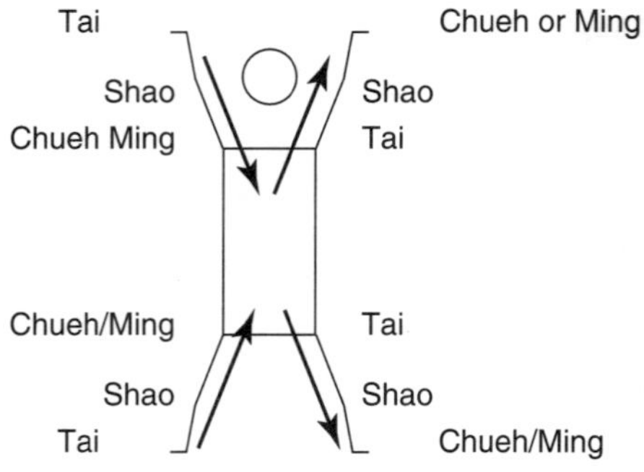

Figure 45

CLASSIFICATION OF QI

The Qi is classified according to its *origin*. We say that:

- Tai Yang or Tai Yin is the most *original* Qi, because it is nearest to the origin.
- Shao Yang or Shao Yin is the *middle* Qi.
- Yang Ming or Chueh Yin is the end or *terminal* Qi (Figure 45).

In describing Qi flowing **out** of the body, the Qi is classified as:

- Tai – shoulder/hip (joint),
- Shao – elbow/knee (joint),
- Chueh or Ming – wrist/foot (joint).

In describing Qi flowing **into** the body, the classification is reversed.

- Tai – wrist/food (joint),
- Shao – elbow/knee (joint),
- Chueh or Ming – shoulder/hip joint.

When the Qi does not **enter** the body properly, there is an accumulation of Qi at the articulation (joint); hence, a fullness of Qi in that area.

When the Qi does not freely **flow out** of the body, there will be an emptiness at the joint (Figure 46).

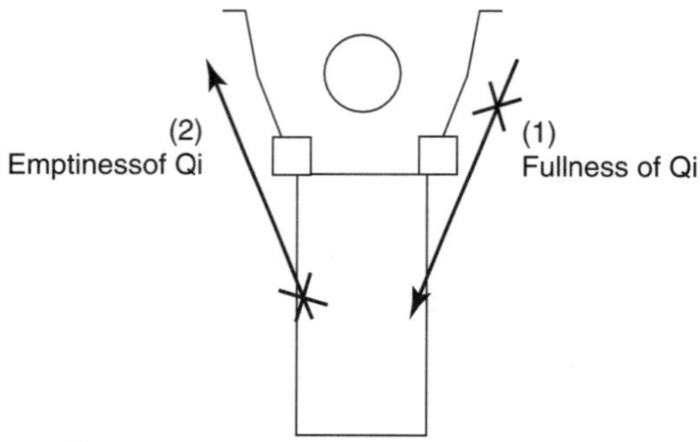

Figure 46

To clarify the application of the barrier points, we will describe the different possibilities of the *flow of the Qi at the level of the shoulder joint*. In Western medicine, this condition is known as "Peri-arthritis Humero Scapularis" (PHS) or "Frozen Shoulder".

According to the *Eight Conditions*, we will have four different clinical situations:

- Fullness of Yang or Yin
- Emptiness of Yang or Yin

Emptiness of Yang at the Shoulder

According to the law expressed in Figure 45, this means that the Yang Qi is not coming out of the body. The Yang Qi does not penetrate into the articulation of the shoulder, hence we have an emptiness of Yang at this joint.

How do we find the barrier point?

Upper extremity is CHEOU, lower extremity is often expressed at TSOU, ZU. The Yang Qi at the shoulder (our example) is the most original one, the nearest to the origin, therefore named TAI YANG (Figure 45).

The command point or barrier point in this case is located on CHEOU TAI YANG, or Small Intestine, specifically **SI2**.

What are the symptoms in this case?

Since there is an emptiness of Yang Qi, the symptoms at the shoulder will be Yin in nature. Weakness of Yang leads to a preponderance of Yin (Cold syndrome of Xu type). The type of pain will be one which is:

- Improved by pressure.
- Improved by Heat (Yang).
- Deep and not sharp (Yin).

In this case, the Yang needs to be strengthened. Dispersing of the Yin will not improve the patient, since this is a case of apparent Yin Excess (Figure 47).

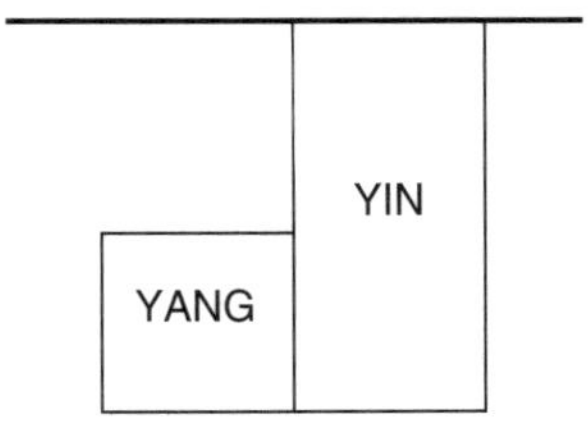

Figure 47

Emptiness of Yin at the Shoulder

According to the law expressed in Figure 46, this means that the Yin Qi is not coming out of the body and is not penetrating into the articulation; hence, we have an emptiness of Yin in this area.

How do we find the barrier point? It is the upper extremity, Cheou. It is the beginning of the Qi or original Qi, Tai Yin. The barrier point is found on CHEOU TAI YIN or LUNG: **L2**.

Symptoms: since there is an emptiness of Yin, the symptoms at this joint will be Yang, since weakness of Yin leads to preponderance of Yang (Heat syndrome of the Xu type).

The pain will have these characteristics:

- Improved by pressure.
- Improved by Cold (Yin).
- Sharp and superficial.

In this case, the Yin must be strengthened. Dispersing of the Yang Qi will aggravate the patient's condition, since this is a case of apparent Yang excess (Figure 48).

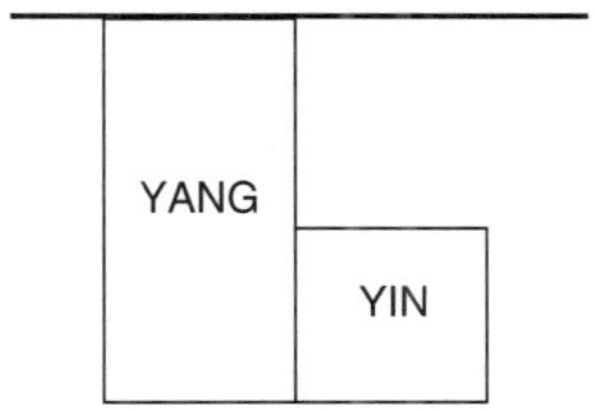

Figure 48

Fullness of Yang at the Shoulder

This means that the Yang Qi is not penetrating from the extremity into the body, but stagnates in the articulation. Now there is a preponderance of Yang, consuming the Yin.

What is the barrier point? It is the upper extremity, Cheou.It is the terminal Qi, Ming or Chueh, but Ming since it is Yang.The barrier point is found on CHEOU YANG MING or LARGE INTESTINE: **LI15**.

Symptoms: this time there is a real Yang excess (Heat syndrome of the Shi type). Characteristics of the pain:

- Worse with pressure.
- Worse with Heat.
- Improving with Cold.
- Sharp and superficial.

In this case, we will disperse the Yang (Figure 49).

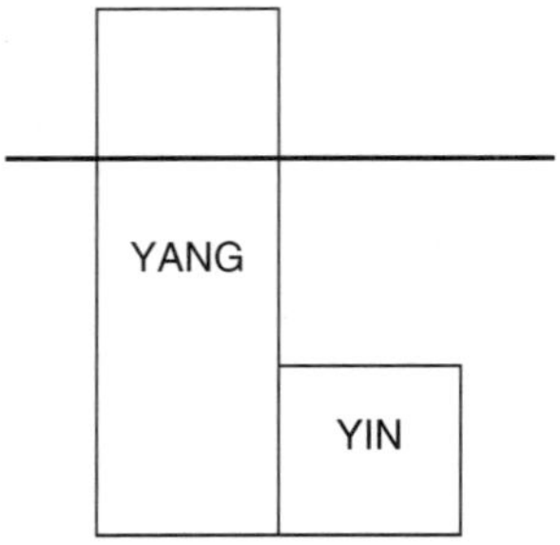

Figure 49

Fullness of Yin at the Shoulder

This means that the Yin Qi does not penetrate into the body, but stagnates in the articulation. This preponderance of Yin leads to a consuming of the Yang.

What is the barrier point? It is the upper extremity, Cheou. It is the terminal Qi, Chueh, since it is Yin.

The barrier point is found on CHEOU CHUEH YIN or PERICARDIUM: **PC2.**

There is a real Yin Excess (Cold syndrome of the Shi type).

Characteristics of the pain:

- Worse with pressure.
- Worse when exposed to Cold.
- Improves with Heat.
- Deep and dull.

In this case we will strengthen the Yang. We could disperse the Yin, but the Yin is less mobile; hence, the result will come at a later moment. For a fast result, mobilize the Yang with LI4 and TB5[t] (Figure 50).

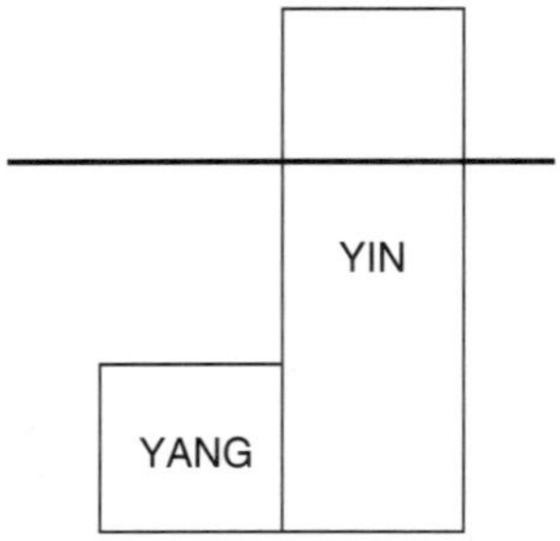

Figure 50

CONCLUSION

The barrier points are important points for the diagnosis as well as for the therapy. Diagnostic: the points become painful spontaneously or upon pressure, indicating to us the right point to puncture. Therapeutic: without any doubt, use of these points gives faster and more permanent results for the patient.

APPENDIX: THE BARRIER POINTS

EMPTINESS OF YANG

Shoulder:	SI11	Hip:	B129
Elbow:	TB13	Knee:	GB3
Wrist:	LI8	Foot:	St37

EMPTINESS OF YIN

Shoulder:	L2	Hip:	Sp1
Elbow:	H6*	Knee:	K5 *
Wrist:	PC4 *	Foot	Li6*

FULLNESS OF YANG

Shoulder:	L15	Hip:	St31*
Elbow:	TB7	Knee:	GB36*
Wrist:	LI6	Foot:	BL63

FULLNESS OF YIN

Shoulder:	PC6	Hip:	Li2
Elbow:	H6*	Knee:	K5*
Wrist:	LI6*	Foot:	Sp8*

* For the unknown barrier points, the accumulation point of the involved meridian is used.

Diseases of the Pei (Bi) or Rheumatic Diseases 12

INTRODUCTION

Even today with our sophisticated medicine, arthritic diseases are one of the most crippling illnesses afflicting people. Every year hundreds of thousands are newly affected. Hundreds of different medications have not been successful in eliminating the terrible deformations. However, arthritis is not a new disease but apparently well-known long before this era. In the ancient Chinese textbooks, the Pei diseases, as they are called, are described extensively. For the Chinese, Pei or Bi designates *"all illnesses characterized by pain and numbness of joints and muscles."*

In Chapter 43 of the *Su Wenn*, the causes and types of rheumatic diseases are presented:

"... they are caused by the combined effect of Wind, Cold and Dampness."

We have the following categories of Pei diseases according to the Pernicious Qi that is deemed to be the cause:

- ❑ Pei with predominance of Wind, or "erratic" or "wandering" Pei.
- ❑ Pei with predominance of Cold, or "painful" Pei;
- ❑ Pei with predominance of Dampness, or "fixed" Pei.

Another classification is according to the Five Elements. We have "five Pei diseases": Pei of the Heart, Spleen, Lung, Kidney and Liver. As long as the disease is of recent origin and not serious, the Pei will be localized in one of the tissues of these organs. This is the case when the so-called "perverse" or External" Energies have not had the opportunity to attack the system repeatedly. However, if the attacks continue, with the patient continuing to show less resistance, the disease will evolve to deeper levels. By this process, it will eventually invade the organs.

EVOLUTION OF THE PEI

There are various External Energies that can attack and invade the body. These Qi's, or so-called "perverse" Energies, are:

Cold—Heat—Wind (Fong)—Summer Heat—Dampness—Dryness

These are also referred to as the *"Six Excesses or Pernicious Influences."*

Through a detailed study of nature, the Chinese have learned that these Six Excesses have a predilection in the body as to where they may most easily invade. For instance, cold initially attacks the Small Intestine and Bladder meridians, which form the level Tai Yang. Figure 28 illustrates the meridians where these Six Excesses attack. It also illustrates that Tai Yin and Tai Yang form a first obstacle or barrier against Cold or Dampness. If the barrier is relatively strong, the attack will be stopped in the exterior. "Pei of the Skin" might develop and would have the most favorable resolution. *"When Pei is in the skin, then the cure will be easy."* (Su Wen, Chapter 43)

What prevents the disease of the Pei from evolving to deeper levels? In other words, what is needed for the first barrier or level to be strong enough to resist the exterior aggression? To resist further evolution of the disease, the organism must fulfill two conditions:

- ❏ The Tai Yang must have enough Yang. If this is the case, then the Yang of Tai Yang will be able to absorb the excesses of Dampness and Cold, which are both Yin. This is why a Yang constitution can resist a Yin disease very easily, but not a Yang affliction, and why a Yin constitution will resist a Yang disease.
- ❏ The body must have enough Wei Qi so that it can resist the exterior aggression. It is known that the Wei energy is produced in the superior Triple Burner and Inferior Triple Burner. Therefore, it is important that both of these are functioning well. Also, since Tchong Mo forms an elevator through the three Triple Burners to spread the Qi in all the Zang and Fu organs, it is important that Tchong Mo is functioning at its normal levels of capabilities.

If these two conditions are not met, the Excesses will then be able to penetrate into the depth and reach the second barrier, which is formed by the Chueh Yin and Shao Yang. At this level, Pei of the Fong (attacking the muscles and tendons) can develop. If the Pei penetrates deeper, the third barrier formed by Yang Ming and Shao Yin is reached. Here the first symptoms of the "bone Pei" appear. Once this barrier is penetrated, the Perverse Energy will penetrate into the organs. (figure 29)

DIFFERENT FORMS OF THE PEI

PEI CAUSED BY COLD OR PEI OF THE BONES.

1. Characteristics.

Pei caused by Cold is painful, sharply defined and located in the joints. This is described in Chapter 43 of the "Su Wenn":

"There is pain when Cold is the aggressive factor. The Cold can attack if there is an abundance of Yin in the organism, in contrast with the Yang. The Cold of the disease combines with the Yin of the body. If the body possesses enough Yang, then the Yang will defeat the aggressor Yin in the meeting between the Yin and Yang."

Most of the time, a patient will not seek treatment until the Cold has reached the third level or Shao Yin. Usually, the previous stages are not recognized by the patient as symptoms of disease. We have to stress the fact that the symptoms of the Pei *do not conform* with the Eight Conditions, which facilitates the differential diagnosis with other diseases.

2. Therapy.

To facilitate an understanding of the therapy, an example of Pei of the *Cold in the shoulder joint* will be discussed.

❏ Pathogenesis

Pei pain is almost always a Yin pain: worse at rest, improving with warmth and movement, night pain, continuous, and stiffness in the morning. As stated previously, the patient most of often seeks treatment when Excess Cold has penetrated the level of Shao Yin.

The first measures to be taken are directed toward keeping the disease at this level in order to inhibit the Cold from penetrating the organs. At the level of Shao Yin, there is more Qi than Xue, more Yang than Yin. The difference in Qi and Xue at the progressive levels (the so-called "Great Meridians") are mentioned in the "Su Wenn", Chapter 24. They are illustrated in Figure 50.

Xue > Qi	Tai Yang
Qi > Xue	Shao Yang
Qi = Xue	Yang Ming
Qi > Xue	Tai Yin
Xue > Qi	Tsiue Yin
Qi > Xue	Shao Yin

Figure 50

The practical application of this knowledge is of great value and is demonstrated in the therapy of the Pei diseases. For instance, when we wish to "obtain" Yang from somewhere in the organism, it would be incorrect to look for it in Tai Yang: this Great Meridian has more Xue (Yin) than Qi (Yang). Shao Yang, full of Qi, will be a better choice!

Returning to our example, we see that Shao Yin normally has more Yang than Yin. Because our patient presents Pei symptoms, it means that the Perverse Qi Cold has been able to penetrate this Shao Yin level. In normal circumstances the abundant Yang of Shao Yin withstands the Cold or Yin attack. This was not the case with our patient, which can only mean that Shao Yin did not have enough Yang Qi! Hence, the first logical step in our therapy: increase the Yang Qi in Shao Yang or in the Kidney, most important organ of this Great Meridian. This will be only one of four steps as explained below.

- ❏ Therapeutic steps.
- · Sending Yang to the Kidney.

In general, there are four excellent points for bringing warmth or Yang to the body. These points were found through extensive clinical experience. They are: **St36, GV4, St30 and K3**. Our first step is puncturing K3 with a golden needle and heating it for a few seconds.

- · Sending Yang to the area of pain.

We return to our example of Pei of the Cold in the shoulder joint. How do we bring more Yang Qi to the Shoulder? We use the centripetal or "entering meridians", which are the Yang meridians of the arm: Small Intestine, Large Intestine and Triple Burner.

According to figure 50, only one of these meridians will fulfill the purpose of bringing Yang Qi locally: this meridian is the Triple Burner, having *more Qi than Xue*. The SI contains more Xue than Qi while the LI has equal amounts of Qi and Xue!

The next step is to determine which point on TB is the best one to select. The junction between the superficial and deep part of the Primary Meridian is the Ho point. From here, the Qi of the arm Yang meridians travels from the surface to the Interior. (See Chapter 4) We will disperse this Ho point, which is like opening a faucet to the shoulder: this means TB10[(d)].

An alternate technique of sending Yang locally involves manipulation of the system of small blood vessels traveling to and from the meridians. These are the *"efferent"* vessels (those traveling away from the meridians) and *"afferent"* vessels (those traveling toward the meridians). The proper ones to use in this case are the efferent vessels. For the shoulder joint, this point is TB15[(d)].

- · Puncturing the Jin point (River-Traversing point).

The Jing point is either the Fire point of the Yang or Fu organs, or the Metal point of the Yin or Yang organs. Inasmuch as Fire and Dryness are both Yang, the Jing point is a favorable point to use in any treatment of rheumatism, which is a Yin disease. Specifically, our therapy here is puncturing the Jing point of the involved meridian in tonification: TB6[(t)].

- · Puncturing an important point locally.

For Pei of the Cold, this last therapeutic gesture must be given very careful consideration. This point needs to be determined by a process of elimination: it may *not* be an opening point, a confluent point of an Extra meridian, or a crossing point or meeting point. For instance, LI15 is an important point of the shoulder, but it is also a meeting point with Yang Tsiao Mo. In other words, dispersing this point (which will be done for this kind of pain) would disperse or drain the Yang, just the opposite of what *should* be done. Instead, SI19[(d)] can be used to disperse the pain.

PEI CAUSED BY WIND (FONG) OR PEI OF THE MUSCLES.

1. Pathogenesis.

This form of Pei is also called the *"wandering"* Pei: the disease wanders just as the Wind does not remain in one place. The Excess Fong has a predilection for the Shao Yang/Chiueh level. Once the patient shows the muscle pain associated with this Pei, we know that the Fong has been able to penetrate the Tai Yang level, normally rich in Xue or Yin (*Figure 50*). Since the Excess Fong has a Yang nature (Wind is moving, and thus Yang), it means that there was not enough Yin Qi in Tai Yang to counter the Yang Fong. Of course, it is of no use to increase the Yin in Tai Yang once the patient already demonstrates the Pei symptoms. We have to concentrate our therapy on the second level, Shao Yang/ Chiueh Yin, in order to prevent the Fong from going deeper.

2. Therapy.

The most effective weapon against Fong is Fire. This natural defense mechanism is well demonstrated in infectious diseases where the Wind (catching a cold on a chilly, windy day) will trigger fever in the patient. The fever is indeed a favorable sign, proof that our Vital Qi is still strong enough to fight a Pernicious Excess.

· Increase the Fire.

As explained above, the first step will be to send Heat or Fire into Fong: GB44[d]. This is part of the therapy of the roots, which explanation is beyond the scope of this work.

· Increase Heat and Wei Qi in the joints.

The Heat points or Fire points are the Jing (river, traversing) points which are tonified. Cutaneous stimulation can be applied along the Tendino-Muscular Meridians to increase the Wei Qi.

· Puncture the Fong point.

All these points are formed from the point Wind or Feng:

Feng Shi (GB 20)
Feng FU (GV 16)

The puncturing of these points chases the Wind and makes the body sweat.

CASE HISTORIES.

1. *Patient:* Alice, 55 years old, with hypertension, Pei of the shoulder and hip.

a. Treatment of hypertension.

Hypertension is Excess of Fire, Excess of Yang in the Heart, and consequently, Emptiness of Yang in the Kidneys. Therapy is tonification of the Fire point of the Kidneys (K2) and warming it up; also heating the Inferior Triple Burner where the Kidneys are located: St36[(t)], St37[(t)] and St39[(t)].

b. Treatment of the shoulder.

As explained previously, K3[(t)], TB10[(d)], TB6[(t)] and SI19[(d)].

c. Treatment of the hip.

Repeat first step: K3[(t)]. Second step is dispersing the Ho point of the entering meridian with much Qi: K10[(d)]. However, an exception must be made in this case, as this patient has hypertension or lack of Yang in the Kidneys. At this stage of the disease, this point should not be punctured. Only after subsequent treatment (after sufficient Yang has entered the Kidneys by treating K2), will it be possible to utilize K10. Thirdly, the Jing point of the involved meridian is tonified: GB 8[(t)]. Finally, we disperse an important point in the region of the pain: GB30[(d)].

2. *Pei of the spinal column.*

Step 1: bring Yang into the K: K3[(t)].

Step 2: disperse the H point of the involved meridian. However, in this case if B40 is punctured, the meridian will be opened and Qi will flow out from the Interior. B40 drains the Heat (Yang) out of the body and therefore should not be punctured.

Step 3: treat the Jing point of the involved meridian. Since the Governing Vessel has no Jing point, the question is, "How can Yang be brought into *the spinal column*?"

Three different points are used:

- Yang in the inferior part of the column (GV4; GV1) is actually the most powerful point; however, for patient comfort, GV4 can be substituted.
- Yang in the middle part of the column: GV10.
- Yang in the inferior part: GV16.

The above points can be tonified by heating. With treatment of these points, the Governing Vessel is filled with Yang. The GV will now fulfill its normal function.

Step 4: Sedate an important point in the region of the pain. Sedating B11, an important point in the spinal column, may cause a dispersal of the Yang, which is to be avoided, since we want to increase the Yang.

APPENDIX ONE: IMPORTANT POINTS OF THE MAJOR JOINTS

A. UPPER EXTREMITIES.

- Shoulder: LI15, LI 5. LI14, TB14, TB15, SI9, 10 and 11.
- Elbow: TB10, SI8, SI11, PC3, L5 and H3.
- Wrist: PC7, H7, L9, TB4, LI15 and TB5.

B. LOWER EXTREMITIES.

- Hip: GB30, St35, GB34, Sp9, Sp10, GB35, B40, Li8, and K10.
- Knee: St36, St35, GB34, Sp9, Sp10, GB35, B40, Li8 and K10.
- Ankle: St41, B60, K6, Sp5, Li4 and GB41.

C. GENERAL POINTS.

- TB5: called "the arthritis point.
- Sp5: influential point for the articulations.
- Genital point: in ear acupuncture, with gold needle.

Causes of Disease 13

THE CLUE TO CURE CHRONIC DISEASES

For a practitioner, every investigation into an illness starts with a good history. Getting the facts together, the symptoms with their modalities and the different factors in the patient's life-style contributing to the disease are essential if we want to be successful in restoring the patient's health. Yet, most of the time, the most important question is often neglected by the physician: "What happened in your life when you became sick or just before you became sick?" I see enough doctors' reports from my patients. They are explicit enough in the description of symptoms and the enumeration of the different illnesses, but they rarely link the onset of the disease to a meaningful event in the patient's life. Yet, it is most often the clue to the solution. Our lives are a succession of events, some more traumatic than others. A human being is like an onion wrapped in many different layers. Each time a person is subjected to a physical or emotional injury *strong enough to create symptoms*, we have a new layer to treat. A person suffering with a chronic ailment usually has a long medical story encompassing a number of ailments which have been manifested at different periods in the patient's life. To the holistic practitioner, the entire history is a connected sequence of different initiating causes. In order to accomplish a real "cure," it is necessary not only to eliminate the ailment from which the patient is currently complaining, but also the entire background of disease. This means that a well-chosen therapy (homeopathic or acupuncture) will have the result of regressing the patient (though often in a less aggravated form) through every illness that has been suffered in his or her life. This is mainly because all those previous illness were **suppressed,** not cured!

This is completely different from what we do in modern medicine. Ask a so-called "mainstream" physician what constitutes a cure, and he is apt to say that the results of the disease must be removed. If there is a tumor, cut it out. If there is an abscess, drain it. If digestion is disordered and intestines clogged, use a purge. If there is fever, use a medicine to lower the temperature. Sounds easy, doesn't it? But are such treatments real and complete? Far from it. This attempt to treat disease solely on the basis of tissue changes ignores the person who lives in his or her body as a house. Such treatment removes external expressions of disorder itself, and so sends the expression deeper into more vital centers, the organs. It will make the patient incurable and is partly responsible for the increase in nervous disorders, cancers, TB and mental disease.

Why is this happening? Most of us are probably under the impression that the medical profession has arrived at a zenith of scientific achievement, from which it will go on from triumph to triumph. But medicine suffers from a defect which, unless remedied, may halt its future progress. The defect is that

Western medicine is NOT a science in the sense in which mathematics, chemistry and physics are sciences. What makes a science is not the collection of data, but the organization and generalization of those facts according to the formulation and understanding of laws. Medicine will not achieve the stature of a science until the basic laws of health and disease have been disclosed. But the search for these laws still has to begun. We may not make the same mistake as a holistic practitioner because we don't have an excuse: we have laws and principles in homeopathy and acupuncture. We have the Sheng-cycle, the Ko-and anti Ko-cycle, the Five Elements, the Eight Conditions, etc. Treating acute diseases is mostly easy, and frankly, most of those illnesses would be cured if not faster, at least as fast if the physician would not interfere with Nature. But Western medicine suppresses superficial symptoms like rashes, discharges, warts, and cysts and pushes the disease back against the natural direction of cure, provided by Nature. "Nature heals while the physician amuses the patient" is so much the truth in many acute illnesses. The real practitioner, alternative or not, stands out who can alter and eradicate true chronic diseases.

Why is it that traditional Western medicine is so ill at ease with the treatment of chronic disease? Why are those patients with chronic illness so often referred to a psychiatrist? Why is it that a homeopathic physician and acupuncturist can be very successful in treating chronically ill patients? Psychiatry, acupuncture and homeopathy share a common premise: that the patient is an individual, different and unique. For both the psychiatrist and the alternative physician, the whole of the patient is greater than the sum of all of his or her parts. A patient who assumes a chronically ill role needs to be evaluated as a person with physical and emotional needs, instead of being labeled "neurotic." For the alert physician, it means doing more than just jotting down a diagnosis of pathology and then giving out a prescription. A chronically ill person has anxieties, anger and depression because of built-up tensions. If the physician does not find a way to help that person release tension, to build up his or her self-worth, then the physician has not helped at all. Mankind has major needs which, if not fulfilled, either directly cause his illness or are certainly major contributing factors to his dis-ease. Practitioners must consider these major needs of each individual at each interview. Failure to do so inevitably leads to the lingering on of the diseased state. If any practitioner wants to understand the clue to the solution of chronic diseases, his full attention has to be turned to the pathogenic factors known to cause illness. Only by treating the *beginning* of the disease can we rightfully expect to cure the endings of the disease. Anything less is a folly, that is unworthy of the name of healing! The next paragraph will have an in-depth look at these different factors.

THE DIFFERENT PATHOGENIC FACTORS

It is ironic that Chinese medicine established the different groups of disease provoking factors already 5,000 years ago, where Western medicine still struggles with the cause of many "mystery" diseases. Of course, names are established for these conditions, and sometimes a defective gene or chromosome is found, or a state of pathology is described, but the answer to the question, : "What are you going to do for this condition?" draws often a blank. The Chinese, through diligent observation of Nature (and it is my sincere opinion that in Nature all answers lie), made all the connections as we have described them in the previous chapters with emotions, colors, tastes, foods, functions, tissues, etc. linked to a *specific* organ. What a pity of Western medicine not to have looked into this matter more closely. For Traditional Chinese Medicine, anything that will disrupt the flow of the body "blood-Qi" will affect the meridian and function of the organ or the collective functions of the organs. These factors are classified in:

INTERNAL: "Seven Emotions"
EXTERNAL: "Six Pernicious Qi's"
NOT INTERNAL—NOT EXTERNAL:
"Injury"
"Diet"
"Poisons"

This was 5,000 years ago. Some of these terms definitely have to be extended to be adjusted to modern times. The "Seven Emotions", in my opinion one of the most important, if not the most important causes of disease, are discussed in a different chapter (chapter 14).

POISONS

I guess the term *"poison"* has to be much more extended now. We have the pollution in the air, the indoor-pollution (the well-known "Sick-Building Syndrome"), the poisoning of our food through additives, hormones, antibiotics and coloring substances, the poisoning of our ground waters, and the "iatrogenic" poisoning. Lately, an outcry about suppressing effects of different medical substances have been submerging in the literature: the silicone breast implants, the experiments on sick and dying people with radio active materials without their consent as happened in the 60s', mercury dental fillings, the misuse of antibiotics which has lead to the creation of "super bugs" resistant to any antibiotic with the comeback of "cured" diseases like TB, syphilis, and gonorrhea. In my opinion, it is not even the tip of the iceberg. One of these days, Western medicine will have to deal with their constant acts of *suppression* through cortisone ointments, cauterization or lasering of warts, cysts, tumors, chemotherapy, radiation, etc. No wonder the task of a practitioner today is much more difficult then it was thousands of years ago. One issue deserves special attention: the *mercury issue* in dental fillings.

In December 1990, *60 Minutes*, CBS's nationally televised feature program, aired an excellent survey of the mercury dental filling controversy. The American Dental Association is adamant that mercury fillings are non-toxic and completely safe. However, many countries in Europe (Sweden, Germany) have banned the use of mercury after clinical reports indicated that mercury fillings are toxic and may lead to brain damage. The big question is: how can you know in advance whether removal of your mercury fillings will benefit you? Removal of mercury, depending on the amount you have in your mouth, can cost you thousands of dollars. And indiscriminate removal of mercury fillings is as much a disservice to the patient as putting it in.

Homeopathy has the answer. Don't forget that mercury was a medication used in Hahnemann's time by his contemporary physicians in the treatment of syphilis. They used it in gross toxic doses so that the keen Hahnemann got "provings" of this remedy just by watching the results on the poorly treated patients. Through the poisonous effects of mercury, which is one way to know the effects of it, and through Hahnemann's own provings (which is given a dose of Mercury 30C daily till the appearance of symptoms without nefast effects of health on the individual) we know that mercury fillings *are* a problem if you have some of the following symptoms:

- Foul-smelling breath with metallic taste.
- Presence of a geographic tongue.
- Imprints of teeth on sides of tongue (liver sign!).
- Recurrent presence of canker sores/ herpes sores within the mouth.
- Bleeding, receding gums with tendency to ulceration.
- Heavy salivation with intense thirst.
- Abscessed teeth.
- Trembling tongue: quivering (again Liver sign!).
- Recurrent pharyngitis and swollen glands.

Notice that all of the above symptoms listed are located in the mouth. It is precisely here that we have the highest concentration of mercury in the dental fillings, causing many of the above mentioned symptoms. But there are others:

- Severe weakness and fatigue.
- Recurrent colds: because of lack of adequate Wei Qi.
- Great sensitivity to warmth and cold: the patient is a human barometer.
- Excessive sweating at night.

- Brainfag and weak memory.
- Chills and fever.
- Volatile nature—changeable, impulsive.
- Worries and has great anxiety about health.
- Highly sensitive to the environment.

Is extraction the only therapy possible? In case you have doubts and hesitate to spend thousands of dollars to change all your mercury fillings, you could take Mercury Solubilis 6C, 3 pellets twice a day for at least one month and see if your symptoms improve. If they improve, this means you have mercury poisoning and would benefit from extraction. The dentist should take this mercury out in different stages to avoid aggravation from too much released mercury in the blood stream. As usual, prevention is the best therapy. In case your patient needs a new filling, advise him to ask the dentist to use inorganic cement or porcelain. You will save yourself and your patient a lot of trouble!

THE SIX PERNICIOUS QI'S

We already discussed some in Chapter 4 on the "Great Meridians" and further in the chapter on the Pei diseases. The Chinese sometimes call them the Six Evil Winds. What are they?

Wind–Cold–Damp–Summer Heat–Fire–Dryness

These Pernicious Qi's usually attack the body in combination: Heat-Dampness, Cold-Dampness, Wind-Heat, etc. Again through great observation the Chinese figured out what level in the body would be attacked and what organ by each of those exterior evils. We have discussed this in figure 28.

WIND

Diseases caused by "Wind or Fong" have characteristics inherent to the swirling wind itself: rapidly moving, changes from place to place, comes and goes quickly, and speedy changes. So pains move around the body, dizzy feelings, spasms, convulsions, jerky movements, involuntary contractions (fibrillations and fasciculations) are all an expression of Wind-involvement. As you can see, these are hard to control diseases, they appear from nowhere suddenly and then stop. The Wind is light and has therefore a tendency to go upwards towards the head creating headaches, insomnia, strokes (internal Wind creation). What are symptoms of "Internal and External" Wind?

Internal Wind causes dizziness, ringing in the ears, numbness in limbs, spasms, sudden stroke, Bell's palsy, dyspnoe, narcolepsy and unconsciousness.

External Wind will provoke fever, fear and sensitivity to Wind, stuffy nose, itchy throat, nasal discharge (clear or yellow), chills, coldness in limbs, edema of face, thirst, dry cough, epistaxis, hoarse voice, headaches and a floating pulse.

General Wind-points are B12 and LI18 (a Sky-Window point) while the Ting points of the Yin meridians and the Iu points of the Yang points can be used to dispel the Wind (Chapter 4-I-C on the Penn points or protection points). Fong has a predilection for Chiueh Yin but can of course attack any level of the "Great Meridians or Six Levels" as long as the circumstances are right. I.e. Fong (Yin) attacks Tai Yang (contains more Qi than Blood) and can penetrate it when there is a deficiency of Qi only, otherwise the excess Yang will "drown" the Yin (Fong).

COLD

Cold makes us think of frozen, ice-like, hence immovable. Cold will always stagnate or slow down. We can use this therapeutically to slow down the excessive Yang Qi, traveling along a meridian.

Symptoms of *external cold* are fear of cold, fever, no sweating, body aches, sore joints (like a flu with deep bone pains, especially in the long bones), clear sputum, clear runny nose, clear urine, and watery stools.

Symptoms of *internal cold* (Yang Qi weak especially in K and Sp) demonstrate a white face, fear of cold, cold limbs, watery stools, abdominal pains, vomiting of clear fluids and a slow and deep pulse.

FIRE/HEAT

Fire is more extreme than heat. Heat means acceleration of Qi. The entire body is warm, there is high fever, a craving for cold drinks, red eyes, red urine, canker sores, carbuncles, a tongue with a yellow fur and a fast pulse. The fire can dry up the liquids, causing extreme thirst and dry stools. It can also affect the spirit or Chenn and cause delirium, fits or craziness in patients with high fever. Speech can be incoherent, the urine yellow, nose bleeds and vomiting blood. These are all signs of true Yang (Fire) excess.

This is different from the apparent or empty fire: there is a deficient Yin, causing false Yang excess symptoms like intermittent fevers, insomnia, dry tongue, dry cough, red cheeks and red tongue. Diseases are TB and diabetes.

DAMPNESS

Another Yin evil, resembling "puddles being stuck" or a "moist cloth." It is sticky and greasy, it "does not go away easily", it stands still and stagnates and illness caused by dampness will last long and is difficult to recover. This exterior dampness is caused by the environment, damp air, living in a damp place, and damp cloths by increased sweating.

Symptoms of *external dampness* are a feeling of a heavy and tired body, the head especially is heavy "as if a bag is sitting on the top of it." The joints feel sore, the chest is full, there is loss of appetite, afternoon fever, a white sticky fur on the tongue and a slow pulse.

Symptoms of *internal dampness* are a distended abdomen and chest, with loss of appetite, nausea, lack of taste, edema, leucorrhea, little urination, watery stool, and a dirty, greasy for especially in middle of tongue.

SUMMER HEAT

This Yang evil easily injures the liquids and wastes the Qi. Usually it is accompanied by Dampness.

Symptoms are high fever, thirst, irritability, sweating, easily tired, dry lips and skin, and nausea.

DRYNESS

Most common in the Fall. It is a Yang evil, causing dry skin and mucosae (lips, mouth, nose, etc.), epistaxis, painful throat, dry cough, and dry tongue with little fur are all signs of *external dryness. Internal* dryness is a sign of empty Yin which is reflected in infectious diseases with little expectoration.

PERNICIOUS QI ATTACK ON THE GREAT MERIDIANS

ATTACK ON THE EXTERIOR LAYER, TAI YANG

We already discussed the attack of Fong on Tai Yang (See Wind above).

Cold attack

Since Tai Yang contains more Qi than Blood, in order for the cold to penetrate, there has to be a deficiency of Yang in Tai Yang. This will be a chilly patient who fears the cold and does not transpire. The treatment is described in the old books: bringing heat to the surface by dispersing the root point of Shao Yin, or more accurately, the major season point of Shao Yin: K1 in spring, K2 in Summer, K3 in Long Summer, etc. Figure 51.

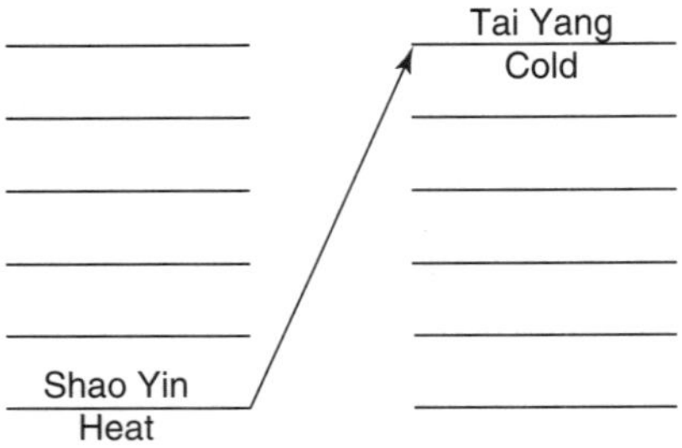

Figure 51

Heat attack

An external attack from heat (like in a sunstroke) will be successful if there is very little Yin in Tai Yang to fight the massive amount of Yang provided by the Pernicious Qi. As we know, since Tai Yang has already less Blood than Qi, long time exposure to extreme heat temperatures will revoke this situation. There will be great thirst and fear for heat. Therapy will be the *perspiration* technique (chapter 4, VI-G). We have to bring more Yin to the surface to counter the excessive Yang. The lack of Yin at the surface is caused by an imbalance in Tai Yin. The Yin of the superficial layer is represented by Tai Yin (the Sp.). The Sp. is Dampness, so the Sp is Tonified and disperse the L, which is too yang.

ATTACK ON THE MIDDLE LAYER, SHAO YANG

The middle layer is the second defense barrier of our body. Fong, heat or cold will all bring the same symptoms when TB-GB is attacked: chills and fever, nausea, bitter taste, pain in the sides and heart pain (Midday-midnight connection of GB and H!). The treatment is explained in chapter 62 of the *"So Ouenn": regularization* (Chapter 4, VI-G).

ATTACK ON THE DEEP LAYER, YANG MING

This is the last "Yang" barrier with symptoms of fever, thirst, constipation, bad taste in mouth, swollen glands and an ever changing pulse. Treatment is described in "Nei King" , Chapter 23: *purging* (chapter 4, VI-G). For the meridians, disperse the Ting points. For the organs, disperse the root points of LI-St.

ATTACK ON THE FIRST YIN LEVEL, TAI YIN

According to figure 50, Tai Yin contains more Qi than Blood. When the dampness of the Sp is in excess (an external fullness), then Tai Yin will be attacked. Anorexia, distention and diarrhea are common symptoms. Again, the So Ouenn gives the solution: *harmonization*. We will send Yang to Tai Yin, in fullness of yin, by dispersing the root point of the St. Since St is coupled organ to the Sp, we accentuate this action by dispersing the Lo point of the St. (Figure 52).

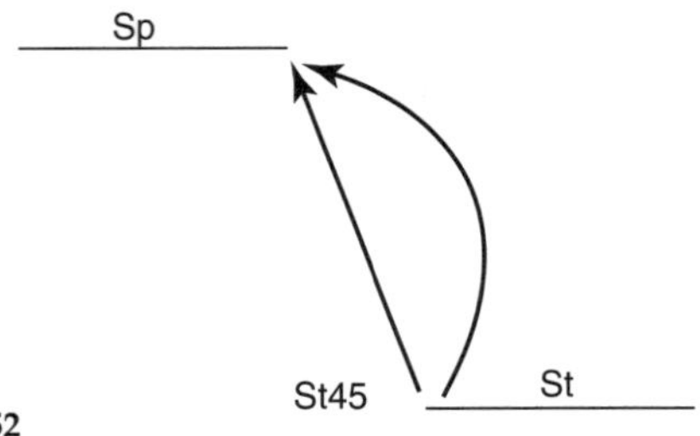

Figure 52

ATTACK ON MIDDLE YIN, CHUEH YIN

According to Figure 50, Chueh Yin contains more Blood (Yin) than Qi. An attack of *Cold* is successful when TB-PC is full with Yin and lacks Yang. To remedy the situation, we bring Yang in general (St36, GV4, LI4) and the Iong (fire) points of the organs involved. An attack of *Heat* is successful when this axis has a deficiency of Yin. Therapy is dispersing the Pernicious Heat by dispersing the Iong point of the organs or to tonify the Iu (Dampness) of the organs. (Dampness is son of Fire, tonifying Dampness will drain the Heat).

ATTACK ON DEEPEST YIN, SHAO YIN

Shao Yin has more Qi than Blood. An emptiness of Yang will allow an attack of a Pernicious Qi. The main attack will come from Cold (excess Yin) creating the picture of arthritis with a patient who is chilly, fears the cold and has cold limbs. Therapy consists in tonifying all the Yang: St36, GV4, GV14, LI4, K3, B25.

Summary of Great meridians in Figure 53.

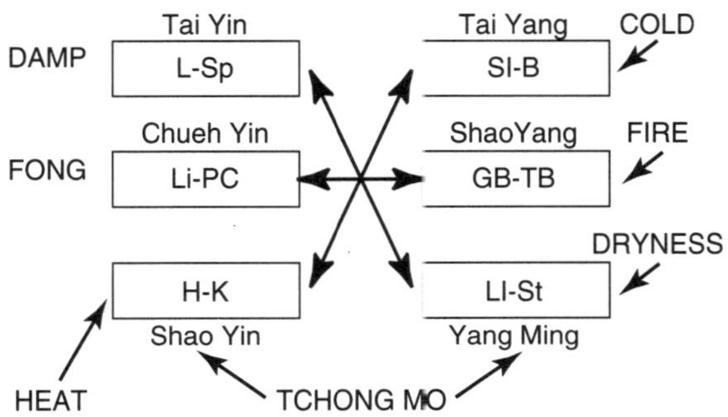

Figure 53

AFFAIRS OF THE BEDROOM

The ancient Chinese believe that a person is capable of living for at least 110 years. To reach longevity however, a person has to avoid the attacks of Pernicious Qi as well as those of diet and emotions. The latter two belong to the internal causes of which sexual habits also constitute an important part of. The arts of bedroom affairs became a well-established branch of Chinese medicine whose ideas were mainly derived from the famous Yellow Emperor (2698 BC.) in his conversations with the Pure Lady. The Yellow Emperor had a total of more than 1,000 women in his palace. For him, sex is like the three legged stool: there is a triple purpose of ensuring the continuity of the human race, satisfying his personal sensual desire and achieving personal longevity. The latter he achieved by having intercourse with as many as ten young women a day without ejaculating himself while capturing the orgasm of the woman. The most damaging effect of intercourse for the man is the act of ejaculation, because each ejaculation will cost him some precious K Qi, eventually depriving him of his sex power (impotence). Men, like the heaven must be on the top, while women like the earth receives him from the bottom, which represents the most common sexual position.

According to the Chinese, sexual intercourse is compared to an interaction between Fire and Water. Indeed, the penis may be fully erected and hot, but the fluids of the vagina (the Water) are always able to put out the fire of the penis, subduing the man sexually. The weaker sexually man is put out by "water" too easily and loses his erection quickly, before the woman reaches an orgasm which will weaken the K Qi of the man considerably. As it takes time to boil water once we have lit the fire, it will take time to boil the "water" of the woman: a woman's sexual response takes place much more slowly than the man's. So ideally, a man's penis should be inserted in the vagina slowly and remain in the vagina for a prolonged period of time (some Chinese Masters could achieve erection in the vagina without ejaculation for hours!).

The Chinese compare sexual intercourse also to an act between an obedient, nice mare (pure Yin) and a dominating dragon, symbol of heaven and pure Yang. But especially during sexual intercourse, this mare is aroused and can't control herself anymore. This is where a lot of man lose self-confidence and are subjected to performance anxiety. So the key is for the man not too get overexcited and reach his orgasm too soon or he will be merely a non-active participant, losing control over the entire situation. Man should restrict deep penetrations and perform more shallow ones, alternated by an *occasional* deep penetration. Too many forceful deep penetrations will numb the vaginal walls and defeat the intended stimulating effects. Since intercourse is a Yang action, the best periods for intercourse are in those months where there is the most Yang: the spring. But ejaculation in the winter, when mostly Yin is present, will consume much more sex energy than in the spring, leading to an exhaustion of this energy.

It does not mean that man should refrain from having sexual intercourse all together. That would mean that there would be no outlet for his sex energy which is like breaking communication between Yin and Yang. The penis must be used like a tool, to make it stronger and to absorb the energy from the opposite sex for the nourishment of the body. According to our basic laws in Chinese medicine, Yin and Yang interact and are complementary: one needs the other constantly to be "alive." So for man, absorbing the Yin Qi for the nourishment of the Yang Qi is a supreme sex tonic. Old Chinese emperors who did not follow these rules of the bedroom affairs, and indulged excessively in sexual intercourse, did not live over fifty years old, quite to the contrary with the Yellow Emperor, who enjoyed longevity because of his knowledge about sex life acquired from his sexual consultants. This is a well-known rule in Homeopathy as well, where a "loss of fluids" can be the onset of many diseases. *"Never well since (nws) loss of fluids"* is covered in the repertory of homeopathy by several remedies, aimed at restoring the initial cause of imbalance or disease. Sexual intercourse with ejaculation means the same as sedation in acupuncture for the man and tonification for the woman; on the other hand, sexual intercourse without ejaculation means the same as sedation for woman and tonification for man.

A Chinese medical classic said: *"The Kidneys are in shape before the fetus has a body."* The Chinese consider the kidneys as the roots of life, and its weakness and strength have great bearings on the life span of a person. Hence, the kidneys are the most important organs and should be constantly nourished. Strong kidneys will benefit other organs as they come into existence prior to the other organs. As a rule, we have to examine one's physical condition in relation to sex power, and if there are signs of premature ejaculation, nocturnal seminal emission and softening of the penis in the middle of intercourse, they should be corrected not by sexual tonics which work only temporary but by appropriate measures. Building up the kidney energy is essential in the art of human sexuality. But abstaining from sexual intercourse completely is as bad as to indulge in sex excessively: "the birth of Yang or Yin will not take place in isolation." The right kidney is fire, the left is water. Fire is responsible for the erection while water is responsible for the act of ejaculation, but a balance of fire and water is essential for a normal sexual intercourse in which a strong erection is supported by a timely ejaculation. Deficient fire leads to impotence while deficient water causes inability to ejaculate. More on how to correct problems with infertility and impotence in Chapter 16 on OB/GYN.

DIET

The subject of nutrition is as old as man's search for food, but the science of nutrition is relatively new. Diet plays an important part in the studies and experiments of modern medicine. The subject of diet is not new to alternative medicines. Hahnemann stated in his master book, "The Organon", Par. 77:

"Those diseases are inappropriately named chronic which persons incur who expose themselves continually to avoidable noxious influences, who are in the habit of indulging in injurious liquors or aliments..."

This truthful statement won't be music to the ears of those patients who ask me on a daily basis: "Is it enough to have the acupuncture treatments and to take this homeopathic remedy, or do I have to follow a good diet, too?" When it comes to food intake, many of us abandon our inborn common sense. Often, because food supplies more than just fuel for the body– i.e., comfort when depressed, a "lift" when tired– we fool ourselves about what we eating and how much. The alternative practitioner understands the value of proper diet to combat diseases. When patients follow desires for certain foods, rather than choosing a variety of food which includes plenty of fruit and vegetables, he recognizes that these strong desires or aversions for foods are indicative of certain disease tendencies. Often these tendencies will be an important factor in selecting the acupuncture points (according to the tastes) or homeopathic remedy.

Practitioners of modern medicine often speak to us in black and white terms: "Don't eat salt, don't eat sugar or sweets." While these blanket instructions may contain a kernel of truth, they provide no insight into what Chinese medicine called "Yin-Yang," or the tenet of homeopathy that "Like Cures Like"—that a substance can be either a poison *or* a medicine. This bipolar character of food substances is expressed in the observations of acupuncturists 5,000 years ago. Each organ has a taste to its name as we have seen in chapter 4. This means that a certain quantity of a food containing that "taste" is required for the normal functioning of the corresponding organ. Recognizing the deficiency or excess of an organ by an acupuncturist has to be followed by diet advise or the acupuncturist will be disappointed in his results. Just keep in mind. The chronic sufferer often desires the very food which has been the greatest single factor in producing his distress. The graver the condition, the less the patient can be trusted to avoid his cravings. Humans are endowed with an accurate sense of when it is time to partake (or not) of food and drink. During illness, we are averse to certain foods and crave others. As usual, we should faithfully obey the internal voice of our digestive organs relative to the proper quantity of nutrients we should take in. Then you will see that the combination of acupuncture and a balanced diet will yield results.

Acupuncture and Psychological Diseases 14

"Before puncturing, the practitioner should know the role of the psyche." NEI KING

INTRODUCTION

More than in any other form of medicine except homeopathy, acupuncture looks at the psyche of the patient, knowing and recognizing its importance to restore health in mankind. In fact, as far as the Chinese are concerned, any disease starts with a psychological disturbance. Psychosomatic Chinese medicine studies the relationship between the organs and the mind. All of the organs have specific psychological reactions. There are *seven emotional factors:* anger, joy, pensiveness, grief, melancholy, terror and fear.

There will be no psychological disorder when these emotions are under control. An excess of one of these emotions will injure the corresponding organ (Chapter 8, Nei King):

Too much anger (or irritability and long-term frustration) will injure the Liver and causes death.

Too much joy will injure the Heart: an excess of joy will disperse the spirit.

Too much pensiveness or worry will injure the Spleen: there is an impact on the H-Sp axis. A lack of joy leads to a Xu of H, too much worry to a Xu of Sp.

Too much grief and melancholy will injure the lung and obstruct the flow of the Qi.

Too much fear or terror will injure the Kidneys and cause insanity.

The Chinese used their knowledge of the emotions and their influence on the organs, to predict the season in which the patient would die. The patient who worries too much will die in the winter. Too much depletes the Qi of the Sp which leads to a less control of the K (Ko cycle). The uncontrolled excessive K Qi, made stronger by the winter season, will suppress the H Qi, leading to the patient's death.

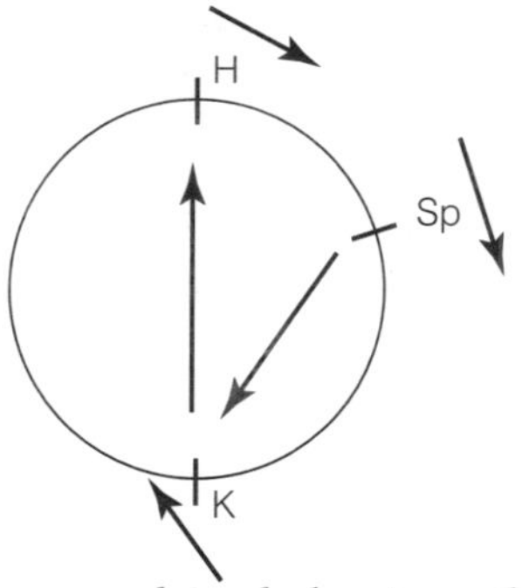

Obsessive compulsive behavior will lead to Shi Qi of the Sp, hence it cannot controlled the K (Ko cycle); Shi K will lead to Fullness of the Li (Sheng cycle)and Xu of the H (Ko cycle). The Xu H cannot give enough Qi to the Sp which is dominated according to the Ko cycle in the spring when the patient will die.

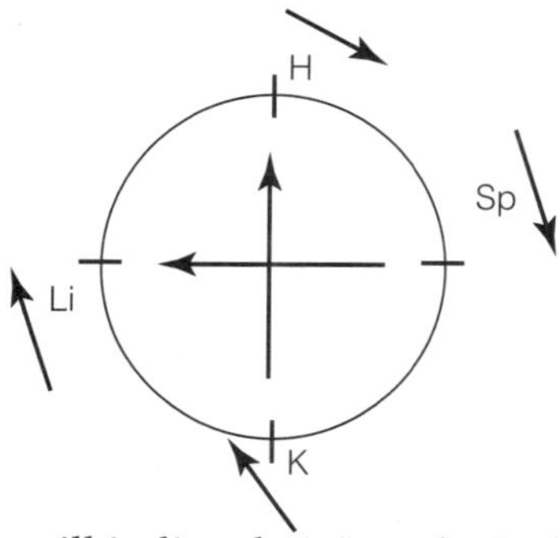

Sadness will indirectly injure the Li (Ko cycle): sadness leads to a Xu of H Qi, which stops controlling the L. The Shi L will dominate the Li more, especially in the fall when the patient will die.

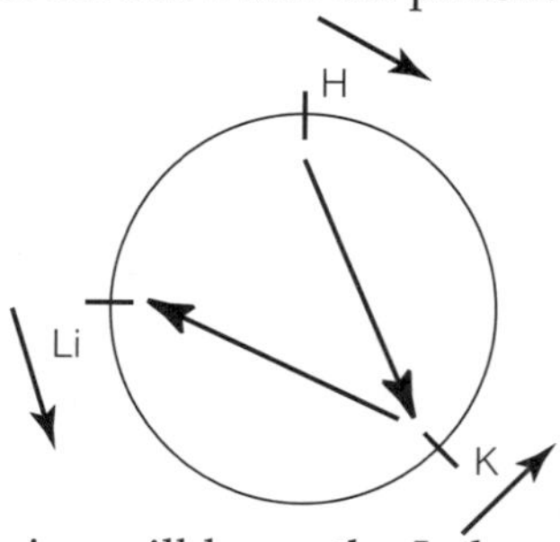

Excessive joy will harm the L through a Shi H and can cause insanity. The patient will die in the summer when the H has most Qi.

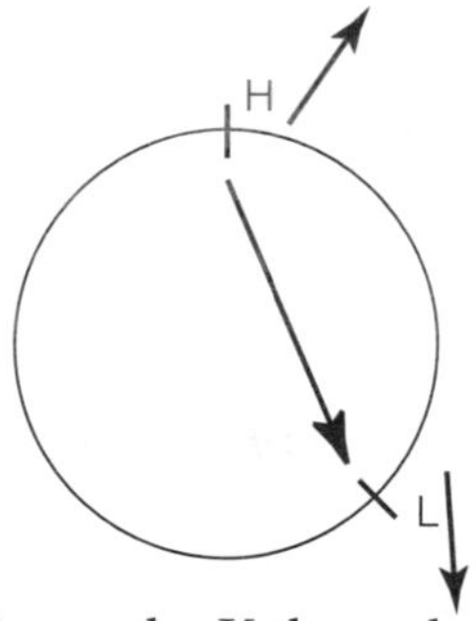

Anger will harm the K through a Yin Xu Li. A Xu Li leads to a Xu H. The patient will die in the 5th season or Long Summer when the Sp Qi is the strongest.

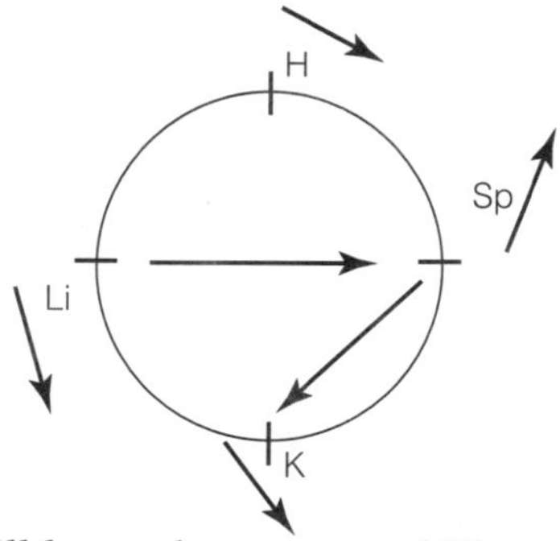

Fear will harm the essence of life or Ancestral Qi, leading to a decrease of this Ancestral Qi preserved in all the organs, but especially in the K.

Emotions also influence energy in general as is expressed in the Su Wen, Chapter 5:

Anger makes Qi rise to the upper body.
Joy renders it harmonious.
Sadness disperses it.
Reflection concentrates it.
Fear makes it descend to the lower body.

The mental/emotional Qi is one of the 5 energies of man:

YONG—WEI—ANCESTRAL—
ESSENTIAL (food+respiratory Qi)—
MENTAL/EMOTIONAL.

This mental/emotional Qi manifests itself through the conscience and thought process and is responsible for all the physical and psychological actions. This mental Qi is formed on the moment life starts, in other words at the conception. The ancestral Qi of the father coupled to the ancestral Qi of the mother forms a certain quantity of ancestral Qi of the fetus, a quantity that only can decrease during its life span. This mental Qi, called *CHENN* is situated in the center of man or in the heart. This Chenn is nourished by the Essential Qi. Of course, the mental Qi has also an influence on the production and circulation of other energies. Su Ouenn says: *"To know how to conserve the Mental Qi is Life, losing it is Death,"* and further:

> *"The Heart conserves the mental Qi (CHENN), the Lung protects the vital fluid (PRO), the Liver safeguards the soul (ROUN), the Spleen preserves the thought (I) and the Kidney maintains the will (TCHE).*

This is discussed further in this chapter. Although the Chenn is inactive before birth, the practitioner has to keep in mind the influence on the fetus during his intra-uterine life. Emotional traumas of the mother during pregnancy, can have a direct influence on the newborn. For instance, in homeopathy we know that if the mother had a heartbreak during pregnancy, it is quite possible that the child is born a Natrum muriaticum constitutionally. Nat. mur. relates to this heartbreak and the baby is born as if he underwent the heartbreak himself!

In chapter 8 of the "Nei King", it says: *"Life is formed by the reunion of the energy of Earth and the energy of Heaven."* This corresponds to the maternal (Yin=Earth) and paternal (Yang=Heaven) Qi. Life preserves the essence of this combination, an essence which is composed of 2 elements, one providing food (from the Earth), the other air (from the cosmos or Heaven). These two elements produce the spirit and the soul living with the spirit.

We will discuss each organ and its emotion separately, followed by the characteristics of what the Chinese call *"The Five Psychological Entities"*.

THE ORGANS AND THEIR EMOTIONS: KNOW WHO YOU ARE

LIVER

An excess of *anger, frustration and irritability* injures the liver and, more specifically, the Yin Qi. If the patient holds a state of continuous anger, or is a person who cannot tolerate contradiction, then this depression of the Qi will lead to Endogenous Heat, turning into fire with an ascending tendency. But other circumstances are fueling anger. Among these are suppressed anger from *indignation*, following emotional, physical, and verbal abuse often encountered in modern life. We think about abusive marriages, abusive work relationships in which the victim cannot stand up for her right because the abuser is the boss, and rape which is the culmination of all forms of abuse. The victim in these circumstances cannot express his/her anger and will suppress it. This leads to indignation (their dignity is taken away), low self confidence, low self esteem, anorexia nervosa and bulimia, and performance anxiety, especially male sexual performance anxiety with a lack of erections. Children and adults alike will dread new situations or tasks because of an extreme low self confidence which stops them from finishing their task. They are *wonderful beginners and bad finishers.* They have started in their lives many projects but failed to finish any of them! Often they need a short nap which refreshes them. Besides the previous mental/emotional symptoms, other physical "liver" symptoms appear: red and burning eyes, hiccough, stomach burning, dizziness, insomnia, bitter taste and dryness of the mouth, migraine, hypoglycemia, unrefreshed sleep, waking up between 1-3 a.m., quick fermentation and bloating after a mouthful of food or immediately after food intake, sour cravings and cravings for warm foods and drinks, constipation in which they have an ineffective and frequent urge with an impression of impacted stool left in the rectum, and pain in the sides and at the lower angle of the right shoulder blade. Another emotion harming the liver is *disappointment*. A strong disappointment, especially in the career-oriented liver patient (this is the typical high powered executive of our modern times or *Nux Vomica type* in homeopathy), will inevitably lead to a depression of the Li Qi causing a burn-out patient, who will change from the hardworking, brilliant leader he once was into the lazy, philosopher who becomes indifferent to his own person and people around him. He changes into a person who neglects his own hygiene, his food intake (which consists only of fast foods) and he hates exercise, preferring to sit in an easy rocking chair, philosophizing about pertinent events in the world. As you can see, low self-esteem, a highly motivated executive living the fast lane and the disgusted philosopher, are all liver people.

If the Endogenous Heat stirs up the Wind, convulsions and unconsciousness can occur (Wind of Liver added to the Fire of the Liver). Differential diagnosis may be assisted by pulse investigation:

> Fire plus wind of liver: pulse is fast, wiry and short
>
> Wind of liver: pulse is weak and wiry.

The same reasoning can be applied to the Five Elements. Anger injures the liver and depression results. According to the KO-cycle, the Emptiness of the Li Qi causes an excess of Qi in the element Earth (or spleen), especially the Yang Earth (the stomach is affected, with formation of rebellious Qi or vomiting). This Earth excess in turn will increase the control of the kidney, spreading a feeling of fear in the patient. This emptiness of the kidney aggravates an Emptiness of the liver (according to the Sheng-cycle) and results in the initial symptom of anger. This shows the correlation between the feeling of fear and anger (fear is a source of anger), and hence the circle of disease becomes a closed one.

In China, many women are the victims of forced marriage. As they are taught to accept this without protest, these women recede into silence, harboring an inner anger. This is a prime example of indignation or suppressed anger as mentioned before. It is not surprising to see symptoms such as headaches, eye trouble, side pains, emotional instability and irregular menstruation in these women. An excellent therapy for this state of mind is:

- Sp6, reunion of the three-leg Yin.
- Li2, Li3, to put the liver Qi into motion and extinguish the Fire.
- B18, associated point of the liver, disperses the Interior Wind.
- TB6, GB34, alleviates intercostal pain.
- GV16, GB20, disperses the Interior Wind.

If there is continued harbored anger, Cold may enter the liver. The illness in these patients has become chronic and they hardly feel anger anymore (they resigned, they can't stand up for themselves anymore). In an advanced stage, tendons and ligaments will lose their function and become rigid. These women typically experience headaches on the vertex, are nauseous and vomit water. The lower abdomen is swollen and painful. The pulse is wiry, deep and slow.

HEART

The heart is the seat of joy. A well-balanced fire patient is jovial, social-oriented, outgoing, optimistic and laughs easily. He has a great sense of humor and is a real sunshine in people's life. He is very excitable and impressionable and darts around like a little butterfly. He is very talkative and laughs all the time, even for little things or nothing at all. They like moving around and are always on the go (the super shoppers among the seniors). But there is a certain fragility in this people. Certain events, like *heartbreak* situations can bring them out of balance and one must consider first a heart disorder in any mental disorder. This can lead to extreme fire with hysteria and incoherent speech. Between these extremes we see sighing, with a sinking feeling in the stomach, a sense of suffocation, confused mind, vertigo, lots of anxiety about the future, guilt feelings, despair and tendency to nervous breakdown. So *excessive joy* leads to an imbalance! This mental irritation first causes a depression of the H Qi, leading to a stagnation of this Qi. This stagnation turns into an Endogenous Fire which will exhaust the liquids of the body and form Phlegm. This Phlegm-Fire will block and injure the heart orifice and the channels and produce symptoms such as insomnia and palpitations. In a later state, the Endogenous Heat stirs up the Internal Wind which can lead to derangement of the mind with incoherent speech, mania, laughing and weeping without reason. If, at this moment, there is an attack of an Exterior nature, delirium may result.

What are other *physical symptoms* felt when the H Qi is imbalanced? Easily fatigued, mentally and physically. Water retention in the ankles as the day goes on. These patients fall asleep easily but wake up any hour of the night. They crave bitter things and are sensitive to odors. They grasp for air especially at night, and can show chest pain with palpitations. Their face is reddish and plethoric, they are hot patients and dread Heat-Dampness. They love the cool, open air and will throw the windows open. They don't like the darkness of the winter and are prone to seasonal affective disorder (SAD). Stuttering is a heart problem (the tongue is the opening to the heart, the heart commands the speech). Nocturnal perspiration indicates an emptiness of H Yin Qi (H commands the perspiration). There is a bitter taste in the mouth and either the whole tongue is red or just the tip. Their favorite color: red of course!

SPLEEN

This is the *5 F's type:* fair, flabby, fat, fears and faint. They are the mother types, always ready to listen and give good advice. Everyone comes with their problems to them, unload them and feels better since the earth type is such a good listener. This earth type does not get burned out easily, they can burden themselves with the problems of others. They act like super moms. They worry about everything and have a tendency to broad over little things, especially about things in the PAST! (L or metal patients worry about the future). But they are down to earth and practical. They are very sensitive to bad news and tend to cry when they see sad things on TV or in the newspaper because they put themselves in the place of victims and have great empathy for them. They are obsessed with bookshelves, drawers and files and they are obsessive list writers (they never leave home without them!). They can be very tidy and obsessive compulsive and tend to overeat and be inactive. There are a lot of fears and anxiety in this person and children typically have nightmares. Typically too, these children will inundate you with questions about God and death.

What are physical symptoms? They tend to go to bed with their socks on (they are very chilly). They hate physical exercise, especially going upstairs which leaves them grasping for air. They sweat profusely and easily, even without physical effort, especially on the forehead, in the neck and hair. They have cold clammy hands. Women show the 3 P's in their menstrual cycle: premature, prolonged and profuse! Three organs have a role in the distribution of the blood. The Liver stores the blood, the heart pumps the blood while the spleen controls the blood. If the Qi of the spleen is blocked and its functions decreased, the spleen loses control over the blood and we get hemorrhaging with no apparent reason, as in abundant menstruation. Therapy: Sp6(t), Sp10(t). Their stools are large and dry, and RARE but they are happy with their constipation: they can go days without having a bowel movement without feeling discomfort. There is an intense desire for eggs (boiled ones), sweets and ice cream. A bad odor in the mouth can be present. The tongue shows typically a yellow white fur in the middle. Favorite colors: yellow and brown, the earth colors. The causality of this spleen dysfunction is grief, overwork, overlifting, too much worry about the past, too many spicy foods and sweets.

LUNG

Mentally this is the depressed person, the "hard-to-live-with. This person does not know the pleasure of giving, all they do is take. They want all the attention turned and geared toward them but don't want to give any to others. They are people who like routine, they are very dogmatic, everything is according to the book, they have a strong sense of duty. They have issues about control and can be narrow-minded people with a rigid thinking. They maintain tight control over their emotions and will ignore their symptoms or tend to minimize them. Internally they are emotionally but they don't show it externally (everything is CONTROL!). They deny their feelings and suppress their anger. They are very absent-minded (they do not hear it in the first place <> forgetful) and very pre-occupied. They easily exaggerate and even the most insignificant event becomes a major trauma. They worry about the future, their health and get easily discouraged. They have anxiety which they describe as "anxiety in the pit of the stomach."

They are hypersensitive to everything: noise, touch (L = skin) and the slightest draft.

Physically they have symptoms related to the fact that the L is the mother of Qi: extreme fatigue, especially expressed in the voice which becomes weak. They are sensitive to dry weather especially, which gives easily constipation and hemorrhoids. The L has an important function in the skin and body hair. Because the L produces the Wei Qi, these people have a tendency to recurrent colds and ear infections. Their worst time is between 2-5 a.m.. Men show weakness after sexual intercourse while women have lower back pains with a feeling of a broken back, just before the menses. Persistent lumbar pains are possible after pregnancies, deliveries and menopause. They have great insomnia with especially problems about falling asleep. Their favorite color is white.

KIDNEY

The main emotion is *fear* and *sadness*. They are very fearful and have all kinds of phobias (claustrophobia, agoraphobia, fear for crowds, public speaking, flying, heights, etc.). They are very indecisive and can't make up their minds. They are closed up people with a stiff upper lip. They will not talk freely but rather hand you a list with their symptoms because they don't like the attention turned to themselves. They don't cry in public: silent grief is a main symptom, they are the ones who will say, "My husband died two years ago but I haven't shed a tear yet." They can be hypochondriac and very fearful for robbers. There is a lot of guilt and resentment in them. They can't let go of things in the past, they dwell over the past and can be unforgiving. They love their psychotherapists (many are K types themselves!) and always choose to pursue the unobtainable partner or knowingly stay with the wrong partner. They show indifference towards others but deep down they do care, they just have a hard time showing it. They are very sentimental especially before the menses. They are cautious people and take everything with a grain of salt. They are nice people to know but not nice people to live with! They only have sex out of obligation and there is tendency to frigidity and impotence.

Physically they crave salt, have herpes simplex attacks, are sensitive to the sun, have greasy face with dry skin everywhere else, brittle hair and dry hard stools. Very thirsty for cold drinks which they tend to drink in big gulps. There is tendency to bulimia and anorexia nervosa. These patients don't want to go to other people's bathroom and prefer to wait till they are home. They are always worse at the seaside, around 10 a.m. and premenstrual. There is loss of teeth, backaches, tinnitus, deafness and night sweats.

Sweating—the sweat itself is Yin. Day sweating is due to an insufficiency of Yang, since the Yang is not able to hold the Yin which will escape in the form of sweat. Therapy for day sweating consists of strengthening the Yang (LI4(t) - K7(s)). Night sweating is due to insufficiency of Yin (SI3(s): confluent point of GV, master of the Yang meridians, disperses the Yang. Perspiration is the fluid of the Yin; when there is an increase of internal heat, the Wei Qi cannot maintain its protective function and does not close the pores. The fluid of the Yin cannot be held in the body, therefore, Yin becomes deficient. Therapy: B35: good equilibration point; B23(t) (left): to strengthen Kidney Yin; H7: to drain the Fire of the Heart (Imperial Fire). Tonification of Liver, Heart, and Lung meridians.

The pulse in the case of *Kidney Yin* deficiency will be thin, empty, weak, but a little fast rather than slow. Deficiency (Xu) of the *Kidney Yang* may also be due to a long-time illness or overindulgence in sex (as mentioned in the previous chapter). The responsibility of the Yang of the kidney is to warm the body, and it also plays an active role in dividing the clear fluids from the turbid fluids. Symptoms of this deficiency include:

- Chilliness
- Sensitivity to cold
- Cold limbs
- Morning diarrhea (approximately 5 a.m.)
- Impotence

This resulting weakness means that the Qi of the Kidney cannot receive the Qi descending from the lung. This will cause a blockage of the descending Chen Qi, with symptoms such as shortness of breath, asthmatic breathing (a low-sounding wheeze),* oliguria and edema.

* **NOTE:** There are two types of dyspnea, wheezing and shortness of breath:

- Type Lung: high-sounding wheezing, with forced exhalations.
- Type kidney: low-sounding wheezing, with difficult inhalations.

Therapy of Xu Yang K:

- GV4(t) Both of these
- B23(t) (right) tonify Kidney Yang

In case both Kidney Yang and Kidney Yin are deficient, the Kidney Yang needs to be strengthened first. It is more difficult to strengthen the Yin (Yin = slow). In order to maintain health, one should proceed as when starting a fire. First, we light the fire (tonifying the Yang), then we add more wood (tonifying the Yin afterwards).

Excessive K Yang will cause: sexual mania, dreams, excessive thirst and oliguria.

THE FIVE PSYCHOLOGICAL ENTITIES

The psyche is not alone represented in the Five Elements. After long-lasting psychological problems, what can be called a *visceral entity,* appears. As there are five elements, there are also Five Visceral Entities. There is an absolute law that says, *"Each psychological entity occurred because the organ Tsang was not strong enough in its season."* As the law explains, it is a Tsang (Yin organ) that is disturbed and not a Fu (Yang organ). A disturbance of a Yang organ or Fu organ will not cause psychological symptoms. The disturbance will go to the Tsang; e.g., a patient with gallstones who becomes aggressive. It is not the gall bladder but the liver that needs to be treated. Before each of the Five Visceral Entities are described, it is important to remember some vital aspects:

- The seven emotions must be present in a certain level in a normal human being.
  One has to have a certain amount of anger, fear, joy, etc.
- Acupuncture therapy will not help with severe psychological entities such as schizophrenia.
- When a patient is being treated for a psychological problem, it is valuable to first work on the heart.

PRO (PO)

PRO relates to the lung and is the *least important* of these entities. The PRO represents anything that is automatic and vegetative (e.g., Babinski, patellar reflexes). The PRO represents all the features or characteristics obtained through heredity. For Soulié De Morant, the PRO is "the deep animal intelligence of the cells, with their essentially hereditary components" (although there are also acquired components). The PRO is also responsible for the movement of the Yang to the Yin or interiorization. But the L meridian, belonging to the level Tae Yin, opens to the exterior. Hence the point commanding the PRO must be situated on the exteriorization of the L or on the level Yang Ming, opening to the interior. This point must be an axis-point, opening to the interior and the lower part of the body. There is only one point responding to this definition: St25 (called "Celestial axis").

We can speak of disturbance of the PRO when there is a perturbation of the automatic life. For example, a person who seemingly accidentally pushes over a glass of water when his intention was to pick it up. A person who has too much PRO may have the following appearance: a person who is large in stature, doesn't think too much, appears to have no problems, lives life automatically, the perfect employee doing everything according to routine, with no spontaneity and originality. Excessive PRO leads to sadness, sighing and fear for *future* events. Emptiness also causes weeping, a weak voice, indifference toward life and others, fragility, vulnerability and sentimentality in the person. An example of automation of the PRO is the growing of hair and nails after death. In China, the dead are buried eight days after decease. It is the PRO which disappears last. In summary, the PRO has an impulsive tendency to action. It is the *instinctive cellular intelligence.*

PRO

Automatic behavior, natural instincts, worries for future, regrets, vital reflexes, fragility, sentimentality.

ROUN (HUN)

The ROUN resides in the liver. It is the collector of information without giving an interpretation. There is indeed very little reasoning in the ROUN. It passes the information to the CHENN, although the ROUN helps to make a distinction between relevant and non-relevant information. It is the experience of the past and is not at all automatic. But the ROUN is responsible for the imagination, the memory of images (Li=eyesight!), dreams, dynamism, violence and jealousy. The putting into movement of Qi, happens in the spring, corresponding to the Li where we will have the transformation of the Yin in the Yang. The Chinese called this "the muscled soul" which leaves the body (Yin) when death occurs to ascend to heaven (Yang). Excessive ROUN leads to abundant dreaming, agitation, irritability and insomnia.

A person who has little ROUN is one who cannot gather information, who has to read everything ten times before he knows what he has read. The ROUN is smaller and less developed in children, and, as they have had little experience, it is necessary for an adult to repeat instructions and directions to them in detail. The ROUN is not the same as memory which is part of the I. Dreams are nothing less than ROUN traveling. Dreams are information: nightmares demonstrate an excess of ROUN (Shi), indicating that the Qi of the Liver is disturbed. According to the control (KO) cycle, grief and worry will injure the ROUN. If the ROUN is not functioning, the PRO will take over. An excess of grief will inhibit the ROUN from accepting the information; for example, a patient whose awareness becomes internalized, as he has blocked out his environment. This patient becomes morose, hesitant, frequent sighing with an evolution to depression. Furthermore, Xu of ROUN leads to apathy, lack of imagination, and physical inactivity. Delirium, and excessive imagination disconnected from the emotional balance fall under the domain of the ROUN disturbance. Discontentment and irritation cause a Shi of Li. This discontentment can cure obsession, while grief can suppress discontentment.

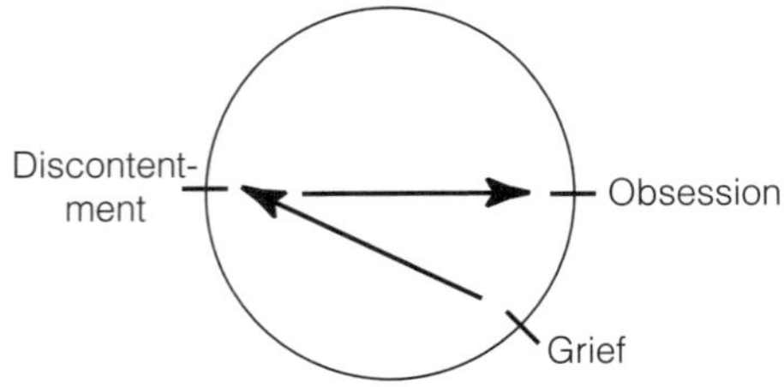

ROUN

Imagination, image memory, dreams, spirit of enterprise,violence, jealousy, emotivity, collector of information.

THE "I"

The "I" resides in the Spleen. The "I" represents *idea and thought.* It is also the reasoning power, meditation, concentration, memory, habits, and sense of perfectionism. The person whose "I" is well-developed has total recall of events experienced in the past. Such persons are able to memorize very easily. An excess of "I" will lead to pensiveness and obsession for the present and past, a tendency to repeat things, mania, rigidity and sterile rumination. This patient has trouble to "produce intellectually." This excess was beautifully demonstrated by a patient of mine.

The patient came to me after being confined in several hospitals. Psychiatrists could not help him; and if were not for the coincidence that the poor man was a classmate of my older brother, I doubt that he would have come to me. What made it even more interesting was the fact that this patient was, at the age of three, a student in my mother's class where she was a teacher in a kindergarten. The chief complaint was a compulsion for cleanliness. He cleaned his car in the middle of the night, simply because there was not time left in the day. Indeed, his habits became an ordeal for his wife and two little children. They were not allowed to come into the living room, as he could not tolerate any dirt. Laid off from work, he would hang the coats of his wife and children on hangers for hours before he was pleased with the result. If somebody used the phone, he had to clean it immediately with a towel. Everything had to stay in exactly the same place: even a vase on the table could not be moved. This poor family had to live in the kitchen and never dare take a vacation. When I mentioned him to my mother, she immediately recalled that as a little boy, he always was super-clean in his personal appearance and punctilious in his school behavior. He refused to participate in any normal children's games for fear of getting himself dirty. Gradually, this obsession became worse, until it reached the point that he had stopped working at the age of 32.

This is a perfect example of derangement of the "I" and, according to Freud, a fixation in the anal stage. It took me a full year to reverse the situation, but it was one of the cases that gave me the most satisfaction.

A *deficiency* (Xu) of "I" will lead to inattentive acts (absent-mindedness), in loss of memory, concentration and inattention, anxiety (especially for past and present events) and an aversion for all activity. The "I" can be compared to a cupboard with many drawers, which are filled with information from the past and present. With each new piece of information or every sensation, a drawer is filled; however, some drawers remain empty on purpose. When a person is experiencing a dangerous or life-threatening situation, the "I" loses control and command is taken up by the ROUN and the PRO. The "I" becomes disconnected, and, therefore, memory of these dangerous situations is not filled with the "I." Physical pain is registered in the PRO, psychological pain is registered in the ROUN. Only the memory of the pain registers with the "I."

Suppose a person is drowning. Since the "I" tends to take in this information, reason it through and try to assist in the survival of the organism, the powers of this element will take too much time, and in fact, may even decrease the chances of survival for the organism. The mechanism(s) [or element(s)] called for are the ROUN and the PRO — working cooperatively for immediate action, acting automatically and spontaneously. This kind of cooperation can also lead to abnormal and non-understandable behavior. For example, a person is skiing downhill on a bright, sunny day. He takes a fall and breaks his shoulder. At the moment he falls, he hears laughter, the sound of a helicopter overhead and experiences the pain from the shoulder injury. The sound of the laughter and the helicopter sounds are registered in the "I", the pain of the shoulder registers with the PRO. All of these sensations (visual, olfactory, auditory) are connected with this ski-laughter-sunny-day-helicopter-pain-experience and become part of the person's memory. If at some later time in the person's life, he experiences a similar situation (sunny day, laughter, skiing, helicopter sounds), he may associate this with pain, even when that situation is without danger. The conditions have changed, but the person may possibly show the same defense reaction shown in the original situation. To a second individual, observing the behavior and not understanding the previous experience, this reaction will seem totally incomprehensible, and he will regard the behavior as strange. The Chinese call this totally of information, together with the automatic reaction, a *KOUEI*. Western culture has no common word for this phenomenon.

I

Thought process, reasoning, meditation, concentration, memory, habits, perfectionism, reflection.

THE TCHE

The TCHE resides in the Kidney. It is demonstrated by the quality of *decisiveness.* Characteristics of the person who has much TCHE are determination and resoluteness. It is will, perseverance, and tenacity to complete what one has begun. Smokers or obese patients almost always lack TCHE. For their treatment it is necessary to strengthen the points of the TCHE. Shi of the TCHE will lead to authoritarianism, dictatorship and ability to influence others. Xu of the TCHE will cause fear, lack of libido and indecisiveness in patients.

The ideogram of TCHE is formed by "heart and counselor", showing the importance of the principal axis kidney/heart. Without the TCHE there can be no action, even with all the information available which the person acquired through ROUN, PRO and I.

TCHE

Decisiveness, will power, determination, libido, courage, tenacity, realization.

THE CHENN

The CHENN is an important psychological entity: the *capacity to judge.* The CHENN is the synthesis of all mental activities. The CHENN residing in the heart, is the most important of the five entities. It represents the general psyche and the spiritual soul. There are two kinds of CHENN: organic (the psyche, the heart), and generic (this is hereditary and cannot be influenced by treatment). CHENN means *intelligence.* It is the "lamp that lights up the brain". One who has CHENN in abundance comprehends immediately. Not only does this person comprehend, but he can also apply what he has learned. The generic CHENN is a gift. One has this kind of CHENN or not. The remainder of the CHENN (organic) is obtained through experience. The CHENN represents also conscience, reasoning, morality, serenity, spirituality, human love and the love for life. Two sources "feed the CHENN": dreams (unconscious information coming through from the liver), and the spleen (the spleen must feed the CHENN — this is not related to the Shen cycle). The heart, the emperor who holds the fire, is situated in the south and symbolizes the harmony, the balance between the movements of the Yin to the Yang in the east, and of the Yang to the Yin in the west. The CHENN is the first visceral entity to appear in the embryo and will participate with the Ancestral Qi in the build-up of the other entities. Therefore, the CHENN is present not only in the heart, but in all the organs to coordinate their functions and allow to judge the received information .

CHENN

Intellect, love for mankind and life, morality, spirituality, serenity, conscience, reasoning, harmony

Following is a remarkable example that shows the feeding of the CHENN by the "I". A 5-year-old child, basically of a sweet disposition, had done something very cruel. She had two little rabbits as pets, whose eyes she had picked out. Asked for the reason, she said: "I love them very much and this way they cannot run away." The act was thus a logical one for this child, but this was due to a disturbance of her "I".

Once the ROUN and the "I" have given enough information, it is time to act. This is the role of the TCHE. The "automatic life" (habit formation) must be good (the PRO). When these four sources work harmoniously, a good CHENN will result.

EXAMPLES OF CURRENT PSYCHOLOGICAL FORMS

WHAT DISTURBANCES CAUSES ONE TO WEEP ALL THE TIME AND BE DEPRESSED?

It is not the PRO that is responsible, because depression is not an automatic response. It is a disturbance of ROUN: this is the entity that collects information, but does not interpret it, and transmits it unchanged to the CHENN. On the level of Chueh Yin, there is normally more Yin (Xue) than Yang (Qi). In the case of a depressed patient, there is too much Yin in the liver. Because of the lack of Yang, the patient cannot interpret the information coming to him.

WHERE WOULD PATIENTS WHO ARE PHYSICALLY, MENTALLY OR EMOTIONALLY ABUSED FIT IN THESE ENTITIES?

The main emotion is suppressed anger caused by this indignation leading to too little ROUN (anger injures the Qi of the liver). Consequently, the ROUN is replaced by the PRO (with its regrets, worries for the future and automatic behavior as presented in their lack of confidence and self-worth). What therapy can be given to these persons? ROUN = LIVER. Normally, there is more Yin than Yang (XUE> Qi). The ROUN is deficient; this means that there is too little Yin. Because the Yin is deficient, this type of person often craves alcoholic drinks. This is because the water, sugar, ice and alcohol are all very Yin in nature.

THERAPY

The idea expressed in therapy is to give the patient a maximum qualitative and quantitative equilibrium to this energy. Any limitation of the results are due primarily to limitations of the acupuncturist. But make sure to take into account the temperament or constitution of the patient (ancestral aspect) and the influence of the environment (family or work stress, pernicious factors, food factors, medications, toxins, etc.)

DIET

For example, if CHENN is in excess, we have to strengthen the TCHE (Ko cycle) by prescribing a diet of extra salt and pork. In the following table, the psychological entities are listed, along with corresponding dietary prescriptions.

Entity	Strengthening Food
ROUN	Sour food, sheep meat, buckwheat, barley
CHENN	Bitter food, chicken, millet
I	Sugar, beef, rye
PRO	Pungent foods, horse meat, rice
TCHE	Salt, pork, beans

THERAPY THROUGH THE FIVE ELEMENTS (SHENG AND KO CYCLE)

1. Fire (CHENN) in excess injures the PRO.—L10 (fire point of the lung) in dispersion, and dispersion of the heart using the season dispersion point.
2. Wood (ROUN) in excess injures the I—Sp1 (wood point of Sp) in dispersion, dispersion of the liver season point.
3. Water (Tche in excess injures the CHENN.—K3 (water point of H) in dispersion, dispersion of the kidney season point.
4. Metal (PRO) in excess injures the ROUN.—Li4 (metal point of Li) in dispersion, dispersion of the lung season point.
5. Earth ("I") in excess injures the Tche.—K3 (earth point of K) in dispersion, dispersion of the spleen season point.

A special technique for therapy of the KOUEI is described in the Nei King. It is called the "*Liberation of the Seven Dragons*" (looking for the KOUEI in the Interior). Six needles must be placed as follows:

CV15(t), St25(t) (bilateral), St36(t), St37(t) (bilateral).

ACCORDING TO ANCIENT CHINESE LITERATURE (TA TCHRENG)

"All mental diseases should be treated by the Mo points and St36."

"Mental diseases are Yang diseases caused by too

much worry and grief (heartbreak!) which weakens the blood of the heart, leading to an illness of emptiness in the interior. We will have to tonifie. Obsessions, worries, discontentment will form mucus and obstruct the Qi causing fullness which we have to disperse."

"All illnesses stemming from one of the Seven Emotions cause a dysfunction of the Stomach Qi. Tonify St36 and the Mo points of all the organs."

"Think also of using the points of GV (sedation or tonification) and the Back Shu points."

Diseases of the Blood 15

PHYSIOLOGY OF THE BLOOD

Three organs are involved in the production of the Blood:

- The Heart, "master" of the Blood, has a pumping function and disperses it throughout the body.
- The Liver stores and receives the Blood.
- The Spleen governs, transports and guides it from the center to the periphery.

The Blood has two fundamental functions. The first is a *nourishing* one, provided by its perpetual movement. The second is a *transporting* function, since the Blood transports the Qi. On the other hand, the Qi moves the Blood. This close relationship is expressed in Chinese by *"Qi Xue"*. This relationship is found at four different levels:

- ❑ The Blood "Xue" is Yin, compared to the Qi, which is Yang.
- ❑ The Blood itself has a Yin component (liquids and solids) and a Yang one (the Energy of the Blood).
- ❑ The Blood level is the Yin of the Yin in comparison with the Wei Qi (Yang of the Yang), the Qi (Yin of the Yang) and the Ying (Yang of the Yin). This is expressed in Figure 54.
- ❑ Quantity of Qi and Blood in the three levels (Figure 50).

Yang of Yang	WEI = SKIN
Yin of Yang	QI = MUSCLES
Yang of Yin	YING = BONES
Yin of Yin	ANCESTRAL QI = BLOOD

Figure 54

Very important in the relationship between the Yin and the Yang is that the Yin follows the fluctuations of the Yang.

- Deceleration of Qi implies deceleration of Blood.
- Stagnation of Yang leads to stagnation of Yin; and
- Acceleration of the Yang leads to acceleration of the Yin.

These rules will have important consequences for the therapy. For instance, when we have a stagnation of Yin in the lower part of the body (heavy feeling in the legs, varicose veins, menstrual disturbances, etc.), besides stimulating the Yin, we tonify the Yang.

PATHOLOGY OF THE BLOOD

The Blood level is the Yin of the Yin or the deepest layer, which indicates that the etiology is essentially internal. The internal pathology shows four different aspects: Xu of Blood, stagnation of Blood, Heat in the Blood and formation of Internal Wind.

EMPTINESS OF BLOOD

This is due to a deficiency of Yin or Yang Qi in the Spleen and Heart. The patient shows physical and psychological asthenia. This Xu of Yin will liberate the Yang, causing the same pathology as Heat in the Blood.

HEAT IN THE BLOOD

The Xue of Yin leads to the liberation of Yang causing this Heat in the Blood. Another pathology is a heating process in the Burners due to fat food, shellfish, etc. The symptoms are bleedings due to non-traumatic internal causes.

STAGNATION OF THE BLOOD

The principal mechanism is the stagnation of the Qi of the liver, which is responsible for the free flow of the Qi. If this stagnation is chronic, the heart, spleen and lung get involved with formation of Internal Heat, phlegm and dysfunction of Tchong Mo/Ren Mo. The symptoms vary, but psychological troubles and depression will predominate. It is interesting to note that the ideogram for stagnation "Yu" means stagnation as well as depression!

ACTIVATION OF THE INTERNAL WIND

The Internal Fong disturbs the Blood, causing skin diseases when the orifices are "open". (When they are closed, epilepsy will be the consequence.)

The External pathology is due to the Six Excesses, but the principal agent is the External Wind. Syndromes are eczema, psoriasis, urticaria, etc.

THERAPEUTICAL ASPECTS IN FUNCTION OF THE ETIOLOGY

TREATMENT OF THE HEAT IN THE BLOOD

We act on the Heat directly:

- Purify: Sp10.
- Disperse the Fire: H7 and
- Cool the Blood by bleeding the Ting points: L11, St45, H9 and Li1.

We neutralize the Yang by increasing the Yin:

K1, Sp6 and CV4.

We also fight the Heat indirectly:

- Make the Wind circulate to fight the Heat: B12 and GB41.
- Make the Yang descend: St37 and GB39; and
- Drain the Fire: K2 and St36.

TREATMENT OF THE EMPTINESS OF THE BLOOD

Principal axis:

- Tonify the Sp: Li13, B17, Sp2 and B20 (moxa),
- Increase the Yin in general: CV4 and CV6.

Secondary axis:

- Tonify the K: K3, B23 and K14.

TREATMENT OF THE STAGNATIONS OF BLOOD

- Circulate the Li: Li2 and Li3 (acceleration and transporting point);
- Unblock the Stagnation of the Qi, of the Li with Li6; in general with CV12 and CV6 and the Tsri point in case of blockage.

TREATMENT OF CUTANEOUS REACTIONS

- Circulate the Internal Wind: B12 and GV16.
- Circulate the External Wind: Li1 and GB41.
- Humidify and "dry": Sp7 and Sp3.
- Tonify the Qi: CV6, mobilizes the Blood.

CLINICAL EXAMPLES

PSORIASIS

Pathogenesis

In TCM, this disease is called Bai Bi. It is a skin disease characterized by white, squamous lesions, especially in the region of the elbows and knees, itching in about 30% of the cases. It is the most widespread skin disease (60% of all skin diseases), affecting people in various degrees. This resistant disease has two important etiologic factors: Excess Wind (Xie Fong), an External factor and dried Blood (Internal factor). While the etiology is still somewhat mysterious, some factors are outstanding. Among these are hereditary factors, diabetes alternating with psoriasis or rheumatism with psoriasis, and a mental picture of obsessive compulsive behavior as well as hypersensitivity (exhibited in the O.S. and P. S. nervous system.

(a) Dried Blood.

The appearance of Heat in the Blood has an internal origin, linked to the physical constitution, the Seven Emotions and imbalance in food intake. For instance, anger and frustration lead to a blocking of the Qi; the Qi stagnates and transforms into Heat, leading to an Excess of Heat in the heart. On the other hand, excess of fatty foods and seafood disturbs the equilibrium between stomach and spleen. The spleen cannot transform and transport the food, and the stagnation leads to a transformation in Heat, drying up the liquids. Hence this imbalance of internal origin is provoked by food intake (especially the excess intake of pungent foods, acting on the lung) or by emotions disrupting the axis heart-lung.

(b) Xie Fong.

This External factor combines with the Heat and Dryness at the level of the skin. The Perverse Qi of the Interior (Nei Xie) combines with the Exterior one (Wai Xie) and the disease appears. The Fong and excessive Dryness cause malnutrition at the level of the skin and are responsible for the white, dry squamous lesions.

The patient has a spontaneous tendency of remissions and aggravations. Remissions occur when the perverse Qi is weak (summer, in sun, heat) or when internal causes abate: less worry, less intoxication through food and alcohol. Aggravations are revealed in the winter (predominance of perverse Qi) and when the Vital Qi is diminished because of a disturbed psyche and intoxication by alcohol especially.

The topographic distribution of the lesions is denotative of the level attacked; in progressive order they are:

- back and head hair: Tae Yang.
- elbows and knees: Cheou Yang Ming and Tsou Yang Ming.
- finally attack of the Triple Burner: generalized psoriasis.
- reaches Tae Yin showing psoriasis pustulosa.
- reaches Shao Yin with rheumatic psoriasis.

Categories

When the Wind, Heat and Dryness persist for a long period they exhaust the Blood Yin and the liquids in general. The Blood cannot feed the skin anymore, it has become "dry" and hot. According to the pathological characteristics, the disease is divided in two categories:

- Type Heat in the Blood
- Type Dryness in the Blood

(a) Psoriasis type Heat in the Blood

This corresponds to the active stage of the disease. The eruptions appear and spread very fast. Large parts of the body are covered with reddish, scaly lesions; new lesions appear constantly from which the superficial layer is easily scratched away while the basal layer is adherent.

Other "Heat symptoms" are predominant: itching, dryness of the mouth and tongue, constipation, anxiety and irritability. There are small amounts of urine, the tongue is red and shows cracks with a dry, yellow fur.

The *therapy* eliminates the Heat, cools and activates the Blood:

- Drain the Heat with the Ting points (especially L11) and GV14, St45 and St44, all in dispersion.
- Cool the Blood with the Yang Ming level, that drains the Heat of the Interior: LI4 and 11.
- Activate the Blood with B17 (Influential point of the Blood) and PC7 (Source point or Shu point), that will guide this Blood where it is needed.

(b) Psoriasis type Dryness in the Blood

This is the phase of psoriasis between the acute stages. The eruptions are hard plaques, more widespread and less numerous. Formation of new lesions occurs seldom in this stage. The tongue is rather pale with a white, thin fur. There is a deep, slow pulse.

Therapy feeds the Blood, irrigates the skin and disperses the Wind:

- Nourish the Blood with B20, stimulate the metabolism of the liquids with Sp7 to fight Dryness.
- Irrigate the skin with the Lo point that commands the skin, SI7. The SI meridian is part of Tai Yang, the Exterior part of the Yang; the Shu point or SI7 rules the Qi outside the meridians.
- Activate the Blood with B17, make the Blood circulate with CV6 (Sea of Qi) and CV17.
- Disperse the Wind with GV16, B20 and GB20.

Other treatment plans

- According to the topography: *a localized* form (one Yang meridian Tsou or Cheou), use Ho points and Lo points of affected meridian; in a more *extensive* form (2 or more Yang meridians affected) use the previous points and add the Yang Oe treatment (TB5 coupled with GB41); in the *generalized* form tonify the essential Qi and balance the Yin and Yang through CV6, 12, 13, 17, B17 and 22, GV14, LI4, St36, 41, Sp6 and 10.
- According to the cause: *food*, tonify the Sp, *mental/emotional* treat according to the 5 elements, depending on the organ attacked (see chapter on "Acupuncture and Psychology"), *perverse Qi attack* treat the Iu (Shu) points of the affected meridian and use Penn or protection points (see Chapter 4).
- A complicated form such as Psoriasis *pustulosa* is treated by the Yu-Mo technique of the Sp (B20-Sp13) coupled with toxin elimination points (LI4 and 11, Li3); the *rheumatic* psoriasis is treated by the tonification of the K (B23-GB25, Yu-Mo), coupled with the tonification of the K meridian [K7 and K4 (Lo)]. Add Influential points of the bones, tendons and the rheumatic master point: B11, GB34 and TB5.

Conclusion

Psoriasis is a disease of internal origin, affecting the Blood. The chronicity is due to numerous factors, responsible for a vicious cycle. Acupuncture has a success rate of about fifty percent in this difficult treatable disease. While we know that Western Medicine is almost helpless, acupuncture is a safe and successful alternative. It is evident again, that we have to treat the patient with a disease and not the disease! Only by individualizing the case can we expect to make a difference.

HEADACHES

Pathogenesis

There are two types of headache, linked to a disturbance of Blood:

- Headaches due to a local disturbance of Blood, in other words due to an emptiness, fullness, or stagnation of Blood.
- Headaches secondary to a disturbance in general (for instance, headache in the menstrual cycle).

We limit ourselves to the first category. How do these headaches present? When an acupuncturist is confronted with headaches, the most important aspect is to determine whether it is an *endo-cranial* or *exo-cranial* headache.

In case of an exo-cranial headache, the patient "feels the headache under his finger". The pain is accessible to palpation and goes to the face and neck.

On the other hand, in an endo-cranial headache, the pain is deep and located in the "orifices" of the skull. These are the eyes, the ears, the occipital barrier GV16 and GV20, which sends a branch into the brain.

The pathology "Headaches and Blood Disorders" is always an endo-cranial one. After eliminating the headaches due to disturbances of the Qi and invasion of Perverse Qi (Wind, Cold and Heat), we distinguish headaches due to an emptiness, fullness and stagnation of the Blood.

Types of "Blood" headaches

(a) Headaches due to an Emptiness of Blood

Symptoms: Blood is Yin in comparison with Qi; so these are headaches due to an emptiness of Yin, responding to the Eight Conditions: internal, deep, improved with Cold and aggravated with Heat, improved upon pressure on the eyes. The patient has a feeling of "emptiness in the head", he cannot concentrate. How do we know if this emptiness of Yin is an emptiness of Blood? Because we have signs of emptiness of Blood: vertigo, fatigue, cerebral fatigue and difficulty in concentrating. A very important notion is that this type of headache becomes aggravated with alcohol or wine intake: both create Liver Fire Ascending Yang and Interior Heat, exhausting the already Deficient Yin.

Causes: we can find three possibilities:

- A non-distribution of Blood by the chest.
- A blockage of Blood in the lower part of the body, especially in the pelvis, the Yin of the Yin.
- A total Emptiness of Blood.

The Blood is not distributed by the chest.

The Qi and Blood assimilated by our food intake arrive at the chest. Here the Qi is distributed by the Lung (master of the Qi), the Blood by the Heart. To distribute the Blood by the heart, we act on the Shu point (distribution or transport point), PC7. At the same time, we increase the amount of Blood with B15 and 17 (Influential point of the Blood and Back Shu point of the heart). Another point is B43, command point of the Envelope of the H.

The Blood is blocked in the pelvis

The Blood or Yin will not ascend to the upper part of the body, resulting in an emptiness of Blood in the head. For the stagnation of Blood in the pelvis, we puncture the command point of the Envelope of the uterus, B53. To circulate the Blood, we need the Qi (the Yang moves the Yin). Two Yang points move the Blood of the pelvis: GB28 and B32.

Total Emptiness of Blood

This will aggravate the local emptiness (at the head). Tiredness, night sweats, insomnia and little menstrual blood loss are clear indications of this syndrome. We act on the quality of the Blood with Sp10, while B17 puts it into movement. To correct the problem completely, we look for the cause of emptiness of the Blood, which can be at the level of the heart, liver or the spleen.

(b) Headaches due to a Fullness of Blood

The patient has a feeling of fullness, that his head may "explode". There is aggravation by pressure on the eyeball and improvement by Heat. The patient has a plethoric, red face. Treatment is PC1, a Sky-window point that makes the Blood descend from the head to the body.

NOTE: two pairs of points rule the movements of Qi and Xue at the head

- GV21, brings Yang to the head.
- G 22, brings Yin to the head.
- L3, makes the Qi descend.
- PC1, makes the Blood descend.

(c) Headaches due to a stagnation of Blood

This is a dull headache, unchanged upon pressure but improved by massage and Heat. Both accelerate the circulation of the Blood. What is the cause of the stagnation?

There is no stagnation of Blood without stagnation of Qi, they go hand in hand. Therefore, treatment must include the movement of the Yang. The first step in therapy is the stimulation of a Wind point, which puts into movement the Endo-cranial Qi and Xue: GV16. Two points move the Yang and therefore the Yin: TB16 and GB15.

Acupuncture and OB/Gyn 16

PREGNANCY AND DELIVERY

Is there ever a greater need for safe and effective medical help than at the moment we bring a new human being into this world? There is no doubt that there cannot be a safer method than acupuncture to alleviate the pain during this — let's face it — enjoyable but difficult process. There is no suppression of the respiratory system of the unborn, no rhythm disturbances and no cyanosis, as can happen with regular medication. Furthermore, acupuncture is extremely helpful in preparing the mother and the baby for delivery. Pregnancy is putting into movement the whole Yin of the woman, not only at the level of the pelvis, but in the whole body.

CONTRA-INDICATIONS OF ACUPUNCTURE DURING PREGNANCY

More than in any other area, it is important to mention the contra-indications of acupuncture during pregnancy. Forbidden points to use in pregnant women are well known, but in general, any points that add too much Yang should not be punctured. All they can do is bring Yang or movement to a fetus which needs rest during nine months. No wonder that large Yang energetic points, such as LI4 and St36, are forbidden during the whole pregnancy.

Some acupuncturists go as far as refusing to accept a pregnant woman as a patient. Although it is essential to be very cautious, there are great points that can benefit the mother-to-be, especially in the weeks prior to delivery.

All the Ting points, strongly energetic in nature, Li3, LI4, St36 and Sp6, are contra-indicated during the entire pregnancy. Puncturing these points may lead to a spontaneous abortion!

During pregnancy, certain points cannot be punctured in certain months, for fear of disturbing the pregnancy:

1st month: Sp2, Li2.

2nd month: GB34.

3rd month: PC8.

4th month: TB4-TB10, PC6.

5th month: Li9.

6th month: St40-St25, LI10.

7th month: L7 - L11.

8th month: Li1-L12-LI10-LI11.

9th month: Li4-K1, K2-K7.

It is also no surprise that we do not puncture points of the lower abdomen. The pelvic zone will be one of rest and growth; no exterior intervention is needed during these months.

If these rules are applied, acupuncture can be regarded as safe and helpful for any pregnant woman.

PREPARATION FOR THE DELIVERY

An important point that can be punctured at the third and sixth months of pregnancy is K9, the accumulation point of the Yin Wei Mo (Yin linking channel). K9 is the point that governs the mutations of the conception. Soulié de Morant said that puncturing this point creates a "child with a nice color, immune to diseases and healthy in body and mind!"

Another important point indicated is K16, a point that governs the closure of the nourishing maternal Yin to the fetus. It is indicated in the case of recurrent miscarriages due to a lack of fetal nutrition, or to maternal malnutrition, alimentary or affective. There is a lack of warmth (Heat/Yang), leading to Cold symptoms: gastric spasms, diarrhea, aggravated by exterior Cold or food.

In addition, three weeks prior to the delivery date, an energetic equilibrium therapy for the pregnant woman can begin. First, differentiation is made between primipara (first birth) and multipara (second or later birth), as the needs will be different for these women.

Primipara will often encounter anxiety, fear and nervousness. A simple therapy, once a week, will suppress these feelings.

- H3(d) and H7(d), pacify the mind.
- CV6(d) and CV12(d), alleviate nausea and vomiting.
- CV3, intersection of the three leg Yin meridians, increases the Yin and suppresses these Yang symptoms.

Multipara suffer more from fatigue and lassitude, with potential danger of rupture of the uterus muscles. Our therapy, therefore, will be directed to these causes:

- CV6, Sea of Qi, with moxa to increase the energy.
- GB34(t), influential point of the muscles, to avoid rupture during the delivery.
- GV1(t), confluent point of all the Yang meridians to bring Yang Qi to the patient.

ACUPUNCTURE DURING THE DELIVERY

Delivery under acupuncture-induced anesthesia is becoming increasingly accepted by the public. Two advantages of this method are: total atoxic anesthesia for mother and child and total reversibility. At any moment the treatment can be reversed and classical Western methods can be started.

According to traditional Chinese medicine, pregnancy is a concentration of Yin in the uterus. The Yin grows in the Shao Yin. The delivery is an expulsion or a movement to the exterior and therefore, Yang. The pain in the delivery is due to concentration of Qi in the pelvis. Qi needs to be brought upward. One possibility for therapy is:

GV2 and GV5: GV2 is theacceleration point of the pelvis

B31 and B34: to aid the sacrum.

LI4 and St25: to improve contractions.

Acupuncture is also very helpful in inducing labor. Since the uterus is an Extra organ, we use the Extra meridians that pass through the uterus:

- Yin Chiao Mo and Jenn Mo: K6, L7 and B67 (Moxa). The latter point is often used in case of malposition of the fetus.
- Dilation of the uterus: St36, Li3 and LI4. To cause dilation of the cervix, it is necessary to bring Qi or Yang to the muscles, as Yin has a tendency to contract and Yang a tendency to dilate. The Qi corresponds to the Liver, the Blood to the Spleen. Tonify Sp6 and the Yung point of the Li, Li2. CV3 and are

also punctured, since they bring the Qi of the lower Yin channels to the uterus.

- Progressive dilation: B60, LI4 and Sp6. Once complete dilation is achieved, take all the needles out and use L7, confluent point of Jenn Mo.

Other techniques for inducing labor are known. Among them is a modern Chinese approach using electro-stimulation on LI4, GB26 and St36, or, GB34 (Influential point of the muscles), CV4 or 3, points of intersection of the three Yin leg channels on the Conception channel. By using these points, Qi is brought to the pelvis and the uterus in particular. Sp6, intersection of the three leg Yin channels in the spleen channel activates the Blood and the Qi.

POST-PARTUM AND PREGNANCY COMPLICATIONS

Prolapsus of the uterus

This is caused by deficient Sp. Qi, which is the energy for uplifting the tissues and strengthening the muscles. Therapy:

- Li13 and Sp6 strengthen the spleen.
- St30 over the Fallopian ligament, assures support to the uterus.
- GV20, draws the uterus upward.

Mastitis and deficient lactation

Therapy is very effective:

- L7, confluent point of Jenn Mo.
- St18, located under the breast, stimulates the Qi circulation.
- CV17, source of Qi, to stimulate lactation.
- SI1, proved clinically effective for these conditions.

Abnormal uterine bleeding

In TCM they are called, "abnormal movements of the fetus." Different causes are possible.

* *Weakness of Blood and Qi:* in patients with weak constitution, prolonged diseases, loss of fluids before, and emptiness of Sp-St all lead to a deficiency of Blood and a malnourishment of the fetus. Treatment consists in puncturing L7, CV12, St36, Sp10 and B17.

* *Emptiness of K Qi:* after recurrent abortions or sexual abuses (excessive masturbation or sexual intercourse). Tonify the K with B23, CV4, K2 and B52.

* *Heat of Blood:* after conception, the Blood accumulate in the sea of Blood or Xue Hai to nourish the fetus. Perverse Heat can disturb the Qi of the fetus, causing abnormal movements of the fetus. Clinical symptoms are anxiety, agitation, dry lips and mouth, hot flushes, oliguria, and red tongue with a yellow fur. Treatment: eliminate the heat, nourish the Yin through LI11, St36, CV4, K11, K7 and Sp10.

* *Trauma:* a fall, intense physical labor or sports, a physical shock can damage the Qi and Blood. Tonify the Blood and Qi through Sp10, B17 and PC6 and calm the fetus through Sp4.

DISEASES DECREASING DURING PREGNANCY

During pregnancy, a woman is in a state of Yin in the Yin, a stage of absolute Yin: the amount of Yin Qi and Blood increases and reaches a maximum during the last trimester. Points such as LI4 and St36 are bringing much Yang to the organism and are for this reason contraindicated during the whole pregnancy. On the other hand, as stated before, they are punctured during the active process of dilation and expulsion where the Yin in the Yin goes to the Yin in the Yang, and to the Yang in the Yang (total expulsion of the neonatus).

As can be deduced from the previous characteristics, any disease due to a LACK OF YIN AND/OR BLOOD will be improved during pregnancy. Examples are: headaches due to deficient blood in the upper part of the body, psoriasis, alopecia areata, etc. Headaches and psoriasis were discussed in Chapter 4. That leaves us with the discussion of alopecia.

The chapter on Tchong Mo states: "*Where there is a lot of Blood there will be a lot of hair growth.*" Alopecia can be caused by Emptiness of Yin, either local or total. It is well-known in Western Medicine that more hair growth is seen during pregnancy. After delivery, that same hair falls out. Pregnancy brings more Yin to the mother, increasing the amount of hair follicles, bringing relief in diseases such as alopecia areata ("exclamation-point" hairs, thick at the top and thin at the base). No treatment can be prescribed for baldness: a clinical example will demonstrate the approach to the difficult problem of alopecia.

Mrs. B. comes to consult for total baldness, existing for 10 years. It started with a small spot. Six months earlier, she had experienced great fear: she witnessed two car accidents. This hair loss made us think of:

- Origin Kidney (fear !).
- An Emptiness of Blood and/or a stagnation of Qi at the level of the hair.
- A general skin problem (there was also a loss of eyebrows).
- An even more general problem of nutrition at all levels (teeth, nails, skin and lips).

INQUIRY:

- Sleep: the patient falls asleep easily, but the sleep is easily disturbed by nightmares and dreams of deportation (her father had been deported).
- Fatigue: she is often tired; she also noted that for ten years, she has not strength and no desire to do anything. She describes moments of lightheadedness, "as if there were no blood in her head," with tinnitus and loss of memory.
- Perspiration: she perspires a lot during the day (deficiency of Qi).
- Headaches: three times a week, violent in nature, located at the temples, improved by Cold and accompanied by lightheadedness and dizziness. Pressure on the eyes alleviates. This headache is of the type emptiness of Yin, either total or local, due to an obstruction of the Blood that is not distributed to the periphery.
- No vertigo, no ENT problems, no eye or back problems.
- Limbs: she often has cold hands and feet with a feeling of numbness; no cramps in the legs, but a sensation of heaviness at the end of the day.
- Thorax: morning cough (smokes two packs a day); tachycardy and feeling of fear and anxiety.
- Abdomen: good digestion, no gas or gastritis.
- Pelvis: no constipation or diarrhea, urination normal. Menarche at 17, oligo menorrhea (32 to 45 days), lasting 15 days.
- Blood: two normal pregnancies with no headaches during these periods (the fullness of Yin during the pregnancy corrected the otherwise existing emptiness of Yin). Frequent leucorrhea. Good harmonious sex life.
- Psychological structure: strong morale, but she has become very anxious and sensitive.

ANALYSIS:

There are two possible causes: An emptiness of the K or an emptiness of the H, both causing an emptiness of Blood. This patient definitely has signs of emptiness of Blood: headaches, type Xu of Yin, cold hands and feet, fatigue, loss of memory and tachycardy. It is not an emptiness of the Upper Burner: there would be oppression and signs of the H and L pulse.

Could this headache be due to a local problem, type obstruction of passage of Blood from the trunk to the head (type Sky-Window point, SI17)? No! There would be more a cerebral fatigue and not a total physical fatigue. This patient mentioned another important aspect: she did not like to have clothes around her neck (sign of Fullness!). This symptom is found when St11 is blocked. This is a barrier problem: the Yang does not descend, and there is a sensation of Fullness. Conclusion: there is Emptiness of Yin, combined with a local Yang Excess.

This creates a vicious circle for the head hair:

- Emptiness of Blood due to a K or H problem.
- A local Yang Fullness, that cannot descend to the thorax.

TREATMENT

There is an alternative between treating H or K. Treatment was started with the H central, according to the pulses:

- B15 and K23.
- B14 (Yu of PC).
- B17, Influential point of the Blood.
- GV22, draws the Blood to the superior part,once it has been put into movement.
- PC7, Shu point, transports and delivers the Blood, once it is put into movement.

Leave the needles in for a long time. Treat once a week for four weeks, then once every 14 days for two months.

MENOPAUSE

Menopause is not a disease but a certain moment, a certain inevitable stage in the life of women. Women's life is dominated by the Figure "7" (Chapter 1, Su Ouenn*). There are two important physiological stages, "2 times 7"* which is the menarche and *"7 times 7"* or menopause. So the Chinese have an exact idea when women should reach menopause: at age 49, not earlier. Quite a difference with modern doctors who perform hysterecomies ad lib from age 40 on.

The Su Ouenn describes these two stages as follows:

"At the age of 14, Ren mo circulates abundantly, Tchong Mo is prosperous, the menses manifest themselves according to a determined cycle."

After puberty, women enter in a period dominated by the figure 7 as is evident in : "7 times 4" or 28 days for the menstrual cycle and "7 times 4 times 10" or 280 days of gestation.

"At the age of 49, Ren Mo is empty, Tchong Mo weakens, the body is exhausted and the woman is not fertile anymore."

From then on, women and men, can concentrate on the second stage in their life, the quest for spirituality which is true life. While puberty represents the passage of the child to a human being sexually well-differentiated, menopause is the passage of the adult, confirmed in her sexuality, to a less distinctive sexual being. Men go through a similar stage except that their "sacred" number is "8." For the Chinese, menopause and andropause, so much feared in Western culture, is a period to celebrate as intimacy will be strengthened, while they enter a period of retreat, preparing themselves to die.

WHAT IS THE TREATMENT OF MENOPAUSE?

Treatment is aimed at facilitating its mutation. The most important point is Li14, the end of Yin, the pass of Tai Yin to Chiueh Yin. Similar points are K9 during pregnancy and Sp15 at the moment of puberty. Other points are K4 and B31: menopause is an emptiness of Qi with a stagnation of Blood at the level of the pelvis and an escape of heat or Qi from the Blood, causing hot flushes. K4, Lo point, commands the Inferior Triple Burner (place of menopausal disturbances) and B31 is a point that stimulates the penetration of the Yang in the pelvis, it is the Yang that puts the Yin into movement. Puncture also GB29, "door of the hips".

In function of certain symptoms, other points

will be added. In case of hypertension and severe hot flushes which indicates a strong obstruction of Blood in the pelvis with ascending of the Yang (wind, heat) of the Blood to the head, add PC7 (stimulates the circulation of Blood) and H7 (calms the mind). To avoid osteoporosis, add B11, master point of the bones. For emotional imbalance such as logorrhea, agitation, dreams about death and jealous episodes, puncture points of the SHENN, B15 (point Shu H) and GV11, "voice of SHENN."

It is important for the acupuncturist to assist women in their menopause, especially to aid women in reaching their "spiritual embryo" and assure their survival.

STERILITY AND AMENORRHEA

Immediate after pelvic pains, amenorrhea and sterility are among our daily gynecological problems. Clinical symptoms are different, treatments are never the same, and results are uncertain. Restoring the menstrual cycle, symbol of femininity, is joyful to the physician and the patient. In Traditional Chinese Medicine, a woman is considered sterile if she stays three years married without bearing a child (of course, if pregnancy is desired).

What is ovulation? It is the liberation of an ova, corresponding to an exteriorization from within the ovary. The ovary is anatomically the deepest, most hidden of all the organs, attached energetically to the "kidney system." In comparison to the ovary, the uterus , "wonder organ," is external since it is an opening to the exterior, allowing the introduction of spermatozoa and nine months later the exit of a child. The Chinese call the uterus the "palace" of the child. So the ova exits from the Yin of the Yin. This movement of the Yin of the Yin to the exterior must be a very special movement of Yin since the Yin in general has the tendency to stagnate, to take refuge in the deepest and lower part of the body. The only Yin which opens to the exterior is the Tai Yin level, hinge of the Yin, opening to the exterior Yang. Hence, Tai Yin is treated in case of menstrual and ovulation deficiencies or blocks. The main cause of these anomalies is psychological since most modern people are free of hygienic problems, malnutrition and hard labor conditions. The major cause is inherent to modern life with its fast pace style. There is the worry (which correspond to the "Earth movement or Sp.) in meticulous women, obsessed with their work and ambitions, as well as the sadness of the Metal movement or Lung. Thus the totality of Tai Yin is affected. Emotionally, often we perceive in these women a difficulty of opening themselves to the "exterior, "to their friends and gentlemen friends. Besides changing these women psychologically (psychotherapy and homeopathy!), the treating physician has to open the Tai Yin of these patients "physically." The technique used is the "knot and root" treatment. K1, CV, CV3 and St29 and the extra meridian point Zi Gong ("Palace of the Son").

The causes of sterility in women are: Xu Yin K, Xu Yang K, Xu Yin and Yang K, stagnation of Blood, accumulation of mucus and emptiness of Ren Mo. In men we have a Xu Yin K, Xu Yang K and accumulation of Dampness.

WOMEN

Emptiness of K Yang

Because of Xu Yang K, the internal cold accumulates at the level of the uterus. Normally, the spleen produces the blood which is filtered and stored by the liver. The blood arrives then at Tchong Mo to descent to the uterus. The uterus is linked to heart and kidney. Both of these, together with Ren Mo and Tchong Mo must be normal.

Symptoms in Xu Yang K are oligomenorrhea, late dark menses with much pain and a broken back feeling or fatigue in lower back and lower extremities. Cold limbs, chilliness and abundant, clear urination. Pale tongue with a small pale fur, deep thin pulse.

Treatment is B23, GV4, K3 (moxa) and CV4.

Emptiness of K Yin

This elicits an "escape" of the Yang K and an internal "fire" in the uterus, preventing pregnancy. Symptoms are abundant menses (profuse), premature or early and prolonged (the 3 "Ps") and bright red. Nocturnal perspiration, and hot palms and soles. Lumbar fatigue, red tongue, with a yellow fur and a thin deep pulse. Treatment is K2, B52, Sp6, St29, CV6, CV12 and K7.

Emptiness of K Yin and Yang

This is caused by abundant chronic bleeding or other chronic conditions consuming blood. Very little bleeding or very long cycle, to the point of amenorrhea. All limbs are ice cold and there is a sensation of cold in the lower abdomen. Evening fever, tinnitus, pale tongue with a light fur and deep and thin pulse, especially in the third position. Treatment is B23, GV4, CV4, K3, St36 and Sp4.

Stagnation of Qi and Blood

Is caused by continuos suppressed anger, frustration, irritability or recurrent disappointment. Irregular cycles, little bleeding with much pain and clotting, with pain in lower abdomen. Painful swelling of the breasts before menses with irritability and depression. Red tongue, white fur, tense pulse. Treatment is St29, Sp10, B18, Li3, Sp6, B17 (Influential point of Blood), and B40.

Accumulation of mucus

Caused by alcohol misuse, alimentary excesses (especially sweets) and obesity will cause a weakness of the spleen with formation of mucus. Symptoms are obesity, pale face, vertigo, palpitations, dyspnoe, rare and little bleeding, often amenorrhea. Anorexia and asthenia. Swollen tongue with dental imprints, yellow fur and slippery pulse. Treatment is St29, PC6, CV12, St40 (anti-mucus point), Sp6, and CV6.

Emptiness of Ren Mo

It is the place that coordinate all the Yin in the body. Symptoms are pelvic signs, prolaps uteri and inflammation of the genital organs. Treatment is CV2.

MEN

Emptiness of K Yang

Causality is chronic disease, physical exhaustion and aging. Symptoms are back pains, fatigue in lower extremities, ejaculatio praecox, decreased libido and frequent urination. The tongue is pale with a white fur and the pulse is deep. Therapy is B23, CV4, GV4, K3, and Sp6, needling and moxa.

Emptiness of K Yin

Causality is bleeding, febrile diseases and medications such as laxatives and anti-fever medication. Symptoms are lumbago, dreams with nocturnal emissions, frequent urination, and decreased libido. Also insomnia, night sweats and tinnitus. Red tongue, with little fur and a rapid thin pulse. Therapy is K2, B52, Sp6, K7 and CV6.

Accumulation of dampness

Caused by alcohol abuse and bad diet habits. There is fatigue in the legs and back, painful, burning urination, a yellow fur on the tongue, and a deep fast pulse. Treatment is K3, Sp6, B23 and Sp9.

URGENCIES IN PREGNANCY AND POST-PARTUM

During pregnancy urgencies can come up rapidly. Decisions either medical or surgical, have to be swiftly. Without forgetting the necessity of Western medicine in many of these cases, it is interesting to view what an acupuncturist can do in these circumstances. In fact, in many cases acupuncture can solidify a medico-surgical act. In this chapter, we are not talking about extra-uterine pregnancy, an uterine rupture, or placenta previa which all necessitate urgent surgical intervention. But what can we do with acupuncture? During the first months, pregnancy vomiting, pain syndromes, certain bleedings and digestive malfunction are responsive to acupuncture treatments. During the following months, oliguria, anuria, fetal malpositions, ecclampsia, convulsions, and the onset of labor. In the post-partum period, acupuncture aides in lactation problems and retention of urine.

PHYSIOLOGY

During pregnancy, the Qi and Blood of the whole organism concentrates in the uterus and pelvis to allow the nutrition of the embryo and fetus. This is under the direction of Ren Mo and Tchong Mo. Thus pregnancy is characterized by a great fullness and an acceleration of the movement of the Yin, diminishing possibly the Yang and slowing down the movement of the Yang. Hence we see during pregnancy aggravation of fullness of Yin states, and improvements of fullness of Yang conditions, empty Yin situations and stagnations of Yin. Also, the accumulation of Blood and Qi in the pelvic envelop can lead to a desequilibrium of Qi/ Blood everywhere in the body: emptiness of Blood in the periphery or fullness of Yang in the organs.

The delivery itself is an exteriorization movement. At the end of forty weeks (40 x 7 days) we are at full term and the Yin fullness is at a maximum and will interact with the Yang, pushing the fetus downwards towards the cervix uteri. The lactation, a physiological consequence of the pregnancy to continue the feeding of the fetus, is under command of Ren Mo and Tchong Mo (Qi/ Blood balance), Dai Mo which controls the circulation of all the genital Yin (menses, lactation) and of the Middle Burner (Sp/St) and Upper Burner where the Lung is the master of Qi and where PC and H disperse the Blood and mental Qi.

PREGNANCY VOMITING

While most of the pregnancy vomiting is benign, although annoying, it can become life threatening in case of complete intolerance to foods and liquids with a total anorexia leading to a disastrous malnutrition (hyperemesis gravidarum). The Chinese called it Zu Bing and it responds to two different mechanisms: a disharmony spleen-stomach or liver-stomach.

Spleen-stomach disharmony

This imbalance is due to a Sp/St Qi deficiency, heat in the stomach and the presence of humidity with formation of mucus.

· *Xu Qi Sp/St.*

The spleen cannot distribute the Qi extracted from foods and air and the impure Qi cannot be directed to the lower part of the body by the stomach. The food Qi and the Qi of Tchong Mo which is very abundant ascend to the upper part of the body, causing nausea and vomiting. The symptoms reflect the Xu Qi of Sp.: vomiting with intolerance to foods, anorexia, abdominal distention, morning diarrhea, a moist tongue with yellow fur and an empty, slippery pulse. We tonify the spleen, harmonize the stomach and regularize the Blood and Qi: St36, PC6, B20, CV12, B21, Sp4.

· *Heat in the stomach*

Occurs in women with excessive Yang-heat. There is a reflux of the stomach Qi, and the recurrent vomiting harms the Yin. There is bitter vomiting with yellow-green liquids, dry mouth, bitter taste, prefers cold drinks but vomits them as soon they reach the stomach (this is a keynote for the homeopathic remedy Phosphorus, indicated in this case of pregnancy vomiting), anxiety, asthenia, insomnia, oliguria, hard stools, red tongue with little fur and a rapid, slippery pulse. Treatment consists in eliminating the heat, harmonize the stomach and increase the Yin through St36, B25, CV12, K11, Sp7, and Sp10.

· *Dampness/mucus formation*

The deficient Sp. Qi allows the invasion of Dampness and the formation of mucus. This mucus takes advantage of the weak stomach Qi to stagnate in the stomach. The vomit is full of mucus, there are palpitations, vertigo, fullness in the chest, damp, white tongue and slippery pulse. Eliminate mucus through St40, CV12, Sp4, St36, B20 and 21.

· *Liver-stomach dysfunction*

After conception, because of Blood accumulation in the pelvis, the Blood (Yin) of the liver is often in deficiency while the Qi or Yang is in excess. Even more so during anger and irritability, the excessive liver Qi and the Qi of Tchong Mo ascend and attack the stomach, with vomiting and nausea as a result. There is clear liquid vomiting, sometimes sour, aerophagy, fullness and a sense of oppression in the chest, pain in the sides, thirst, vertigo, bitter taste in mouth, pale red tongue and a hard, slippery pulse. Calm the liver through Li8, harmonize the stomach through CV12, St36 and Sp4.

· *Hyperemesis gravidarum (Zu Bing)*

Even in this case, often when the patient is hospitalized, acupuncture can help before Western methods with infusions, tranquilizers, isolation, and anti-depressants is instituted. Deep puncture of PC6, CV12, puncturing upwards towards CV15, and Sp4. One session of 30′ daily.

GENITAL BLEEDING

They are often the first signs of abortion and are called "abnormal movements of the fetus" in Chinese medicine. Tchong Mo ("Sea of Blood") and Ren Mo are disturbed and cannot feed the fetus. It is a non-consolidation of Tchong Mo and Ren Mo, called, "non-consolidation of Chong Ren." This is caused by a weakness of Blood and Qi, emptiness of K Qi, heat in the Blood and trauma.

· *Weak Blood and Qi*

Caused by weak constitution—Phosphorus and Calcarea Carbonicum in homeopathy, and long-time illnesses. Treatment is L7, CV12, St36, B17 (Influential point of Blood) and Sp10.

· *Kidney emptiness*

Born out of sexual abuses (frequent masturbation and intercourse) and repetitive abortions. Before pregnancy these women have little bleeding, long cycles, cold limbs and lumbar fatigue. During pregnancy, abnormal movements of the fetus, bleedings, extreme fatigue in lower back, vertigo, tinnitus, pale tongue with white fur, deep and thin pulse in third position. B23, CV4, K2 and B52 will tonify the kidneys and calm the fetus.

· *Heat in Blood*

After conception, because the Blood accumulates in the sea of Blood to nourish the fetus the Yang Qi has a tendency to be in excess. This excessive perverse Qi disturbs the Qi circulation of the fetus. Abnormal movements and bleeding result from it. There is anxiety, agitation, palms and hands are warm, hot flushes, oliguria, dark urine, red tongue with dry yellow fur and a rapid, slippery pulse. Eliminate the heat and nourish the Yin through St36, LI11, CV4, K11, Sp7 and Sp10.

· *Trauma*

A fall, an intense physical effort or a physical shock can damage the Qi/Blood and disturb Chong Ren. Tonify the Blood/Qi: Sp10, B17, CV6 and Sp4.

FETAL MALPOSITIONS

After 30 weeks of gestation, either a transversal position or breech position can be noticed. This is often the case in multiparae with a decreased tone in their muscles or in fearful, frightful patients through an emotional stress. This fetal malposition is due to a stagnation of Qi. Treatment must therefore de block the Qi. The best point is B67 in moxa! Put the patient on her back, and moxa both sides 15′ once or twice a day. Control the position again after one week of treatment. Best results are obtained before the seventh month of pregnancy! Long-term studies have shown a positive result in 95% of the cases!

DYNAMIC DYSTOCIAS

These are problems arising during delivery in the pattern of contractions and dilatation. They will be due either to an emptiness of Qi and Blood or stagnation of Qi and Blood.

· *Emptiness of Blood/Qi*

In women who are weakened by too much work or in case of premature rupture of the membranes. It is often present in multiparae, in cases of large babies or in hydramnios with short and feeble contractions. The labor progresses slowly and one observes a pale face, asthenia, palpitations and often abundant blood loss. Tonify with moxa and needles LI4, Sp6, CV6, Sp10, CV3 and CV4.

· *Stagnation of Blood/Qi*

Lumbar pains, strong but irregular contractions, often loss of dark-red blood, nausea, red tongue with thick fur, hard, irregular pulse. It is often present in case of hypersensitive people, who are very sensitive to pain. Because contractions are very intense and following each other up quickly, the patient fatigues easily and becomes anxious. Eliminate the stagnation to accelerate the delivery: LI4, GB27, Sp6, GB28, B37, and St36. In case of non-dilation of the cervix, puncture Li2 and Li3!

PELVIC PAINS AND DYSMENORRHEA

When confronted with a pelvic pain in absence of an anatomical lesion, the acupuncture diagnostic is systematic: first, an analysis of the pain according the Eight Conditions, followed by an inquiry to discover the global disturbance with this local dysfunction. At last but not least, just like in homeopathy, the acupuncturist must get a sense of the personality of the patient to understand why this patient came down with a pelvic pain (the *totality of the symptoms*).

The *Eight Conditions* are discussed in Chapter 7. According to the energy movements, pelvic pains are caused in order of frequency by stagnations and fullnesses of Yin, emptninesses of Yang, emptinesses of Yin, fullnesses of Yang and rarely by stagnations of Yang.

· *Stagnation of Yin*

A typical Yin pain, spastic and cramping, not changed by pressure, but improved by massage, heat and movement, aggravated by cold and rest. This stagnation reflects on the menses (difficult start and painful the first day), on the stools (constipation) and the urination (oliguria and pollakiuria, necessity of pressing). The Yin of the pelvic area is put into movement by K13 and B31. The stagnation of Yin resonate especially on Tsou Shao Yin (K) and Yin Wei.

· *Fullness of Yin*

Spastic, cramping pains aggravated by pressure, movement and cold, improved by heat, often situated in the right lower part of the pelvis. Often accompanied by constipation, oliguria, and premenstrual pain, diminishing as soon as the flow starts. The blood is often black with a lot of clots. Sp14 dissolves the fullness of Yin in the pelvic area, Sp12 facilitates the movement of the Yin from trunk to the lower extremities, CV4 facilitates the movement of the Yin downwards in general and B34 which empties the pelvic Yin accumulations.

· *Emptiness of Yang*

Spastic, cramping Yin pain, better by pressure and heat, worse by movement which consumes Yang. Usually the pain is located higher than in the case of a fullness of Yin and often the patient is diagnosed with a cystitis or colitis in Western medicine. This emptiness of Yang can be the result of a non-descending of the Yang in the abdomen, which is corrected by St27 or St31 (barrier point, allows the entry of Yang in the pelvis) or by a non-descending of the Yang in the trunk, treated by St25 (closure of yang in the abdomen), St39 and GV20.

· *Emptiness of Yin*

Burning, stinging, electrical Yang pains, improved by cold and pressure and aggravated by heat. Little modified by massage and localized mainly on the left side. Other symptoms are constipation, oliguria and late menses. Sp6 and Li10 allow the penetration of Yin in the pelvis from below while Li12 makes the Yin descend from the trunk or by stimulation of CV3.

· *Fullness of Yang*

Violent, sharp electrical pains, worse upon pressure and heat, improved by cold and movement, using the excess Yang. Menses are abundant and too early (profuse and premature). B29 descends the Yang to the lower extremities or GB24.

· *Stagnation of Yang*

Is a rare clinical picture, more often we see a slipped disc or a lumbar pain picture in these circumstances. Sharp, burning pains, not improved by pressure, but calmed down by massage, exercise and heat. B32 is the main point.

ENDOMETRIOSIS

According to Western medicine, endometriosis is a growth of endometrium outside the uterine cavity. The most common localization is in the ovary, but theoretically it can be anywhere in the body. It is mainly found in women between 30 and 50 years old, mostly childless. Endometriosis is often associated with sterility and in many cases, this will be the reason for consultation. Another frequent symptom is dysmenorrhea, with abdominal pain radiating to the inner side of the thighs. Patients are frequently considered lazy until the diagnosis is made. Beside fatigue, the pain begins two to seven days before the onset of the menstrual cycle and becomes increasingly severe until the flow slackens. The best therapeutic regimen depends on the age of the patient, the severity of symptoms and desire for pregnancy. Hormonal treatment and conservative surgery are the main approaches for this disease.

According To TCM

Endometriosis is the presence of congealed Blood in the pelvis of the woman; in other words, in the Yin of the Yin. The pelvic zone, being the most Yin zone of the body, corresponds with the Lower Burner, the "pelvic envelope" or sexuality.

Different *causes* can be involved: the Yin is not put into movement, an abnormal exchange between the Yin and the Yang or the exteriorization of the Yin is blocked.

· *The Yin is not put into movement*

Two meridians put the Yin into movement: Shao Yin and the Extra meridian, Yin Keo or Tchiao Mo. Differential diagnosis between two is made by the concomitant symptoms. Disturbances of Shao Yin (Tsou) cause backaches, dyspnea and bone diseases. Yin Keo, on the other hand, demonstrates typical symptoms such as insomnia (K6 is a sleeping point), constipation, dry eyes (Yin Tchiao Mo brings tears to the eyes) and palpation of hard masses in the abdomen. Therapy is the use of the command point of the Extra, K6 and K1, Sp6 and K6 for Tsou Shao Yin.

· *Abnormal exchange between the Yin and the Yang or Emptiness of Yang*

There is a Xu of Yang in the Interior and a relative Yang Excess in the Exterior. The problem is located at the level of Yang Ming, which does not open to the Interior. Symptoms are constipation, cervical adenitits, gum bleeding, foul breath and a constant hungry feeling. We open Yang Ming to the Interior by stimulating St25, St36 and LI11.

· *Exteriorization of the Yin is blocked.*

This defective exteriorization of the Yin causes a fullness of Yin in the interior, an emptiness of Yin with a fullness of Yang in the exterior. Since the exteriorization of the Yin happens at the level of Tai Yin (Sp and L), we will see signs of Yang emptiness of the Sp in the patient: morning diarrhea, sensitivity to cold, fatigue, abdominal distention, anorexia and sallow complexion. Sp5[(d)], Sp3, or L2 and Sp8.

Symptomatic, we see that all these endometriosis patients demonstrate a deficient Earth element. Either we note heat in Yang Ming (these Xu Heat symptoms are discussed before) or deficient Blood symptoms: dry eyes, sleep disturbances with dreams, late menstrual cycle, irregular and small amounts of blood, dizziness, night sweats, gray hair, black dots in the eyes, Chueh Yin headaches (vertex), and irritability.

The *tongue picture* shows a narrow red tongue with little fur or with yellow greasy fur in the Middle and Lower Burner.

Therapeutic points are already mentioned in the pathogenesis for the special causes. The following are points that need to be punctured in all cases of endometriosis:

- strengthening of the Middle Burner: St36, B20 and B21.
- production of the Blood: B17, Sp6 and CV4 (moxa).
- the "envelope" of the Yin in the pelvic area: Li9.
- point of the mobilization of the blood at the level of the abdomen, and more particularly in the pelvic area: CV4 (already punctured); CV6 (moxa) will

mobilize the Yin in the pelvic area, as well as Sp6 (already punctured).

- "meeting" point of the menstrual cycle, point of Yin Tsiao Mo, accelerator of the Yin: K6.
- mobilization point of the Ancestral Qi in the pelvic loge: B23.
- command point of the "envelope" of the uterus: B53.
- we also must treat the Yang because the Yang circulates the Yin. Two points circulate the pelvic blood: GB28 and B32.

GENERAL POINTS IN PELVIC PROBLEMS

· *Blocking of the Yin in the pelvis*

The Yin does not ascend, causing a Fullness of Yin in the pelvis. Symptoms are pain, aggravated by pressure and cold, occurring during the night The pain diminishes with Heat (Yang, Moxa) and occurs during the day; it is a deep, dull pain.

- CV14: barrier point of the pelvis.
- K18: barrier point of the trunk.
- Sp13: origin, Tai (see Barrier points, Chapter 11) of the pelvic Yin.

· *Non-circulation of the Yin*

The Yin stagnates in the pelvis. The pain does not change upon pressure, decreases with movement, heat and massage, and worsens with Cold and rest.

- K13: point of Shao Yin, puts the Yin into movement.
- L1: circulation of the pelvic Yin.

· *Non-interiorization of the Yin*

Yang Ming, the terminal Yang, does not open to the interior. As a result, deficient quantities of Yang are moving into the pelvis to move the Yin. Besides symptoms of stagnation of the Yin we find symptoms of stagnation at the Yang Ming level: insomnia, foul breath, diarrhea or constipation, cervical adenitis, etc.

- St25[(t)], St36[(t)] and LI11[(t)], open Yang Ming tothe interior
- GB28: Shao Yang, puts the Yang into movement and circulates the Yin.

· *Symptomatic points, bringing Yang to the pelvic area*

- CV6: "Sea of Qi";
- St31, barrier point, brings Yang in the pelvis;
- B53: rules the "pelvic envelope".

CONCLUSION

There is no doubt that acupuncture is a marvelous tool in gynecological and obstetrical problems. To illustrate this once more, here is the case of a 30-year old woman with oligomenorrhea. At consultation, she had a cycle every nine months, not a very good prognosis for becoming pregnant. The only abnormality was a decrease in the progesterone level. Just having returned from the World Congress of Acupuncture in Paris, I decided to try a treatment that was proposed in one of the lectures. We have to bear in mind that the first fourteen days of the menses are the exteriorization of the Yang. After the ovulation, the Yin grows to its maximum around the 28th day (normal cycle). The maximum Yin concentration produces the Yang (according to the acupuncture law: "*the Yin at its maximum turns into Yang and vice-versa.*"). The Qi moves the Blood and the menses appear. As a solution to the above case, a treatment consisting of four different steps was proposed. For one month, each week the points were changed. They are indicated below:

Days:	lst		7th		14th		21st	
		SI 3		PC 6		PC 6		PC 6
		L 7		K 9		K 9		K 9
		CV 24		Sp 15		Sp 13		CV 22
		CV 4		Sp 16		Li 14		CV 23
		GV 17 & 20						

I must confess, she did not menstruate the next cycle, because she was pregnant! To exclude any coincidence, I did the same thing the year after with the same woman! I can tell you, I made a believer in acupuncture out of her!

Tinnitus and Deafness 17

INTRODUCTION

Tinnitus in an ear is a sign of evolving towards deafness. This condition involves a sclerotic evolution of the middle ear progressing to deafness. Hence, the problem of tinnitus and deafness is treated in a similar way. In the majority of cases, tinnitus is essentially a subjective phenomenon, by most people felt as a constant nuisance. Tinnitus and deafness are often curable, medically or surgically, when the problem is located in the middle or external ear. But the therapy is desperate in case of disturbance of the inner ear, at the level of the cochlea and the semi-circular channels. Every acupuncturist has received patients in his office with this problem, since Western medicine is often unsuccessful in fighting this disease. Tinnitus can exist without deafness and deafness can develop without tinnitus. For the Chinese, these are two phases of the same disease.

PATHOGENESIS

According to the Tsang-Fu theory

Tinnitus and deafness can be attributed primarily to two *causes*:

- Deficient Kidney Yin leading to Deficient Liver Yin, disrupting the Yin-Yang unity, causing an ascending of the Li Yang with stirring up the Internal Wind and formation of phlegm.
- Formation of Fire in the Liver (Endogenous Heat) due to alcohol, smoking and anger.

A good *therapeutic* approach can be found in studying the internal connections of the meridians, particularly those regarding the ear. One big axis in the treatment will be the hinge of the Yang, Shao Yang. Shao Yang is formed by the meridians of TB and GB. The TB meridian starts at the fourth finger and ends at TB23, at the lateral end of the eyebrow, where it forms an internal connection with GB1. Running upward, the Triple Burner ascends to the neck, runs along the posterior border of the ear and on to the superior aspect of the ear. The auricular branch arises from the retroauricular region and enters the ear. However, there is another meridian which brings Qi to the ear and links with the same point (GB1) on the GB meridian: the small intestine meridian. This meridian starts at the fifth finger, brings the Qi up to the ear, and terminates at SI19, in front of the tragus. There is an internal connection between SI17, SI19 and GB1. Thus, there are two meridians (TB and SI) bringing Qi to the ear, where there is one major meridian bringing the Qi away from the ear: GB.

An excellent therapy is stimulating the circulation of the Qi along the meridians of TB and SI, which deliver the Energy to the ear. To activate the circulation on any given meridian, we stimulate points which have an acceleration role, the Yung point and the tonification point. In our case, there are SI2 and 7, TB2 and 10.

Secondly, we focus the Qi on the active points of the ear: TB21, GB2 and SI 9.

Our third action will be one of extraction along the GB meridian. One part of the Shao Yang becomes "Gall Bladder" after TB23. The energetic circulation along this meridian can be activated at GB34, the Ho point, where the deep Qi becomes superficial. The law "One-two" states that *"One additional needle be placed in the direction in which the Qi should go."* Therefore, we look for another point in the distal part of the GB meridian: one point (GB2), in the upper part of the body, requires two points in the distal part of the body. The point GB43 (acceleration point) will be ideal, as it will accelerate the movement of the energy in the proper direction. As the second point, we usually choose a strong energetic point along the meridian, such as the Tsri or accumulation point. Puncturing the Ho point in this case will assure the passage of the Qi to the Liver, maintaining the exterior/interior connection.

ACCORDING TO THE EIGHT CONDITIONS

Two disturbances have to be discussed: a local cause and a disequilibrium in the Yin/Yang unity.

Local cause

We have to bear in mind that the local disturbance is only a manifestation of the disease. Even after disappearance of the pain as a result of puncturing a "barrier point", and in spite of complete satisfaction of the patient, we must look for the root of the disease. We describe the local movements of the Qi to the face and neck and those points commanding these movements. As explained in Chapter 11, movements of the Qi can be classified according to intensity, quality, time and space.

- In intensity, from the lateral to the medial side of the head, SI19, TB23 and LI20.
- In intensity, from the back to the front, B9, GB5 and St1.
- In quality, from the front of the head to the back, B3.
- In time, putting into movement of the Qi from the front of the head to the back, GB1.
- In time, putting into movement of the Qi from the back of the head to the front, GB2.
- In time, putting into movement of Qi of the lateral part of the head to the nose, TB21.
- In space, the hinge of the Yang in the space, TB21.

In general, we can say that a block at one of these points causes fullness before the block, emptiness after this point. Therefore, this block can be responsible for ringing in the ears.

Disequilibrium Ying/Yang

We have to remember that the Yang descends from the head to the legs, the Yin ascends normally from the legs to the head.

(a) Disequilibrium between head and trunk

(1) Barrier trunk-head

Barrier points at this level are SI14, TB15 and St3. Obstruction of one of these points induces a symptomatology, type Fullness at the level of the trunk or thorax and an emptiness at the head. Ringing in the ears and deafness, type "emptiness", are possible symptoms. It is obvious that we mention here the movements of the Yin Qi.

(2) Barrier head-trunk
Barrier points are B 0, GB21 and St11. Obstruction causes a fullness at the head and an emptiness of the thorax. This is a ringing in the ears and deafness, type "fullness".

(b) Disequilibrium between the head and the whole body

(1) Emptiness of Yin at the head

· Deficient production at the source

We will puncture CV 4; it commands the production of the original Yin, and this at the level of the whole body

· Non-ascending of the Yin, due to stagnation inthe lower part of the body

- K6, puts into movement the Yin.
- PC5, brings the Yin to the upper part of the body.
- K18, induces the movement of the Yin of the trunk to the head.

· Blocking of the Yin at the level of the pelvis

This is frequently seen in women, with irregularities of the menses as a consequence.

- CV4 and K18 make the Yin ascend.
- K13, induces heat in the pelvis and makes the Yin circulate.
- B1, 32, 33 and 34, Yang points that mobilize the Yin

(2) Fullness of Yang at the head

· Non-descending of the Yang B10, GB21 and St11 make the Yang descend.

· Non-entering of the Yin into the Yang

This is due to non-opening of Tai-Yin to the Exterior, its natural movement. We use L2 and Sp8.

(3) Stagnation of Yang at the head

· Non-movement of the Yang in the upper part

The point to put the Yang of the Superior part into movement is found on Cheou Shao Yang or TB8.

· Non-movement of the Yang to the lower part of the body

We draw the moving Yang towards the lower part of the body with St37 and GB39.

(c) Pathology of the Blood

This pathology is extensively discussed in Chapter 15 and is only briefly repeated.

(1) The Blood is not distributed by the chest

(2) The Blood is blocked in the pelvis

The Yin or Blood, which normally ascends, does not arrive at the chest and less so at the head. To unblock this Blood, we puncture the point of the envelope of the uterus, B53, together with a stimulation of the Yang to move the Yin: GB28 and B32.

(3) General Deficiency of Blood

Besides ringing in the ears and deafness we find mental and physical fatigue, night sweats and lightheadedness. Therapy is described in Chapter 15

(4) Fullness of Blood at the head

Other symptoms will be headaches, improving with application of heat, worsening with cold and upon pressure. We make the Blood descend with puncturing of the point PC1.

(5) Stagnation of Blood at the head

This time the headaches will diminish with massage, exercise and Heat. Pressure has a negligible effect. The Yang point

GB15 moves the cephalic Yin. Remember, "Shao" means putting into movement; therefore, we take a point of Shao Yang (Tsou). A Wind point, GV16, puts into movement the Qi and Blood of the whole head.

DISEASE OF MENIERE

Meniere's disease consists of a characteristic triad: vertigo, tinnitus, and deafness. Often, the feeling of ear fullness is mentioned by the patient. These attacks are violent, with nausea, vomiting, sweating and decreased hearing. The disease occurs in patients between the ages of 30 and 60, resulting in residual tinnitus and permanent hearing loss. Pathogenesis in Western medicine is unknown, hence the therapy is a symptomatic one.

According to TCM, Meniere's disease is due to a deficient Kidney Yin, leading to a deficient Liver Yin. The unity in the Li Yin/Yang is broken, with an ascending of the Li Yang and stirring up the Interior Wind. The formation of Phlegm will obstruct the channels.

Therapy according to the theory of Tsang Fu is evident:

- GB20, disperses the Interior Wind.
- Li3, calms the Liver.
- St36, Sp4 and PC6, calm the Stomach and control vomiting.
- Li2 drains the Heat.
- St40 and Sp6 dissolve the Phlegm.

Therapy according to the *auriculotherapy* gives the best results in treating of the vertigo, nausea and vomiting. The following points in the ear are common, effective points:

- The point of the superior cervical plexus at the level of C1, C2.
- The point of the 8th cranial nerve (Acoustic nerve) with a golden needle.
- The Sensorial master point.
- The auricular ear point, which can be found inthe cheek, anterior to the lobe.

CASE HISTORY

Mrs. B., 53 years old.

Chief complaint: impairment of hearing on the left side (right-side hearing normal).

History: her hearing problem began 14 years ago and has increased in severity since that time. The loss was now estimated at 60%. During the past several months, she noticed constipation where previously no such problem was evident. Two weeks prior to this consultation, she complained of dysuria: painful urination, urgency and frequency. On her chart, she noted also a long-standing TMJ problem. Her hearing loss was diagnosed as a senso-neural deafness, as opposed to conductive deafness: she hears poorly in a noisy environment and on a telephone; speaks loudly; and air conduction is better than bone conduction.

Past medical history: hysterectomy for myomata uteri, otherwise uneventful.

Familial history: hearing impairment of a brother and a sister.

CONCLUSION 1:

According to TCM, there are two possible causes: a decrease of Yin of the Kidney (the organ related to the ear); and/or an Excess Liver Yang ascending. The first cause can lead to a situation described in the second; but it is important to know what the primary cause was. This patient's primary cause was definitely Xu of Yin of the K. Impairment of hearing was accompanied by tinnitus; she had an arthritis problem at the mandibular joint and complained of recurrent backache. The presence of myomata must have caused menstrual irregularities. The presence of impaired hearing in a brother and a sister indicated an inherited problem. We need to remember that the hereditary or Ancestral Qi is stored in the Yin Kidney. Upon being further questioned, she confessed to having become more irritable in recent years and having an awareness of decreasing memory.

CONCLUSION 2:

The patient has a Xu of Yin of the Kidney with symptoms related to the ascendance of Liver Yang. The constipation and the cystitis problem indicated that the disease was located at the level of the Burners, and even more precisely, at the level of the Lower Burner (as dysfunction of a Burner means involvement of all the organs located in that Burner). At the Lower Burner are the Kidney, Bladder and Intestines. As can be seen by the history, all three organs have been attacked and have caused a blockage at the Lower Burner level. The disease has progressed to a deep level and hence will be difficult to treat with acupuncture.

What else did we find with this patient?

Pulse diagnosis:

- Absent superficial pulses, only deep ones were present.
- Fast (5/1), weak pulse at the left Kidney position.
- Right pulses stronger than left (Yin dominance).
- Pulses in the third position weaker than in the first position (Lower Burner Deficiency).
- Pulse at K 3 position very weak (Deficiency of Qi).

Tongue diagnosis:
Red, especially at the sides and the tip. These symptoms indicate presence of heat in the Heart (Kidney/Heart axis imbalanced) and also heat in the Liver.

Palpation:

- Li4 painful (Mu point of Li).
- GB25 and CV3 painful (Mu points of B and K).
- B28 sensitive (presence of heat in B).

Therapy:

- Sp6$^{(t)}$, CV4$^{(t)}$, B23 R$^{(t)}$ and GB25$^{(t)}$, for the Xu of Yin K.
- Li2, in dispersion, to extinguish the Interior Wind.
- Li3, B18 and Li4, Yu Mo technique.
- CV6$^{(t)}$ and St36$^{(t)}$, for the deficiency in Qi.

Perspiration 18

LIQUIDS OF THE BODY

The Chinese call these liquids the *"JIN YE "* influenced by the foods, climate and even emotions. Deficiency of Jin Ye or blockage of its circulation cause symptoms of hypo or hyperfunction, especially at the level of the digestive, circulatory and nervous system. The body liquids are produced at the level of the Middle Burner and are interrelated with each other. A deficiency of one leads to a repercussion on the others: excessive perspiration, severe vomiting, a bleeding, an excessive urination which can lead to an injure of the Jin Ye. Jin Ye is not an extract that we can isolate from the body (although the urine and sweat are part of the Ye).

According to the Su Ouern JIN , *"...nourishes the external part"*, it is the most fluid form, Yang in nature and circulates outside of the meridians, lubricates the skin and warms the muscles. It is the visible part of the liquids: sweat, tears, urine, etc. Following the path of Wei Qi, JIN facilitates the circulation of Blood at the periphery and participates in the formation of sweat, in relation with the heart, master of XUE LO. JIN plays a role in the thermoregulation, maintaining the Yin-Yang balance.

YE "nourishes the internal world", it is a more dense liquid. The YE nature liquids are those which are invisible: liquids in articulations, CSF, etc. YE locks itself in closed spaces, such as is the case in the cerebrospinal fluids and synovia. It has a nature YIN and follows with the YING Qi the internal tracts of the meridians. It protects the brain, and lubricates the tendons and articulations. YIN YE is a liquid which combines with the YING to form the BLOOD. "Ling Throu", Chapter 30 says: *"YE assures the lubrication and is diverted to the bones which regulate the movements of flexion and extension. YE assures the humidification, and tonification of the brain and marrow, the layers of the skin are lubricated, the liquids of the eyes are increased. These are the YE."*

JIN YE is produced by the foods, transformed at the Middle Burner, Spleen/Stomach. Part of this is transported by the spleen to the lung and becomes BLOOD and Qi. Another part is brought to the small intestine which splits it into pure (QING) and impure (ZUO). The impure liquids are eliminated by the bladder and intestines, while the pure ones follow the pathways of CHEN QI to be distributed throughout the body, manifesting themselves at the level of each organ according to their specificity (*Nei Ching*, Chapter 23):

- For the heart: the sweat (HAN)
- For the lung: mucus (TI)
- For the liver: tears (LEI)
- For the kidneys: fluid saliva (XIAN)
- For the spleen: dense saliva (TUO)

The one we are interested here is the perspiration in connection with the heart.

MECHANISM OF PERSPIRATION

It is mainly established by the action of the SHENN of the heart and its emotions. The emotions contract the SHENN which is housed in the vessels. The latter are contacted themselves and expels and liberate the sweat. The contraction of the SHENN opens the pores of the skin at the same time, allowing the evacuation of the sweat. As we have seen before, the impure liquids are eliminated towards the bladder. If this elimination is excessive and pathological, the pure liquids will not go to the lungs and the skin, but are pulled along with the impure ones. We will have absence of perspiration. The opposite is also true: an excessive pull towards the lung, causes diminished urination.

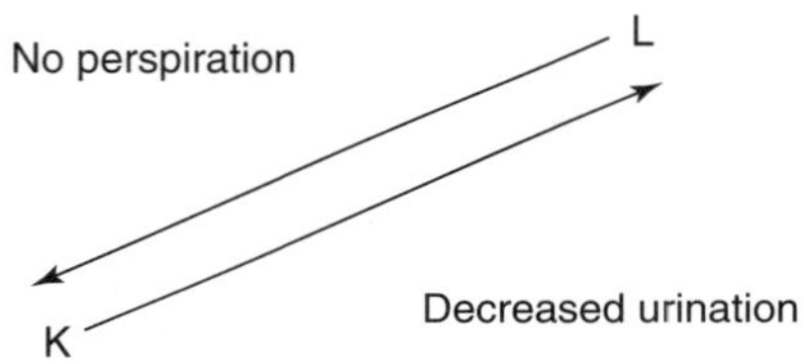

The general control of the perspiration is the responsibility of the kidneys which maintain the Yin-Yang balance between water and respiration on one hand and fire and blood on the other hand. We distinguish external and internal triggering factors.

EXTERNAL PATHOLOGY

It is an attack by the cold, the wind, and the cold wind. The battle between the Wei Qi and these perverse Qi's is translated in fever, chills and perspiration. In certain cases, there will be no perspiration because of blockage of the skin. We may not forget that the perspiration besides a possible loss of liquids, is also a mean to eliminate toxins from the blood!

Spontaneous, generalized perspiration
Occurs especially when Tae Yang is attacked, when the Wei Qi is not strong at the exterior and the Yong Qi is not sufficient on the interior. These patients fear the wind. Pulses are superficial which will require the perspiration technique: Sp1 and 2 in tonification will chase the liquids to the lung, L9 and 10 in dispersion , opens the skin and disperses the liquids. This perverse heat produced by the struggle between the perverse Qi and Wei Qi can penetrate Yang Ming. This heat will chase the liquids to the exterior. Therefore bleed LI1 and St45 to disperse the heat from Yang Ming when the pulses are rapid but not superficial, and do the perspiration technique with L7 and LI4 when the pulses are superficial.

Excessive transpiration
Is observed when Tae Yang is empty, often after a mistake by the acupuncturist. Tonifie Tae Yang with B67, SI3 and disperse first GV14, then tonifie.

Perspiration of feet and hands
Caused by cold attacking the Yin. Cold accumulate at the interior to become apparent Yang, chasing the Yin Ye from palms and soles, mechanism called in Chinese medicine, "*the heat of five hearts.*" The four "hearts" are the two palms and two soles, and the fifth is the center of man where the perverse heat is accumulated. The pathology is here a true cold attack with an apparent or false heat at the level of the spleen. Perform moxa on B20 (activates the Yang of the Sp) and GV14.

Transpiration at the head
Corresponds to a heat-dampness pathology which vaporizes and ascends. A deficient Qi is not able to descend this perverse Qi, hence elimination at the head of sweat. Tonifie GV14 and CV6, as well as L1 and K27.

Incessant transpiration
Sometimes spontaneous, sometimes caused by a wrong therapy. It is linked to a loss of control of

the Yang connections. Disperse TB5.

Blocked perspiration
A mistake in therapy can block the transpiration with a suppression of the perspiration to the deeper parts of the body (goes against the laws of Nature). Restore Yin Ye first with tonifying K7 and Sp7; afterwards free the perspiration as indicated above, according to its etiology.

INTERNAL PATHOLOGY

Perspiration is excessive or deficient according to when the skin pores are open or closed. This results from an emptiness of Qi, Yang or Yin.

Excessive transpiration
In hypersensitive, emotional people. Disperse B15 and H7!

Emptiness of Yang
Cold sweat presents in three different pictures:

- *Xu Yang K*, with lumbago, irregular cycles, sexual disturbances and weak lower limbs. Moxa for a long time B23 and GV4.
- *Heat of Yang and emptiness of Yin*, withheadaches, red eyes and face, oliguria, lumbago, redness of interior corner of the eye (Tae yang), fever, delirium, dry nose and mouth, and hemorrhoids (Yang Ming).

Restore the liquids by tonifying the K with Sp7 and K7, and disperse the Yang with LI4 or bleeding of B67.

Emptiness of Blood
The patient is chilly, pale and fatigued. Tonifie B17 and Sp10.

Emptiness of the lung
Sweating with coughing and dyspnoe. Tonifie L11.

All the above circumstances can cause absence of sweating if the pores of the skin are closed. It is sufficient at that point to "open the skin" and apply the above treatments by changing tonifications in dispersions and vice versa.

Modern Diseases 19

THE FAILURE OF WESTERN MEDICINE

It is obvious that THE principle on which alternative medicines like acupuncture and homeopathy are based, is what Hippocrates, the greatest of Greek physicians wrote centuries ago: *"In order to cure the human body, it is necessary to have a knowledge of the whole of things."* This was echoed later in the dictum and laws of homeopathy by Samuel Hahnemann, M.D. (° 1755-† 1843): *"The chosen remedy is based on the totality of the symptoms, the mental, emotional and physical."* Hahnemann was the first physician to discover and formulate underlying principles of medicine, a haunting thought with great physicians for centuries. How "surprising" then how Hahnemann was castigated and persecuted during his entire life at a time where Western, modern medicine did not amount to much more than blood letting with leeches, purging, fasting, and whipping and teasing the mentally ill for the amusement of visitors, while locking them up in dungeons. Ask any modern physician who Hahnemann is, and you will get a blank stare. Yet, he was the first hygienist, and the first microbiologist able to stop cholera, typhoid fever, scarlatina, TB, gonorrhea and syphilis, and this in the early 1800. The long survival and numerous successes, well-documented of acupuncture and homeopathy, are continuously challenged and ridiculed by a medicine that has not been able to formulate its collection of data in the formulation of general laws and principles. Yet, for the intelligent practice of medicine and the understanding of disease, the simplification of medicine is necessary. The phenomena and mysterious diseases which at present are so difficult to understand, on account of their diversity, are all produced in simple ways as long as the practitioner applies existing Nature laws and formulated ancient principles based on them.

Yet what is the situation in medicine today? Western medicine breaks the human body down into a definite set of facts and drawers. By reducing the body to Gray's *Anatomy*, modern medicine fails to see that the *Vital Energy* or *Qi* has no material existence and, therefore, cannot be dissected like other parts of the body. Health is a harmony of vital processes. Disease has its beginning in the disturbance of this harmony: this is the fundamental law of homeopathy and acupuncture. In modern terms, disease begins in the imbalance of electromagnetic processes, which precipitates a change in body chemistry; this change, if not reversed, results in tissue changes, called pathology—the *end result* of disease. Traditional medicine regards pathology as the disease itself and seeks to remove it, thinking thereby, that they are curing the patient. This folly, rightly criticized by Hahnemann, continues today. Diseases are consequences of a disturbed Qi, and as such are *effects*, not causes. Illnesses are the result of exposure to harmful influences: emotional, mental and physical. (see Chapter 13) If these pernicious triggers are stronger than the present Vital Energy in the person, then disorder or discomfort (dis-ease) will follow. What is worse, Western medicine breeds disorder by introducing vaccines, drugs and invasive harmful techniques, undermining already disturbed energy, leaving behind a greater disorder than before. This is one of the great delusions of Western medicine: *it replaces a small disorder with a greater one.* A typical example is the continued misuse of antibiotics, which were and are prescribed for mere colds and flus. The result: *"Revenge of the Killer Microbes" (Time Magazine, September 12, 1994). "Are we losing the war against infectious diseases?"* I have news for you. We never won the war, if anything we lulled ourselves into believing that Pyrrhus victories scored in the last 40 years were winning the war for us.

Why? Because disease is a conflict between *two parties:* on one side, the provoking agent (microorganism); on the other side, the living subject (the patient) undergoing the aggression. The first part is all too overemphasized in Western medicine, while the second part disappears into oblivion. For any given disease, the search is on for the tiny offender but, reinforcement of the victim is advised all too rarely. Why is it that in some epidemics some people get sick and others do not? Why do some AIDS victims succumb to the disease within a year while others are still around in apparent good health after ten years? This is due to *inherent causes, a morbid receptivity and a lack of natural defense of the individual.* As long as the defense system is intact, we are resistant to most exterior aggressions. *"The virus means nothing, the terrain is everything."* Modern, allopathic medicine has not learned this yet. It is time for them to start paying attention to the recipient instead of the aggressor alone.

Health is the balanced state of the body and mind in an individual. The Vital Energy controls the harmony between body and mind. This normal health and the harmonious Qi depend on *Hygiene* (nutrition or Yong Qi, respiratory Qi, personal and social hygiene, water supply) AND the absence of a hereditary disease dyscrasia or miasm (defective Ancestral Qi). Homeopathy and acupuncture can successfully *prevent* the onset of many chronic diseases by regulation of hygienic measures and constitutional treatment of the present miasma. True jewels of internal Hygiene are diet, Tai Chi, Qigong, meditation, mental hygiene and lucid dreaming. Two hundred years ago, Hahnemann wrote,

"Therefore disease considered, as it is by the allopathists (modern doctors), as a thing separate from the living whole, from the organism and its animating vital force, and hidden in the interior, is an absurdity, that could only be imagined by mind of materialistic stamp, and for thousands of years given to the prevailing system of medicine all those pernicious impulses that have made it a truly non healing art." Paragraph 13, Organon, 6th Edition.

What a condemnation of "modern" medicine by Hahnemann in his time. Alas, not much has been changed in 200 years. Most physicians still practice as if the body and mind are two separate entities. The doctor looks for any subtle anatomical and laboratory change, while the psychiatrist or psychotherapist seem to feel that a human being is only composed of the mind. Therefore, a psychotherapist, not knowing the physical symptoms of the diseased state, will declare the patient "healed" after dwelling long enough on the past. The true physician has to approach the diseased person from a viewpoint which includes all three levels of human expression: mental, emotional and physical.

Of course, people in general and physicians especially, will tell you: "We don't need those old medicines, look at all our successes we have with modern medicine." They say, "we live longer." Yes, but it is undeniable that people are more chronically ill. We *survive* longer. A study in the *Journal of the American Medical Association (July 1994)* showed poor prescribing practices among the elderly. Of course, this is only the tip of the iceberg. Many of these elderly get drugs that are likely to do them more harm than good. It is not uncommon that patients take 4 drugs for different ailments, and another 4 to go against the "accepted" toxic effects of the first 4. Speaking of adding a drug picture to the disease picture! Most of modern medicines (cancer drugs, cortisone, etc.) work *against* the most elementary laws. Instead of raising the individual's defenses, it suppresses them. Every day, we read in our newspapers about the increased incidence of cancer, cardiovascular diseases, infectious diseases, yeast overgrowth, mental diseases and an explosion of allergic conditions. The lack of solution to the immense suffering of the chronically ill patients clearly reveals that modern medicine lacks the adequate therapeutic means to obtain a real cure of the patient. I only have to refer to the resurgence of TB, syphilis and gonorrhea, resistant to present antibiotics. Or do we need to mention, "mystery" diseases like the Gulf War Syndrome, CFIDS, the HANTA virus epidemic and the Multiple Chemical Sensitivity Syndrome (MCS)? After a decade of AIDS research, the taming of this disease is going nowhere and stand to become another unsuccessful war. Genetic medicine and the location of broken genes on chromosomes are taunted as the latest victory for just about everything known to afflict humankind—deadly diseases like colon cancer, breast cancer, manic depression, cystic fibrosis, etc. The virus-of-the-week impression (remember CFIDS and its history of linked viruses!) has been replaced with the gene-of-the-week, with its implication, that we are only a step away of conquering these diseases. What false hope! Those same scientists have to admit that diseased genes do not always make you sick and these genes do not operate the way textbooks claim. Their behavior is changeable and capricious, making some people sick and others not. And then there is the possibility of mutation which was discovered in the cystic fibrosis gene. As a result, the National Academy of Sciences, had to admit that, "Genetic tests are seldom perfect predictors of health risks." And I will go one step further. Despite all the big hoopla around the discovering of these genes, so far, not one disease has been corrected by repairing that defective gene. As usual, Western medicine puts the accent on pathology and diagnosis, and forgets all about therapy! Alternative medicines like acupuncture and homeopathy do not need a name for a disease in order to cure it! Our "names" will sound esoteric and simplistic at the same time, but diagnoses such as Kidney Qi Deficiency, Liver fire Ascending Yang, or Never Well Since (NWS) childbirth are more correctly describing the diseased state of the patient than names such as fibromyositis, colitis ulcerosa, Crohn's disease, olivo-ponto-cerebellar atrophy (OPCA) which describe symptoms in medical jargon or a disease with the name of the scientist who described it for the first time. Has it helped the patient because a name was given? I leave that conclusion to the victims of these diseases. Rather let us look what alternative medicines have to offer in the ever increasing mystery diseases and immuno-suppressed conditions.

CHRONIC FATIGUE AND IMMUNE DYSFUNCTION SYNDROME (CFIDS)

DEFINITION AND ORIGIN

Incline Village, Lake Tahoe, 1983 was roaring with the sound of a "newly" discovered disease: a cluster of people exhibited severe fatigue and brain fag, leaving them in a daze, uncapable of doing some of the simpliest jobs. The name "Chronic Fatigue Syndrome" was obvious and swiftly given. The second step was also predictable: a virus has to be the cause (as it always is when a new disease is discovered). And there was no lack of them. In succession, this disease was linked to the Epstein Barr virus (EBV), the Herpes Simplex Viruses, especially HHV-6, the Cytomegalo virus (CMV), the spuma viruses and finally a broader group of viruses, the retroviruses, more specific, HTLV-1 and 2. Talking about roaming around in the dark! Of course, the medical community took its sweet time to even acknowledge this syndrome, leaving victims in the cold, depressed and abandonned if it was not for alternative medicine. It was not until May 1990 that the Center for Disease Control (CDC) decided to accept this diagnosis and put their own, (incomplete) definition on the market. This definition was put together by a group of mainstream doctors out of Massacuchetts (*HOLMES et al., 1988* Annals of Internal *Medicine),* grouping all these victims in one category. Does this sound familiar? This is one of the big failures of Western medicine: to acknowledge the endstage of the disease or pathology rather than the individual. In other words, all these patients are the same, their disease must be caused by the same triggering factor (a virus) and therefore the therapy must be the same. I can imagine that Hahnemann in his grave throws his hands up in despair at hearing such continued folly. But for what it is worth, here are their criteria:

Two Major ones:

1. Relapsing fatigue or easy fatigability not resolved by bed rest and severe enough to reduce average daily activity by at least 50% for at least 6 months.
2. Any other illness, including psychiatric diseases, leading to fatigue have to be excluded before one can be diagnosed as having CFIDS.

Several minor criteria:

- Neurologic symptoms such as brain fag, dizziness, short-time
- Recurrent sore throats.
- Low-grade fevers and chills.
- Unexplained generalized muscle weakness.
- Myalgia.
- Prolonged (>24 hrs) generalized fatigue following previous tolerable levels of exercise.
- New, generalized headaches.
- Sleeplessness with sleepiness.
- Tender posterior cervical lymphnodes.
- Migratory noninflammatory arthralgias.

Besides the fact that thousands of these victims are treated this way as a disease-group rather than individuals, I have some other objections with these criteria. Looking at the major criteria, if you are not sick yet for 6 months, you are not a CFIDS person. Is it not typically again for Western medicine to wait until the patient is more sick, rather than intervening in the earlier stages? How can we think we do these patients any favor by letting their Vital Energy decrease before we want to accept the diagnosis and intervene, not to mention the emotional abandonment these patients must feel when they are told, "to come back in 6 months, and prey and hope it will go away." The second major criterium is a "cover-all" phrase. In other words, first rule out the thousands of other diseases before you decide on CFIDS, which shows the allopathic medicine standpoint: it is an exclusion diagnosis. But practically again, this means any possible medical specialist has a crack at these patients (and usually does) before CFIDS is accepted. What a waist of time, a waist of money and a waist of Vital Energy of the patient. At the end of this long saga, Western medicine has not too much to offer. Besides drugs that cover *part* of the symptoms, not *all* of them (which is called *suppression* in homeopathy), usually a drug picture (euphemism for side effects or toxic effects) is added to the already tarnished Vital Qi of the patient. Furthermore, some half-concerted effort is done at loaning some therapies from alternative medicine: Vitamin B injections, Liver extract injections, or other supplements like Coenzym Q10 or betacarotene. Alas! All of this is nothing else than pruning the sick branches of the tree while forgetting to treat the sick root. And unfortunately, there are plenty of alternative practitioners out there who practice like they never heard about principles and laws in acupuncture and homeopathy either.

ALTERNATIVE MEDICINE APPROACH

Chapter 13 on Causes, gives the first clue to the right approach. It bears repeating: *"What happens in your life when you got sick?"* is the most important question to be answered. *"What was strong enough in intensity to create new symptoms or aggravate existing symptoms?"* Because all those are possible roots to the problems. Without treating these beginnings, the endings will never be cured. Instead of hopelessly concentrating on an end product, Western medicine would do better at focussing on the initial triggering factor! And of course they are numerous as is explained in Chapter 13. Besides these numerous factors already discussed, there is one class of symptoms which draws our attention and allows the practitioner, acupuncturist or homeopath, to focus on THE etiological factor: *"the never well since" or NWS or "Ailments from."* Quite often, the patient can pinpoint one or several important events in his life preceding immediately his spiraling down of health. I have mentioned some in the table below. What homeopathy especially and acupuncture to a lesser degree is capable of doing, is exactly matching the hole that was punched in the balloon (the triggering factor), sealing it immedialy so that no further decrease of Vital Qi is possible. Western medicine is not capable of doing so and this is probably the main reason that it focusses on a crude end product and suppresses parts of it. In other words, the "NWS" factors are *all possible etiological factors* in CFIDS and allow *secondarily* an overgrowth of micro organisms, not the other way around. Look at some of these NWS factors and we will discuss some of the remedies we have for them in alternative medicine.

TABLE NWS or AILMENTS FROM

"a childhood disease"
"puberty"
"menopause"
"childbirth, miscarriage, birth controll pill"
"grief or death of beloved one"
"mental exertion"
"influenza"
"pneumonia"
"head injury"
"surgery"
"anaesthesia"
" vaccinations"
"Mono"
"hepatitis"
"whiplash"
"allergy shots"
"antibiotics"
"travellers diarrhea"
"trauma"
"emotional shock or fright"
"suppressed sweating"
"suppressed eczema"
"overuse of drugs, medically and street drugs"
"lack of sleep by nursing a loved one"
"overambition"

This list is endless but a lot of CFIDS cases are covered by the above mentioned factors. No matter what practitioner you are, your success will depend on your ability to match a similar therapeutic picture to the disease picture ("Like Cures Like" in homeopathy), since *"Two similar diseases cannot coexist next to one other. The stronger disease will cure the weaker similar one."* This means that if you are curing the beginning root of this disease, no matter what the end product looks like, you will be successful. I have mentioned below some of the solutions in homeopathy and acupuncture.

"Never well since puberty, menopause, childbirth, miscarriage" all indicate hormonal disturbances and are intimately related in acupuncture to a Kidney organ disturbance, most likely a K Yin deficiency, secondarily with a Liver Blood deficiency or "dried up Blood." Your therapy will include B23, B17, Sp6, St36, K3 and 7, GB23 and Li14. In homeopathy "Nws puberty" relates to Pulsatilla while Sepia is the #1 remedy for "Nws menopause, childbirth or miscarriage".

"Nws a grief, heartbreak or death of a beloved one" clearly affects the Heart Qi and disrupts the Kidney-Heart axis. We know that for "mental" factors, we need to use the heart points. B15 and CV14, H3^{t} ("Sea of Joy"), H7^{t}, together with the season tonification point of the Liver will balance this patient. Natrum muriaticum will be one of the front runners in homeopathy.

"Nws mental exertion" as happens in students or driven bussiness people, indicates a decrease of the "bone marrow" and "I" or memory and is linked to a Spleen Qi deficiency. B20 and Li13, Sp6, Sp9, GV14, GV20 and St36 are a possible solution. Homeopathy covers it with remedies such as Sulphur, Kali Phos or Silica.

"Nws influenza" has decreased the Lung Qi (*see* Wind-Cold or Wind-Heat attack, page 61 for symptoms and therapy). These patients still need the same therapy as they needed at that time, even if they consult you years later. The nosode Influenzinum, Gelsemium or Psorinum are possible remedies.

"Nws suppressed sweating or suppressed eczema": especially eczema is suppressed on a routine basis in Western medicine with all the horrible consequences. These drug therapies go against the law of Nature, well-known in acupuncture and home-

opathy, *"cure from the Interior to the Exterior"*. Cortisone therapies and drugs for sweat suppression deliberately go against Nature's advice with asthma, CFIDS and other numerous diseases as a consequence, unfortunately not recognized as such by the patient and doctor alike who keeps on treating then, so ever foolishly, the created, much stronger disease.

We have the *perspiration technique,* page 37 to help Nature in cleansing our body (*see* also Perspiration, Chapter 18). Skin diseases, no matter what their names are, are linked to the Lung organ and to the LI-L unit. It is easy for an acupuncturist to understand the alternation of eczema and asthma since they belong to a disturbance of the same organ, the Lung, except for driving the disease more inwards. Many skindiseases (*see Psoriasis, page 161 and Diseases of the Blood in general, Chapter 15)* are linked to Heat or Wind invasion in the blood. Proper treatments are discussed in those chapters and help the acupuncturist work *with* Nature instead of against it. Sulphur for suppressed eczema and Silica and Sulphur again for suppressed sweating are major remedies in homeopathy.

"Nws travelers' diarrhea" indicates the loss of body fluids which is also possible in the "affairs of bedroom", excessive masturbation, excessive sweating, or vomiting, and excessive bleeding post operatively or in delivery. They cause a mild form of Yin deficiency, preceding a possible Yin deficient state if unchecked. Thus deficiency of fluids affects mostly the Lungs, Stomach, Large Intestine and of course, Kidneys. Therapy will be aimed at restoring these organ imbalances on an individual basis. Don't forget to include B17, and PC 6-7 in most of these cases, while the Lower He Sea points, St 36-37-38 are of great importance in travelers diarrhea. See also the Large Intestine syndromes page 63-4. In homeopathy we can be very specific. Arsenicum for travelers' diarrhea or food poisoning, Phosphoric Acid for excessive masturbation, China for excessive blood loss and Sulphur for excesive sweating, are specifics.

I hope, these few examples will stimulate the practitioner to look at the patient as an individuial whose energy was disturbed at some point in his life and not as just another disease name. Treat the beginnings rather than the endings! Only then will the physician be able to really cure the patient and bring him back to the road of well being. I also hope that practitioners will see the idiocy of searching for an elusive virus in CFIDS. I have seen all of the above cases numerous times and cured. I never needed to know what viruses were involved. And since when has Western medicine anything to offer for viral diseases?

THE GULF WAR SYNDROME (MCS)

January 17, 1991 is a date edged in the American history: Americans went to Kuweit to fight against the Iraqi dictator Sadam Hussein in order to protect the little state Kuweit and their friends in Saudy Arabia. For many veterans, this date is remembered for another , more personal reason: they lost their health in obeying the call from their government. At least 20,000 veterans (and this is a conservative number, in no way close to the actual number) came down with large, red blotches on hands and arms, extreme tiredness, aches in joints, difficullty breathing and chronic diarrhea. This was only the beginning of their illness. Some of them, also in increasing number, exhibit multiple sensitivities to many chemicals in the environment. As usual, Western medicine had no problem giving it a name, dubbing it now, Multiple Chemical Sensitivity or MCS. This is as far as modern medicine has come. Three years later, and after sending American troops to Saudi Arabia again, nobody in Western medicine is anything wiser, leaving to languish its veterans in ill health. Some of them live in a sterile "bubble" and run up high medical bills. I remember seeing one of those early on, way before it was named MCS. As you know, a homeopathic physician does not need a name for a disease in order to treat it. When I finished my inquiry, the matching remedy was Arsenicum. Following the law, "Like Cures Like" I could therefore deduct, that if a poison is the cure, a poison has to be the cause. Therefore, I was not a bit surprised when I read about the experimental drugs and vaccinations given to the departing soldiers without divulging potentially harmful side effects. This does look a lot like "Agent Orange" and the

Plutonium experiments on the military in the 60s'. Combine the drugs and vaccines with the exposure to chemicals released from bombed factories and breathing in of air polluted by burning oil, and you have a major poison "coctail." That no more people got sick is only again a prove of human resilience or what we would call, constitution. But the most sensitive of these individuals will get sick, got sick and will stay sick, unless a medical intervention, according to Nature laws, will be used. Only homeopathy, and to a lesser extent, acupuncture can do this. Of course, other adjuvans will be a clean diet, a clean environment, and a detoxification program through anti-oxidants and colonic therapy. But the major work and solution will come from homeopathy. How will a homeopath go to work? It would be sufficient if a good homeopath could see 20-30 of these victims and note all the common symptoms. This probably would bring up, 2 to 3 different homeopathic remedies which would then be given to the thousands of victims after matching this small amount of remedies to their disease picture. Cost of this process: pennies!! At the time, the minister of defense, Mr. Les Aspin, created a board of inquiry headed by a Nobel-prize winning expert. I have not heard or seen any solution after three years.

What can an acupuncturist do? Most of the symptoms experienced by these veterans seem to be linked to the METAL/WATER group: breathing problems, diarrhea, fatigue (Lung is master of Qi!), skin rashes, all linked to Lung/Large Intestine with the aching joints belonging to the Kidney. From the majority of the symptoms, it seems that the metal group is the primary movement that is disturbed, while the Water group will receive less descending Qi from the Metal group. Again, a balancing of the Metal group will be priority among the treatment of these victims. Strengthening the Lung/Large Intestine group will be done through the Yu-Mo technique (*see* page 24) while the acupuncturist can use appropriate points, corresponding to the individual's case. (again, mainly Metal points). I hope for these victim's sake, that the Government will apply all measures possible, and this has to include alternative medicine! At the same time, it would give clues to the Pentagon officials as how to avoid future tragedies like the Gulf War Syndrome.

THE FOUR CORNERS DISEASE OR THE HANTA VIRUS LINK

It started as a bad case of flu in May 1993 for a 19-year-old Navajo man. Or so they thought. He was rushed to the emergency room and suddenly couldn't breathe anymore. Within hours he was dead. The case was the first but not the last one. Initially, people in the Southwest were affected. They all started as a flu becoming life threatening as tiny blood vessels throughout the lungs began to leak plasma. Gasping for breath, victims literally started to drown in their own body fluids. In more than 50%, the outcome was a quick death, enough to get the attention of the medical world in spite of the low number of victims (about 85 so far). After naming it the Navajo disease and running into trouble with the Navajo tribe, health officials unofficially called it the Four Corners disease, because it was identified in the region around the intersection of Arizona, New Mexico, Colorado and Utah. However, the malady started to show up in many other states (about 15 now) too. As usual, confronted with a deadly "mysterious" disease, Western medicine turned all its attention to a possible virus link. And loh-and-behold, they found one. For them the culprit was the hantavirus, carried by wild deer mice. The next step of course should be the development of an adequate vaccine. And a new name was born: the Hantavirus Pulmonary Syndrome. Treatment consists of course in hospitalizing these victims and administering heavy amounts of IV antibiotics. But still, it is praying and hoping for these victims as the outcome is uncertain.

Many questions remain. The virus is not new in the US. It has been around for a long time. Then why has the disease not shown up earlier and why are not more people affected? Because as usual, we put the horse behind the chart. We should look at what these victims have in common, life style wise, constitutional, and traumatic (physical/emotional) wise? It is obvious that it is the recipient that became different, not the virus. And why are we giving antibiotics to these victims if viruses are the "cause?" What medical book advocates that viruses get killed by antibiotics? If anything, it will prolong the recovery by putting additional strain on the victims' body. Antibiotics for one kill the friendly intestinal flora, a strong weapon in our immunity, and Western medicine has not grasped the importance of a simple step as supplying acidophyllus when administering antibiotics. There are millions of different viruses out there. I am curious which one will be the next one to be blamed for the next "Agatha Christie" disease.

Again, alternative medicine will look at these individuals as unique and try to find common symptoms and triggering factors, which we could call, kinks in their armor of defense. The same tactic as with any epidemic as described above in the MCS will be used. Get the history of 20 victims together and find the common link. Match that disease picture with the existing homeopathic remedy. Again, the main difference between the inquiry of a Western medical trained physician and an alternative physician, will be that where the Western doctor stops asking questions, the alternative physician starts asking questions. The only way I could come to a therapeutic approach, is, if I would have a chance to do an inquiry with about 20 of these victims. Western medicine simply does not go into detail enough to provide any clue.

REVENGE OF THE KILLER MICROBES

The bubonic plague in India, October 1994. Cholera epidemics in Rwanda and Zaire in refugee camps, 1994. Resurgence of TB, gonorrhea and syphilis, 1994. Did we not declare victory in the war against these diseases? Foolishly enough, we did. And those are only the eye-catchers. We might forget that more than 4 million people annually die from acute respiratory diseases, more than 3 million a year from diarrhea, two million from hepatitis and 1 million from malaria. I guess they are common diseases and not sensational enough to get the media's attention. One thing it has achieved. It has shifted again the attention to these tiny microbes as THE culprits of most human diseases. It will only take a few more "new" diseases and the microbe-phobia will be full-blown. Forgotten of course, that most of these diseases reoccur when there is a breakdown of hygiene and a breakdown of the life style of its victims. Forgotten too, that Hahnemann, 200 years ago, was curing all of the above diseases with his inexpensive, non-toxic remedies and that any good homeopath could still do the same. What is the answer of Western medicine? We have to find other drugs, engineer new antibiotics that will act specifically against the targeted microbe. Forgotten again is the patient. When are we going to learn to strengthen the patient?

To the true physician, a cure consists of but one thing, and that is the *eradication of the predisposition* to that disease to be cured. A true remedy does not apply a palliative action which merely deadens the pain somewhat for 15 minutes or so, only to return even more severely and with additional, more annoying symptoms. The homeopath implies a medicinal agent entirely compatible with the malady, which completely eradicates the disease in the course of a few hours or days, so that it does not recur again for a long time, possibly the rest of the patient's life. The cured patient feels better, appears healthier to those close to him, the pathological conditions are eliminated, and he is less susceptible to the development of acute or chronic disease. This type of healing is almost never achieved in Western medicine. Do you want common examples. Look what we do for recurrent ear infections in children and recurrent vaginal yeast infections? The physician continues to prescribe drugs. It does not occur to him that he is contributing to disorder in an already weakened, fragile human being. But if you ask him to do something to prevent the recurrence of this illness, he will shrug his shoulders. Should this physician really take pride in his achievements? Of course not. His allopathic treatments contribute more than their share to the decline of the human species.

What ought to be done in order to stem the outbreak of these killer microbes? After curing the acute attacks of the infection, and after improving hygiene as much as possible, acupuncture and homeopathy can strengthen the patient's constitution. In Chapter 15, I described the different types belonging to the Five Elements. Once you have recognized your patient in one of those classes, strengthen the movement through an appropriate homeopathic remedy or through strengthening of the element movement by stimulating the corresponding acupuncture points. Below are some of the therapeutic solutions.

- *Liver Type (WOOD):* Sulphur, Nux Vomica, B18, Li14, St36, Li8, Li3. The strengthening should be done preferably in the spring.
- *Heart Type (FIRE):* Lachesis, Phosphorus, B15, CV14, PC7, PC6, K3, in the summer.
- *Spleen Type (EARTH):* Calc. carb., Silica, B20, Li13, Sp6, St36 in the intermittent seasons (4 times a year).
- *Lung Type (METAL):* KaliCarb, Sulphur, B13, L1, B12, L7, L9, B67 in the fall.
- *Kidney Type (WATER):* Nat-mur, Arsenicum, B23, GB24, K3, K7, B28 in the winter.

In general we can strengthen the Wei Qi by stimulating: L9, St36, TB3, B67, all in tonification. This will prevent recurrent infectious diseases.

We should keep in mind that the world around us is not always the enemy. More than ever, we ourselves are our biggest enemy. Changes in food, soil, water, air, not to mention the emotional upheavals, are weakening the human race. If one wants to be successful in the war against infectious diseases, start with strengthening the human being!

Index